**This book is to be returned on or before
the last date stamped below.**

Tonsils: A Clinically Oriented Update

Advances in Oto-Rhino-Laryngology

Vol. 47

Series Editor
C.R. Pfaltz, Basel

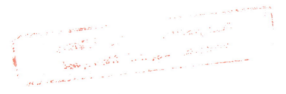

KARGER

Basel · Freiburg · Paris · London · New York · New Delhi · Bangkok · Singapore · Tokyo · Sydney

Tonsils:
A Clinically Oriented Update

Volume Editor: *G.B. Galioto,* Pavia
Volume Co-Editors: *E. Mevio, P. Galioto, M. Benazzo,* Pavia

151 figures, 1 color plate and 57 tables, 1992

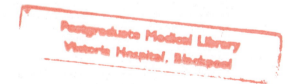
KARGER

Basel · Freiburg · Paris · London · New York · New Delhi · Bangkok · Singapore · Tokyo · Sydney

Advances in Oto-Rhino-Laryngology

Library of Congress Cataloging-in-Publication Data
International Symposium on Tonsils (2nd: 1991: Pavia, Italy)
Tonsils: a clinically oriented update/2nd International Symposium on Tonsils, Pavia,
September 11–13, 1991; volume editor, G.B. Galioto.
(Advances in oto-rhino-laryngology; vol. 47)
Includes bibliographical references and index. (alk. paper)
1. Tonsils – Congresses.   2. Tonsils – Diseases – Congresses.   I. Galioto, G.B.   II. Title.
III. Series.
[DNLM: 1. Tonsil – congresses.   2. Tonsillectomy – congresses.   3. Tonsillitis –
congresses.   W1 AD701 v.47]
RF16.A38 vol. 47 [RF481] 617.5'1 s–dc20 [617.5'32]
ISBN 3–8055–5604–7

Bibliographic Indices
This publication is listed in bibliographic services, including Current Contents® and Index
Medicus.

Drug Dosage
The authors and the publisher have exerted every effort to ensure that drug selection and dosage set forth in this text are in accord with current recommendations and practice at the time
of publication. However, in view of ongoing research, changes in government regulations, and
the constant flow of information relating to drug therapy and drug reactions, the reader is
urged to check the package insert for each drug for any change in indications and dosage and
for added warnings and precautions. This is particularly important when the recommended
agent is a new and/or infrequently employed drug.

Contents

Focal Infection of Tonsils and Related Diseases

Adenoids and Tonsil Hypertrophy and Its Complications

Medical and Surgical Therapy

Preface

I had the pleasure of hosting here in my country the Second International Symposium on Tonsils; the first one was held in 1987 in Kyoto, Japan, and the next one will be held in Japan again, in Sapporo in 1995.

The second edition of the symposium has been very successful and was attended by specialists from all over the world. A prestigious scientific committee and faculty of invited speakers treated the main topics in different areas. Recent developments in functional anatomy and immunology have thrown new light upon the role of tonsils in addition to the clinical significance of pharyngotonsillitis infections and tonsillar foci. The subject of sleep apnea and its correlations with adenotonsillar hypertrophy is now stirring greater interest among pediatricians, neurologists and otorhinolaryngologists. While the relationship between secretory otitis media, adenoids vegetations, and infections of the rhinopharynx still remains open, new trends emerged in the fields of medical and surgical therapy of tonsillar diseases.

The contributions presented during the symposium are collected in this book in order to offer a significant state of the art of the studies on problems of the tonsils. As the editor of this book I would like to acknowledge Prof. T. Tabata who was the president of the first symposium on tonsils and whose cooperation helped make this congress a success.

Prof. *G.B. Galioto*

Galioto GB (ed): Tonsils: A Clinically Oriented Update.
Adv Otorhinolaryngol. Basel, Karger, 1992, vol 47, pp 1–4

The Development and Involution of Tonsils

Jaroslav Slípka

Department of Histology and Embryology, Faculty of Medicine,
Charles University, Plzeň, Czechoslovakia

The development of the human palatine tonsils has been studied many times [1, 2]. The crypts start to develop in the 9th week and the stroma becomes infiltrated by lymphoid elements in the 13th week of pregnancy. The mother region of the crypts forms the epithelial lining of the previous second branchial pouch, whereas the material for the tonsillar stroma comes from the mesenchyme of the second and third branchial arches. There is still lack of knowledge on the origin of the earliest predetermined material which contributes to the tonsillar patterns, as well as on the trigger of their ontogeny, and process of their involution. This paper would like to help to enlighten these problems.

Material and Methods

We used serial sagittal and transversal histological sections of the branchial region of the earliest human embryos, and some representatives of all other vertebrate classes. The germ-free (GF) piglets used for our studies were kept in incubators just after delivery, and were fed with sterile milk only for 15 and 42 days. The relations between thymus and tonsils were studied in 920 thymuses. The findings in thymus were correlated with lymph nodes and spleen, some also with tonsils.

Results

The second branchial membrane in human embryos breaks down at the end of the first month. The border between both linings disappears and both epithelia can mix. The second pouch gradually obliterates during the 6th week and much later forms the mother region of the palatine tonsil.

The tonsil in newborn piglets is situated between two mucous glands. The crypts are branched tubulous with some detritus in their lumina. The stroma is scarcely infiltrated by lymphoid elements (T prevailed over O and B lymphocytes). In 15-day-old GF piglets the situation was very similar to the newborn. Striking was only a larger amount of cellular detritus inside the crypts and a rich proliferation of vessels among them. The crypt epithelium was not reticulated. On the sides of the tonsil the small primary follicles are not bound on crypts but on the surface epithelium with signs of reticulation. Nearly the same situation was seen in the GF piglets at 42 days.

Whereas in thymus the age involution starts in puberty, in tonsils it is shifted to the fourth decade, in which the crypts become wider, the follicles possess no germinal centers and the reticulation of the epithelium gradually disappears.

In cases of 'accidental' involution in the perinatal and early childhood period in which cortex was collapsed and the medulla was crowded with Hassall's corpuscles, the tonsils were also affected and crypt epithelium formed concentric bodies similar to thymic corpuscles.

Discussion

From our observations, as well as from results of previous papers, tonsils develop relatively late in ontogeny of the branchial region, especially its second pouch. This mother region proceeds through a large conversion in very early ontogeny and the epithelial lining of the second pouch which provides material for the crypts most probably also contains ectodermal admixture. We also call our attention to the fact that the connective tissue stroma derives from the mesenchyme of the neural crest. From that point of view the tonsils differ very much from other peripheral lymph organs.

Also in phylogeny the tonsils evolved late as a reaction of the complicated antigenic situation in coevolution with xenobionts (fig. 1). The tonsils of higher organisms bear the memory of the imprinted ontogenies of their ancestors, and do not need to start their development by antigenic stimuli. This has been proved in our observations of GF piglets. Their

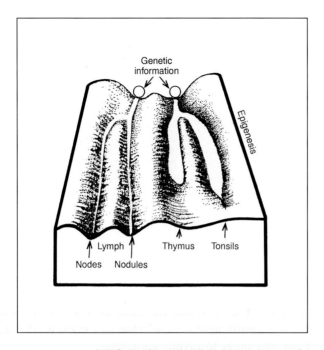

Fig. 1. The genetic information constrains the development in the valleys of a morphogenetic landscape, but the whole scenery can be modified by epigenetic influences, like in the case of transitory development of thymus and tonsils.

tonsils keep together with all lymphatic organs [3] the fetal character. There is no doubt that the exogenous stimulation influences just after birth the differentiation of the lymphatic tissue and the whole immunocompetence of the organism.

The development of such tissue is only a temporary one [4]. The most active structure is reached in human tonsils between 4 and 30 years. The involution begins in the fourth decade and never finishes. In thymus the same process starts much earlier in the age of puberty. The large time difference between both organs corresponds also to the position of these organs in phylogeny. The relation of the thymus to the tonsils is even more conspicuous in our cases of 'accidental' involution not depending on age [5]. In case of predominant Hassall's corpuscles in thymus, the tonsillar epithelium of the newborns also becomes affected. This proves the epithelial homology of both organs.

References

1   Von Gaudecker B, Müller-Hermelink HK: The development of the human tonsilla palatina. Cell Tissue Res 1982;224:579–585.
2   Slípka J: Palatine tonsils – their evolution and ontogeny. Acta Otolaryngol (Stockh) 1988;454:18–22.
3   Kovářů F, Štěpánková R, Kruml J, Mandel L, Kenig E: Development of lymphatic and haemopoietic organs in germ-free models. Folia Microbiol 1979;24:32–43.
4   Favre A, Paoli D, Polleti M, Marzoli A, Pesce G, Giampalmo A, Rossi F: The human palatine tonsil studied from surgical specimens at all ages and various pathological conditions. Z Mikrosk Anat Forsch 1986;100:7–33, 161–188.
5   Von Baarlen J, Schuurman HJ, Huber J: Acute thymus involution in pregnancy and childhood. Hum Pathol 1988;19:1155–1160.

Prof. Jaroslav Slípka, Faculty of Medicine, Charles University,
Department of Histology and Embryology, 48 Karlovarská Str.,
CS–30166 Plzeň (Czechoslovakia)

Galioto GB (ed): Tonsils: A Clinically Oriented Update.
Adv Otorhinolaryngol. Basel, Karger, 1992, vol 47, pp 5–10

Three-Dimensional Ultrastructure of the Secondary Nodule of the Human Palatine Tonsil

Hiroshi Watanabe, Masaya Takumida, Yasuo Harada

Department of Otolaryngology, Hiroshima University, School of Medicine,
Hiroshima, Japan

The structural and functional aspects of the secondary nodule of the palatine tonsil have been intensively studied because of its importance as one of the lymphopoietic organs. Especially, recent progress of the immunological and electron microscopic techniques has provided us with even further knowledge. Yet, stereoscopic study on the human secondary nodule is rather scarce. The present study focuses on three-dimensional ultrastructure of the secondary nodule of the human palatine tonsil. For this purpose, scanning electron microscopy was used in combination with methods of freeze fracture and free cell removal.

Materials and Method

The human palatine tonsils were removed from the patients with chronic tonsillitis or tonsillar hypertrophy. The specimens were processed by two different methods for scanning electron microscopic observation.

For observation of the cracked surface of the germinal center, the specimens were fixed with the mixture of 0.5% glutaraldehyde and 0.5% paraformaldehyde by immersion. After additional fixation with 1% OsO_4, the specimens were immersed in 25% and 50% DMSO. They were then cracked in liquid nitrogen and then macerated in 0.1% OsO_4 for 0–90 h. The specimens were stained by 1% OsO_4 and 2% tannic acid.

For observation of the framework of the lymphatic reticulum, the specimens were fixed with the 2.5% glutaraldehyde by immersion. To remove free cells, ultrasonic vibration and water jet stream were used. The specimens were fixed again for 1 h in 1% OsO_4 and then stained by 1% tannic acid.

Following dehydration with graded ethanol solutions, all specimens were treated with isoamyl acetate, critical-point dried (liquid CO_2) and sputter-coated with platinum. A Hitachi S-800 scanning electron microscope was used for observation of the specimens.

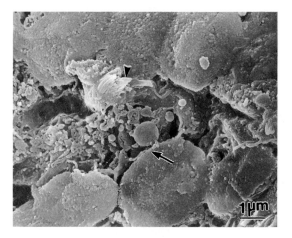

Fig. 1. The mantle zone. A reticular cell (arrow) and collagen fibers (arrowhead) are observed between the lined lymphocytes.

Results

Germinal Center

The framework of the lymphatic reticulum was formed by dense mesh of the fine reticulum. Inside this framework, villous cells and smooth cells were observed, indicating B and T lymphocytes respectively. The cracked surface of the germinal center appeared honeycomb, since the cells and the cytoplasm were lost. In higher magnification, numerous medium-sized or large lymphocytes, plasma cells with well-developed endoplasmic reticulum were observed. Reticular cells and immature lymphocytes with small nucleus and large cytoplasm were also present. There were two kinds of reticular cells. One was a nonphagocytic reticular cell with small cytoplasm. The other one was a phagocytic reticular cell with an inclusion body in its cytoplasm.

Mantle Zone

Medium or small lymphocytes were lining like beads. Collagen fibers and reticular cells were observed between the lined-up lymphocytes (fig. 1).

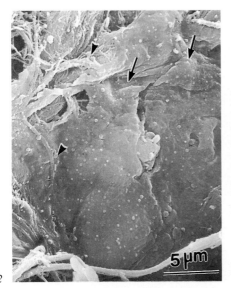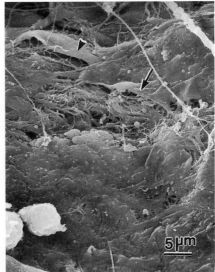

2   3

Fig. 2. The surface of the partition between the germinal center and the mantle zone. The flat and rectangular cells with smooth surface (arrows) are lined up. The collagen fibers (arrowheads) are observed between these cells.

Fig. 3. Clefts and pores on the partition. The cleft (arrow) is about 7 × 14 μm in size. Inside these clefts and pores (arrowhead), a bundle of collagen and reticular fibers are seen.

Border Area between the Germinal Center and the Mantle Zone

After washing out free cells of the germinal center, a structure like a partition was observed in the border. The surface of this partition was formed by the flat and rectangular cells with smooth surface. Collagen fibrils filled between these cells (fig. 2). The mantle zone had similar appearance. On the partition, there were some pores and clefts of various size. Their diameters were more than 7 μm. Inside these pores and clefts, a bundle of the collagen fibers and some reticular fibers were noticed (fig. 3). At the partition far from the basal pole, the collagen and the reticular fibers were very sparse. In some focal areas, the collagen fibers were running curved leaving a large space. The lymphocytes possibly move through this space.

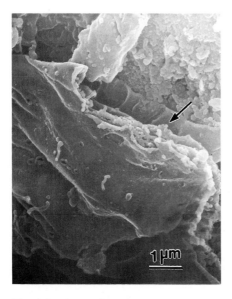

Fig. 4. Cracked surface of the flat cell. The flat cells (arrow) form a partition between the germinal center and the mantle zone. This cell is possibly a dendritic reticular cell.

In the surface of the partition from the mantle zone, the collagen and the reticular fibers densely covered the flat cells. By the freeze fracturing method, a cracked surface of the flat cell was observed (fig. 4). In some focal areas, a small and smooth lymphocyte was recognized inside the network of the reticulum fibers.

Discussion

Recent progress of the immunological techniques allowed close observation of lymphocytes and immunoglobulins of the human palatine tonsil [1–3]. In the germinal center there are immature lymphocytes, reticular cells (phagocyte and nonphagocyte), plasma cells, and a few helper T cells. But, in the mantle zone, there are almost only mature B lymphocytes. It is also known that a B lymphocyte is derived from the germinal center. Kotani [4] suggested the reasons why only B lymphocytes are found in the mantle zone as follows: (1) lymphocytes have a potential of determining their route to move from the germinal center to the mantle zone, and (2) the structure surrounding lymphocytes acts as a lymphocyte inducer. There are many IgG in the border zone between the germinal center and the mantle zone, thus attracting B lymphocytes with IgG receptor, while helper T lymphocytes possibly help the movement of B lymphocytes. The authors could observe a cell resembling a T lymphocyte inside the network of the reticular fibers.

Reticular cells in the mantle zone are named as a dendritic cell, because of its complex process. It is thought that the dendritic cell takes, concentrates, and preserves antigens to take part in the movement of B lymphocytes. Kawabata [5] observed the lamellar structure in the mantle zone and considered that the structure is organized by the dendritic cells. Yet, there is a controversial report that no lamellar structure was observed in the mantle zone [6].

In the present study, the flat cells lining up in the border area between the germinal center and the mantle zone were seen. The mantle zone also showed a similar finding. These flat cells are presumably the dendritic cells. In the partition, some clefts and pores were observed, indicating possible movement of a lymphocyte through this portion. In spite of the dense collagen and reticular fibers outside the flat cells, the surface of the flat cell on the side of the germinal center was smooth. Therefore, we assume the flat cell plays a role in supplying the antigens to allow movement of B lymphocytes.

In summary: (1) The framework of the lymphatic reticulum of the germinal center was dense mesh of fine reticulum. The cracked surface of large and medium-sized lymphocytes, plasma cells, and reticular cells were observed. (2) The border zone between the germinal center and the mantle was formed by flat and rectangular cells with a smooth surface. These cells were surrounded by the dense collagen and the reticular fibers. In some portions of the partition, there were clefts and pores. (3) At the partition far from the basal pole, collagen and reticular fibers were sparse. In some focal areas, the collagen fibers were running curved, leaving a large space.

References

1   Kuki K, Tabata T: Immunohistological studies on tonsils of recurrent tonsillitis and tonsils with focal infections. Acta Otolaryngol 1988(suppl 454):75–82.
2   Kimura T, Kunimoto M, Kuki K, Tabata T: Immunohistochemical study of tonsil,

with special reference to MHC class II antigen and lymphocytes in tonsillar epithelium. Pract Otol (Kyoto) 1989(suppl 33):103–111.

3 Von Gaudecker B: Development and functional anatomy of the human tonsilla palatina. Acta Otolaryngol 1988(suppl 454):28–32.

4 Kotani M: Structure and function of lymphoid follicles. Jpn J Tonsil 1973;12:150–156.

5 Kawabata I: Scanning electron microscopic observation of the human palatine tonsils. Jpn J Tonsil 1977;16:1–7.

6 Yasumoto Y, Soda T: Three-dimensional arrangement of the lymphatic reticulum in the human and canine tonsil. J Otolaryngol Jpn 1988;91:739–750.

Hiroshi Watanabe, MD, Department of Otolaryngology, Hiroshima University School of Medicine, 1-2-3 Kasumi, Minami-ku, Hiroshima 734 (Japan)

Galioto GB (ed): Tonsils: A Clinically Oriented Update.
Adv Otorhinolaryngol. Basel, Karger, 1992, vol 47, pp 11–15

The Microvasculature of the Human Palatine Tonsil and Its Role in the Homing of Lymphocytes

Marta E. Perry[a], *Y. Mustafa*[a], *K. Alun Brown*[b]

[a] Division of Anatomy and Cell Biology, Guy's Hospital, and
[b] Division of Immunology, St. Thomas' Hospital, UMDS,
University of London, UK

The human palatine tonsil receives a rich blood supply from vessels whose distribution is not uniform [1]. This is illustrated by the profuse vascular network within the parafollicular areas which contrasts with the relatively hypovascular lymphoid follicles [2, 3].

It is generally agreed that recirculating lymphocytes migrate into peripheral lymphoid tissue through specialized structures of the microvasculature, the high endothelial venules (HEV) [4]. These venules are present in the parafollicular regions of the palatine tonsil but absent from germinal follicles and the oropharyngeal epithelium [1]. Although lymphocytes recognize HEVs through specific 'homing' receptors [5] their binding to these and other endothelial cells is mediated by their surface expression of leucocyte function antigen-1 (LFA-1) and by its ligand, the intercellular adhesion molecule-1 (ICAM-1), expressed on the endothelium [4, 6].

The aim of the present study was to identify the various types of vessels and their location within the palatine tonsil, and to determine whether vascular areas with a high expression of ICAM-1 were associated with large numbers of LFA-1-bearing lymphocytes. The investigation was undertaken by using light microscopy (LM), scanning (SEM) and transmission electron microscopy (TEM). Immunoelectron microscopy (IEM) using gold-coupled reagents was performed in order to visualize the distribution of LFA-1 and ICAM-1 [7].

Materials and Methods

Material was obtained from patients undergoing tonsillectomy. Tissue samples were prepared for LM using conventional techniques, and stained using routine (haematoxylin and eosin) and special methods (azan, Giemsa, Gordon and Sweet, methylene blue/Azur II and Movat hexachrome stain).

Dissected pieces of tissue were prepared for SEM and TEM using standard techniques, and for the IEM tissue was fixed, cryoprotected and frozen in liquid nitrogen [7]. Subsequently, 30-μm cryostat sections were incubated either with an anti-ICAM-1 (RR/1) or anti-LFA-1 (R7.01.H09) monoclonal antibody, followed by incubation with goat-anti-mouse IgG coupled with 5-nm gold particles (Amersham International plc, UK). After postfixation and silver enhancement, the sections were osmicated, dehydrated and flat embedded in TAAB-resin. The 30-μm sections were examined by light microscope and areas selected from which ultrathin sections were cut and viewed in TEM.

Results

The microvasculature of the human palatine tonsil consisted of a network of capillaries, sinusoids, arterioles, low endothelial venules, HEV, and lymphatic channels, which were present in four distinct areas (fig. 1): (1) the parafollicular area, containing a rich vascular network and most of the HEV (fig. 2); (2) the subepithelial connective tissue band, which was located below the avascular oropharyngeal epithelium and contained numerous capillaries, low endothelial venules and lymphatic channels; (3) the reticulated crypt epithelium, with a network of capillaries and sinusoids arranged in loops, and also HEV, which were seen predominantly in its lower border regions (fig. 3), and (4) the lymphoid follicles, which were supplied by central arterioles but possessed only a few capillaries, hence their relatively hypovascular appearance.

The various LM stains aided the recognition and identification of all blood vessels, including the HEV (fig. 3). The characteristic morphology

---

Fig. 1. Illustration of reticulated epithelium of the human palatine tonsil with suggested locations of lymphocytic infiltration.

Fig. 2. Parafollicular area of the human palatine tonsil showing sectioned lumina of vessels, including an HEV. SEM. × 515.

Fig. 3. An HEV located in the lower border region of reticulated crypt epithelium. c = Crypt lumen; cr = occluded crypt ramus. HE. × 170.

Fig. 4. An HEV showing strongly ICAM-1-positive luminal and lateral surfaces of the high endothelial cells. Immunogold. TEM. × 9,500.

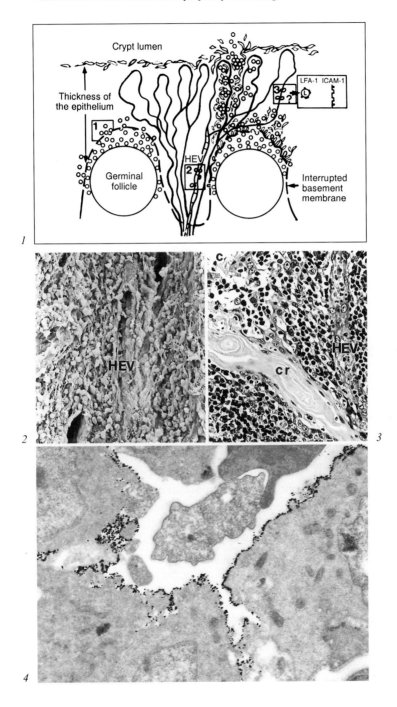

and cobblestone appearance of the HEV was confirmed by SEM (fig. 2) and TEM (fig. 4).

The IEM demonstrated that the staining of ICAM-1 was predominantly confined to the vascular endothelium. However, arterioles, lymphatics and low endothelial venules stained only weakly in comparison with the strongly stained endothelium of the HEV (fig. 4).

The greatest expression of LFA-1 was seen on lymphocytes in both the intra- and extravascular location, especially those in the parafollicular T cell regions, and in the lower border regions of the crypt epithelium, close to HEV.

Discussion

The present study shows the varied distribution of blood vessels in the human palatine tonsil and demonstrates that HEV are located not only in the parafollicular areas, but also within the reticulated crypt epithelium.

Furthermore, vascular areas with a high ICAM-1 expression are often in close proximity to large numbers of LFA-1-positive lymphocytes. Since ICAM-1 is a ligand for LFA-1 [7], and antibodies against ICAM-1 strongly stain the HEV of the parafollicular regions, it is likely that HEV in the tonsil occupy a strategic position in promoting lymphocyte extravasation into this tissue. This view supports the suggestion that all recirculating lymphocytes enter the subepithelial parafollicular areas of the tonsil and pass through the HEV located there [8, 9].

Many LFA-1-positive lymphocytes were also associated with ICAM-1-positive HEV situated in the reticulated crypt epithelium. From these findings it is further proposed that lymphocytes infiltrating this epithelium may originate not only from the subepithelial tissues [2], but also directly from the circulation. Hence, the presence of blood vessels in the reticulated epithelium may have a special role in its local surface protection [10].

Acknowledgements

This investigation was supported by a grant from the Special Trustess of Guy's Hospital and by the Arthritis and Rheumatism Council. The authors appreciate the kind gifts of antibodies from Dr. Springer (Boston, Mass., USA) and Dr. Rothlein (Conn., USA), the excellent technical assistance of Miss S. Smith, Mr. K. Fitzpatrick, Miss F. Winning and Mr. K. Brady, and are grateful to Mrs. D. Paterson who typed the manuscript.

References

1   Perry ME: A study of the microscopical structure of the human palatine tonsil with special reference to the epithelium; PhD thesis, University of London, 1990.

2   Olah I: Structure of the tonsils; in Antoni E, Staub M (eds): Tonsils, Structure, Immunology and Biochemistry. Budapest, Akadémiai Kiadó, 1978, sect I, pp 5–51.

3   Perry ME, Jones MM, Mustafa Y: Structure of the crypt epithelium in human palatine tonsils. Acta Otolaryngol (Stockh) 1988(suppl 454):53–59.

4   Springer TA: Adhesion receptors of the immune system. Nature 1990;346:425–434.

5   Berg EL, Goldstein LA, Jutila MA, Nahacher M, Picker LJ, Streeter PR, Wu NW, Zhon D, Butcher DC: Homing receptors and vascular addressins. Immunol Rev 1989;108:5–18.

6   Pober JS, Cotran RS: What can be learned from the expression of endothelial adhesion molecules in tissues? Lab Invest 1991;64:301–305.

7   Perry ME, von Gaudecker B, Sterry W, Mielke V: Immunoelectron microscopic demonstration of increased intercellular adhesion molecule-1 expression on high endothelial venules in human palatine tonsils; in Imhof BA, Berrih-Aknin S, Ezine S (eds): Lymphatic Tissues and in vivo Immune Responses. New York, Dekker, 1991, pp 877–881.

8   Umetani Y: Postcapillary venule in rabbit tonsil and entry of lymphocytes into its endothelium. Arch Histol Jpn 1977;40:77–94.

9   Crocker J: The T lymphoycte content of the efferent lymphatics of the human palatine tonsil. Clin Otolaryngol 1982;7:331–334.

10 Brandtzaeg P: Immunopathological alterations in tonsillar disease. Acta Otolaryngol (Stockh) 1988(suppl 454):64–69.

Dr. Marta E. Perry, Division of Anatomy and Cell Biology, UMDS,
Guy's Hospital, London Bridge, London SE1 9RT (UK)

Galioto GB (ed): Tonsils: A Clinically Oriented Update.
Adv Otorhinolaryngol. Basel, Karger, 1992, vol 47, pp 16–20

Functional Morphology of Tonsillar Germinal Center

I. Kawabata[a], *M. Nakamura*[b], *H. Tabe*[a]

[a] Department of Otolaryngology, Saitama Medical Center,
Saitama Medical School, Kawagoe, Saitama, and [b] Department of Otolaryngology,
Faculty of Medicine, Hongo Tokyo, University of Tokyo, Japan

The purpose of the present studies was to determine proliferation and migration of lymphocytes in tonsillar tissue using immunohistochemical methods.

The germinal center and crypt epithelium are thought to be the morphological unit of tonsillar function. The outcoming antigens are captured in crypt epithelium, and immunoinformation is transferred to the germinal center, where antibodies are produced. The lymphocytes in the germinal center play an important role in the production of antibodies. Therefore, it is very important to know the cell proliferation and migration of lymphocytes in the germinal center for immunoactivity of the tonsil.

Since Koburg [1] in 1963 reported the cell proliferation and migration of lymphocytes in the germinal center utilizing thymidine-^{3}H, several studies have been done. Recently the immunohistochemical method using anti-bromodeoxyuridine (BrdU, thymidine analogue) monoclonal antibodies has been tried extensively in various fields of medicine [2, 3]. Using this method, we have attempted to detect the cell dynamics of lymphocytes in the germinal center. We report the results of both rabbit in vivo studies and human in vitro studies.

Material and Methods

In vivo Experiments on Rabbit Tonsil

Healthy white rabbits weighing 2.0–2.5 kg were used in this study. The animals received BrdU (Sigma Chemical Co.), 60 mg/kg body weight, as a simple bolus injection administered intravenously. The animals were sacrificed and the tonsils were removed at

15 min, 2 h, 14 h, and 24 h after injection respectively. Tonsils were fixed in Bouin's fluid, dehydrated, embedded in paraffin and sectioned into 5-μm thick slices. The specimens were incubated with the anti-BrdU monoclonal antibody for 1 h at room temperature, washed with PBS, and then incubated again with the anti-mouse IgG peroxidase conjugated for 30 min. The specimens were suspended in PB containing DAB to be stained at the site of BrdU incorporation.

In vitro Experiments on Human Tonsil

Human tonsils taken at tonsillectomy were used for in vitro experiments. The small pieces of tonsillar tissue were incubated in artificial blood (FC-43) containing 0.5 mM BrdU at 37 °C for 30 min under 3 atm pressure of mixed gases. The succeeding procedures were the same as those mentioned above.

Results

Distribution of BrdU-Incorporated Cells in Tonsil

The BrdU-incorporated cells were stained blue-black in the nucleus, and easily distinguished from the other ones. They were located in the basal layer of epithelium of the pharyngeal site, and were scattered mainly in the germinal center, however few in the crypt epithelium. The BrdU-incorporated cells in the germinal center seemed to be the large or medium-sized lymphocytes in their appearance.

Localization of BrdU-Incorporated Cells in Germinal Center

The distribution of BrdU-incorporated cells in the germinal center was changed with increasing time after administration of BrdU. The nuclei of the large or medium-sized lymphocytes in the germinal center were already stained blue-black 15 min after injection of BrdU (fig. 1). The majority of those cells were found in the posterior portion (basal part) of the germinal center. With increasing time, BrdU-incorporated cells appeared in the central and anterior part (near the dark zone) (fig. 2). 14 h after injection, they reached the anterior portion (near the dark zone) (fig. 3). Most of them disappeared within 24 h after injection. Several cells were found in the parafollicular area and crypt epithelium (fig. 4). BrdU-incorporated cells were hardly found in the dark zone. Figure 5 shows the schematic drawing of migration of BrdU-incorporated cells in the germinal center.

The Existence of Germinal Center without BrdU-Incorporated Cells

It is well known that rabbit tonsil has 30–60 germinal centers. Whole germinal centers in one tonsil were examined by serial section to determine

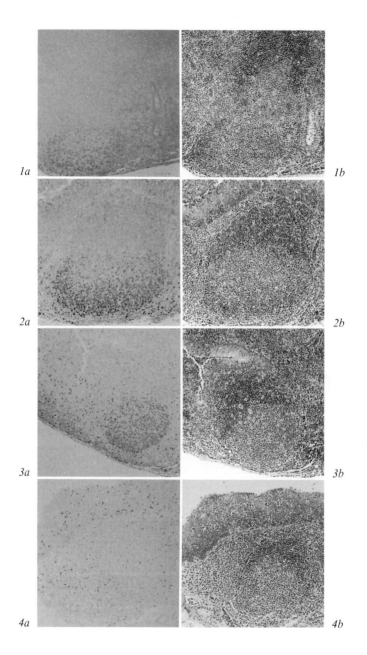

Fig. 1–4. Migration of BrdU-incorporated cells in the germinal center. *1a, 2a, 3a,* and *4a* show the localization of BrdU-incorporated cells at 15 min, 2 h, 14 h, and 24 h after BrdU injection respectively. *1b* is an adjacent HE-stained section of *1a,* as well as *2b, 3b,* and *4b.*

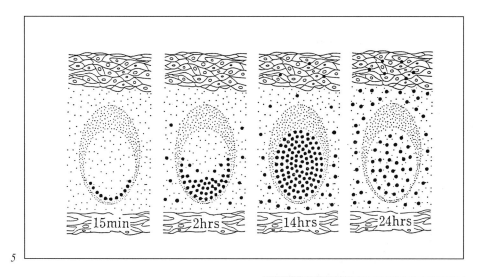

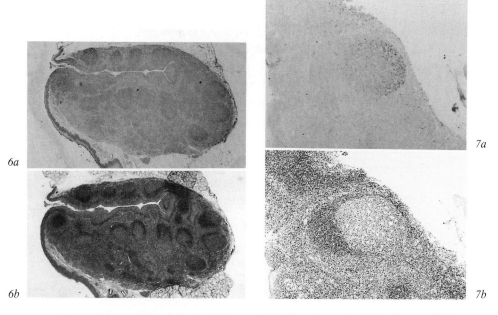

Fig. 5. Schematic drawing of migration of BrdU-incorporated cells in the germinal center.

Fig. 6. a Existence of the germinal center without BrdU-incorporated cells. *b* An adjacent HE-stained section.

Fig. 7. a The distribution of BrdU-incorporated cells in human tonsil. *b* An adjacent HE-stained section.

whether or not all germinal centers have a similar reaction to that mentioned above. We found that 20–30% of the germinal centers did not have any BrdU-incorporated cells (fig. 6).

In vitro Experiments on Human Tonsil

In vitro experiments on human tonsil, BrdU-incorporated cells were found mainly in the germinal center and pharyngeal epithelium. In the germinal center they seemed to be the large or medium-sized lymphocytes and were distributed in the posterior portion as in the findings of in vivo experiments (fig. 7). This finding suggested that the posterior portion of the germinal center in human tonsil is the site of cell proliferation of lymphocytes.

Conclusion

To conclude: (1) the immunohistochemical methods utilizing anti-BrdU monoclonal antibodies were used to examine the cell dynamics of lymphocytes in the tonsillar tissue; (2) the germinal centers in the tonsil have a higher cell proliferation of lymphocytes, and a considerable number of lymphocytes migrate from the posterior to the anterior portion of the germinal center, and (3) the germinal centers without BrdU-incorporated cells are found.

References

1   Koburg E: Zur Lymphocytopoese in den Tonsillen. Arch Ohren Nasen Kehlkopf-heilkd 1965;185:785.
2   Gratzner HG: Monoclonal antibody to 5-bromo and 5-iododeoxyuridine: A new reagent for detection of DNA replication. Science 1982;218:474.
3   Shutte B, et al: Effect of tissue fixation on anti-bromodeoxyuridine immunohisto-chemistry. J Histochem Cytochem 1987;35:1343.

Dr. I. Kawabata, Department of Otolaryngology, Saitama Medical Center, Saitama Medical School, Kawagoe, Saitama 350 (Japan)

Galioto GB (ed): Tonsils: A Clinically Oriented Update.
Adv Otorhinolaryngol. Basel, Karger, 1992, vol 47, pp 21–27

Phylogenic and Ultrastructural Properties of the Primitive Tonsils of Laboratory Suncuses

Michio Kimura[a], *Kazuo Tohya*[a], *Toshihide Tabata*[b]

[a] Department of Anatomy, Kansai Shinkyu College, Kansai Academy of Medical Sciences, Kumatori, Sennan, Osaka, and [b] Department of Otorhinolaryngology, Wakayama Medical College, Wakayama, Japan

Suncus *(Suncus murinus),* recently developed as a new small laboratory animal of Insectivora in Japan, is of special interest in understanding tonsillar evolution since the suncus has a pair of primitive palatine tonsils [1]. Phylogenically, the animal is closer to primates than conventional laboratory rodents – mice, rats and guinea pigs lacking palatine tonsils. The present study deals with the ultrastructural and immunohistochemical characteristics of the suncus tonsils and discusses its phylogenic properties.

Materials and Methods

Suncuses of both sexes, weighing 60–120 g, were used in this study. They were obtained from CLEA Experimental Animals Japan Inc., Tokyo. One group of suncuses was prepared for scanning (SEM) and transmission (TEM) electron microscopies. A second group was intra-abdominally sensitized with an injection of 0.03 ml of horseradish peroxidase (HRP) (3 mg/ml) in Freund's complete adjuvant. Three weeks later, the animals were boostered with 0.01 ml of 1/10 diluted HRP in physiological saline (PBS) into the fauces region using a 27-gauge injection needle. Three to seven days after the booster, the animals were perfused via the left ventricle with a periodate-lysine-paraformaldehyde (PLP) fixative under deep ether anesthesia. The fauces, including tonsillar regions, were removed and prepared for ultrastructural visualization of the HRP-antibody-producing cells in the tonsils. A third group was prepared for an immunohistochemical demonstration of suncus IgM-like monoclonal antibody prepared by our laboratory [2]. They were perfused with a PLP fixative for 30 min. The fauces regions, including tonsils, were removed and kept in the same fixative for 4 h. After washing in PBS, they were frozen in liquid nitrogen, and sectioned at 4–10 μm in a cryostat microtome. The serial sections were incubated in a moist chamber with 1/1,000-diluted monoclonal antibody to suncus

IgM and left overnight at 4 °C. The immunoreacted specimens were rinsed twice in cold PBS, 2–3 min each time and immersed in 1/200-diluted FITC-labeled anti-mouse IgG (Cappel, USA) in PBS for 1 h at room temperature. After a brief rinse, the specific FITC fluorescence was examined under epifluorescence illumination using an Olympus fluorescence microscope.

Results

The average length of an adult suncus is almost the same as that of a young rat. The animal has a pair of palatine tonsils [1] and a tubal tonsil-like lymphoid organ, respectively (fig. 1a, b). The palatine tonsil is oval in shape, approximately 1.2 mm in length and contains a single nodule with a germinal center. The epithelium covering the nodule retains lymphoepithelial symbiotic images. A thin capsule-like demarcation separates the tonsil from the neighboring tissues. On the other hand, the latter tubal tonsils retained lymphoinfiltration images with ciliated epithelium. The epithelium also contained numerous infiltrating mononuclear cells (fig. 1c). They are situated near the pharyngeal opening of the auditory tube. In SEM, the surface of the palatine tonsil revealed a cobblestone-like structure in the crypt region (fig. 2). At higher magnification, few migrating lymphocytes can be seen in the region. In TEM, the crypt epithelium consisted of keratinocytes, lymphocytes, monocytes, plasma cells and nonlymphoid mononuclear cells and revealed the lymphoepithelial symbiosis image (fig. 3). Often, the throat bacteria were found within the keratinocytes and nonlymphoid cells. In the lymphoid parenchyma, numerous lymphocytes were observed. Postcapillary venules were also detected in the paranodular regions. The present HRP sensitization experiment showed the appearance of the HRP-antibody-producing cells both in the lymphoid parenchyma and in the crypt epithelium (fig. 4). The HRP-positive cells revealed lymphoplasma cell properties in the fine structure. The HRP-positive reactions were situated in the perinuclear and cytoplasmic cisterna of the endoplasmic reticulum. Although it has been suggested that suncuses possess IgM and IgG serum antibodies [3], the present immunohistochemical preparations of anti-suncus IgM-like monoclonal antibody [2] revealed that IgM-positive lymphoplasma cells dispersed throughout the parenchyma and the symbiosis (fig. 5).

Figure 6 illustrates bisbenzimide-labeling autospleen lymphocytes in the palatine tonsil. These cells were originally obtained from their spleen tissues and labeled with bisbenzimide in vitro, by the method of Austin et

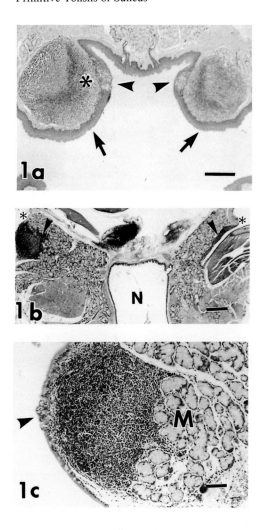

Fig. 1. Light micrographs of the suncus fauces and nasopharynx. *a* Arrows show palatine tonsils. Arrowheads indicate crypt regions. The asterisk shows the mantle zone. Bar = 0.5 mm. *b* Asterisks show auditory tubules. Arrowheads indicate tubal tonsil-like structures. N = Nasopharynx. Bar = 0.5 mm. *c* Enlarged light micrograph of the tubal tonsil-like structure. Arrowhead shows ciliated epithelium with mononuclear cell infiltration. M = Mucous gland. Bar = 100 μm.

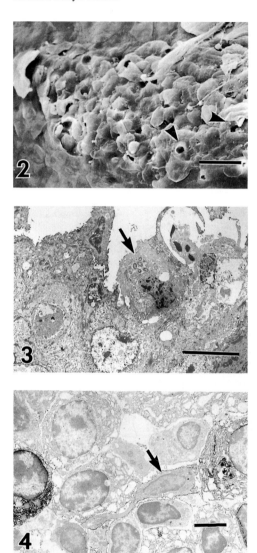

Fig. 2. SEM of the crypt region in the suncus palatine tonsil. Note the peculiar surface images and the small pores (arrowheads). Bar = 40 µm.

Fig. 3. TEM of the lymphoepithelial symbiosis. Arrow shows the throat bacteria. Bar = 10 µm.

Fig. 4. HRP-sensitized tonsil. HRP-antibody-producing plasma cells and a surface HRP-antibody-positive nonlymphoid cell (arrow) located within the paranodular region. Bar = 2 µm.

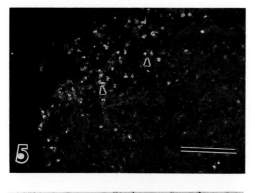

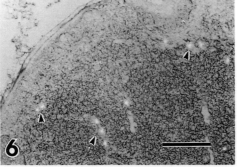

Fig. 5. Immunohistochemical preparation of the palatine tonsil. IgM monoclonal antibody-positive cells (arrowheads) located in the paranodular region. Bar = 100 μm.

Fig. 6. Fluorescence micrograph of bisbenzimide-labeling spleen lymphocytes (arrowheads) in the palatine tonsil. Bar = 100 μm.

al. [4]. Thereafter, the labeling cells were returned into the general circulation via the jugular vein using a 27-gauge injection needle. Sixty to ninety minutes after the injection, the tonsils were removed, sectioned at 10–20 μm and observed under the fluorescence microscope.

Discussion

Although earlier studies have been mostly done with the palatine tonsils [1, 5, 6], the suncus has a pair of tubal tonsil-like structures, in addition to the palatine tonsils. Human tonsils consist of four types: palatine, tubal,

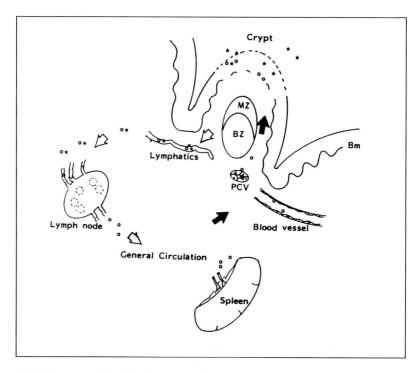

Fig. 7. A presumable migration route of tonsillar lymphocytes. Open arrows show lymphatic routes and black arrows indicate blood circulation. * = Antigen; o = migrating lymphocyte; Bm = basement membrane; BZ = basal zone; MZ = mantle zone.

lingual and phalyngeal, and retain so-called Waldeyer's ring; while the suncus possesses only two primitive types of them. The animal, although phylogenically a lower mammal, is noteworthy as a direct ancestor of primates. From this point of view, the suncus tonsils are critical in understanding tonsillar evolution in mammals. The present study also indicated that the suncus tonsils reacted positively to the exogenous HRP antigen (fig. 4) and selectively received the bisbenzimide-labeling spleen lymphocytes (fig. 6). This data presumes that the suncus tonsils participate in both the regional and systemic immunity. The suncus tonsils probably act as a dynamic lymphoid organ rather than a mere static lymphoid organ (fig. 7). Since the palatine tonsils are located in the alimentary tract, the functions may resemble those of Peyer's patches. Although the present IgM-like monoclonal antibody experiment positively reacted in some lymphoplasma cells within the tonsils, it is uncertain whether the IgM-positive cells produce the HRP antibody or not. T-cell-mediated immunity is very important in understanding tonsil functions. Further research on the suncus T-cell properties is necessary to clarify the pathological mechanism of systemic tonsillar disease including tonsillar focal infection. The peculiar localization of the tubal tonsil-like structure is extremely important since the tonsil-like structure may be utilized as a model of experimental otitis media.

References

1   Kimura M, Tohya K: Scanning, transmission and immunoelectron microscopical studies of the tonsil-like lymphoid organ of normal and horseradish-peroxidase-injected laboratory suncuses. Acta Anat 1989;136:177–184.
2   Tohya K, Kimura M, Kawamata J: Immunohistochemical studies on the distribution of lymphocytes in the peripheral and mucosal lymphoid tissues of laboratory musk shrews *(Suncus murinus).* Dev Comp Immunol 1992; submitted.
3   Sato K: Immune response in the house musk shrew, *Suncus murinus;* in Kondo K, Oda S, Kitoh J, Ota K, Isomura G (eds): *Suncus murinus* (in Japanese with English abstract). Tokyo, JSS Press, 1985, pp 446–451.
4   Austin JM, Kupiec-Weglimki JW, Hankins DF, Morris PJ: Migration patterns of dendritic cells in the mouse. J Exp Med 1988;167:646–651.
5   Takagi T, Nishikawa K, Igarashi H, Nobuki K: Problems on the definition of a palatine tonsil – with special references to the Suncus's tonsil (in Japanese). Jpn J Tonsil 1985;24:202–207.
6   Nishikawa K, Takagi T: Comparative immunobiology of the palatine tonsil. Acta Otolyngol (Stockh) 1988;454:43–47.

Dr. M. Kimura, Department of Anatomy, Kansai Shinkyu College,
Kansai Academy of Medical Sciences, Kumatori, Sennan, Osaka 590-04 (Japan)

Galioto GB (ed): Tonsils: A Clinically Oriented Update.
Adv Otorhinolaryngol. Basel, Karger, 1992, vol 47, pp 28–31

Autonomic Nervous System in the Tonsil

Koichi Tomoda, Norio Maeda, Kageyuki Kozuki, Kazuo Sato,
Nobuo Kubo, Masanori Kitajiri, Toshio Yamashita,
Tadami Kumazawa

Department of Otolaryngology, Kansai Medical University, Fumizonocho,
Moriguchi, Osaka, Japan

Concerning the participation of autonomic nerves in the tonsils, the autonomic nerves have long been assumed to play an important role when the relation between the tonsillar focus and the whole body is considered, or when shock at tonsillectomy is associated with Reilly's phenomenon, and it has attracted a great deal of interest.

In the present study, we investigated the anatomic distribution of autonomic nerve fibers and its terminals in the tonsils.

Material and Methods

Twenty human palatine tonsils, obtained from patients aged from 6 to 8 years who had undergone tonsillectomy, were prepared for the histologic examinations. Adrenergic nerve fibers were observed by the glyoxylic acid method [1], while cholinergic nerves were investigated using acetylcholinesterase (AchE) by the method of Karnovsky and Roots [2]. Neuropeptide-containing nerve fibers, such as tyrosine hydroxylase (TH), vasoactive intestinal polypeptide (VIP), neuropeptide Y (NPY), somatostatin (SOM), substance P (SP) and calcitonin gene-related peptide (CGRP), were immunohistochemically investigated by the ABC method.

Adrenergic nerve terminals innervated in the rabbit's palatine tonsils were observed using an electron microscope with a pretreatment of an injection of 5-hydroxydopamine (5-OHDA).

Results

The distribution of adrenergic, cholinergic and neuropeptide-containing nerve fibers in the tonsil are shown in table 1. Adrenergic nerve fibers

Table 1. Distribution of adrenergic, cholinergic or neuropeptidergic nerve fibers in tonsil

	AD	AchE	TH	NPY	VIP	CGRP	SP	SOM
Capsule	+	+	++	++	++	+	+	+
Septum	++	+	++	++	++	+	+	+
Follicle	+	+	+	+	+			+
Epithelium								
Glands	+	+	+		++			

+ = < 4 fibers; ++ = > 5 fibers in 200 × 200 μm².

with a varicose appearance were seen closely associated with the vessel walls in the hilus and travelled, with a decreasing number, through the septum to the parafollicular region. The strong activity of AchE was found around the vessel walls located in the tonsillar capsule and septum. The fine nerve fibers containing AchE activity distributed to the parafollicular spaces.

Of neuropeptide-containing fibers, a large number of fibers immunoreactive to TH or VIP were dominantly distributed around the vessels in the hilus and septum, and less distributed in the parafollicular spaces. Those individual nerve fibers showed a varicose appearance. An abundant distribution of VIP fibers was specially seen in the para-acinal region of the Weber's glands. The localization of NPY-immunoreactive fibers was similar to those of TH or VIP with an exception of distributing to the glands. The nerve supply of SP, SOM or CGRP was less as compared to those of three fibers mentioned. However, SOM fibers were only seen in the germinal center. None of the fibers were distributed to the epithelium.

Adrenergic nerve terminals were characterized by the presence of small and large dense-cored granular vesicles which contained 5-OHDA, while cholinergic nerve terminals had only small clear synaptic vesicles (agranular vesicles). Both adrenergic or cholinergic nerve terminals were mainly located in the hilus, just beneath the smooth muscle layer of the arteries and in the preacinal region of the Weber's glands (fig. 1). None of the nerve terminals were found in the parafollicular regions or germinal centers.

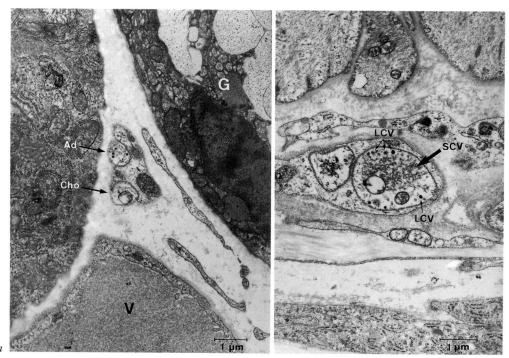

Fig. 1. a Adrenergic (Ad) and cholinergic nerve terminal (Cho) are seen close to the gland (G) and vessel (V). *b* Adrenergic nerve terminals are characterized by the presence of small (SCV) and large dense-cored granular vesicles (LCV) which contained 5-OHDA.

Discussion

The sympathetic nerves containing TH and NPY distributed in the tonsil originate from the superior cervical ganglion, and its neurotransmitter is noradrenaline. The parasympathetic nerves containing VIP distributed in the tonsil originate from the sphenopalatine ganglion, and its neurotransmitter is acetylcholine. They are thought to be involved in direct information transmission from the central nervous system to the tonsils.

Adrenergic or cholinergic receptors are known to be present on thymic, splenic and tonsillar lymphocytes [3–5]. VIP receptors have been reported on specific lymphocytes of the peripheral blood [6]. With these communications, the functional significance of an autonomic nervous system may include not only regulation of blood flow in the tonsils but also of lymphocyte development and immune responses.

The afferent (sensory) nerves containing SP, SOM and CGRP located in the tonsils originate from the trigeminal or the dorsal root of the cervical ganglion and directly transmit information, arising from inflammatory or immune reactions, from lymphoid tissues to the central nervous system. They may participate in the local regulation of blood flow or the vascular permeability by an axonal collateral. The quantitative analysis of norepinephrine in the tonsillar tissues revealed that the value of norepinephrine was higher in the cases of habitual tonsillitis than those of simple hypertrophy [7].

Our results may require further studies on the neural-immune interactions in the tonsils.

References

1 Lindvall O, Björklund A: The glyoxylic acid fluorescence histochemical method: a detailed account of the methodology for the visualization of central catecholamine neurons. Histochemistry 1974;39:97–127.

2 Karnovsky MJ, Roots L: A 'direct coloring' thiocholine method for cholinesterases. J Histochem Cytochem 1964;12:219–221.

3 Felten SY, Felten DL, Bellinger DL, et al: Noradrenergic sympathetic innervation of lymphoid organs. Prog Allergy 1988;43:14–36.

4 Richman DP, Arnason BGW: Nicotinic acetylcholine receptor; evidence for a functional distinct receptor on human lymphocytes. Proc Natl Acad Sci USA 1979;76: 4632–4635.

5 Yamashita T, Kumazawa H, Kozuki K, Amano H, Tomoda K, Kumazawa T: Autonomic nervous system in human palatine tonsil. Acta Otolaryngol 1984(suppl 416): 63–71.

6 O'Dorsio MS, Shannon BT, Fleshman DJ, et al: Identification of high affinity receptors for vasoactive intestinal peptide on human lymphocytes of B cell lineage. J Immunol 1989;142:3533–3536.

7 Kozuki K: Various tonsillitis and sympathetic nerves – A study of chemical neurotransmitters. Pract Otol (Kyoto) 1987;80:299–312.

Dr. Koichi Tomoda, Department of Otolaryngology, Kansai Medical University, Fumizonocho, Moriguchi, Osaka 570 (Japan)

Galioto GB (ed): Tonsils: A Clinically Oriented Update.
Adv Otorhinolaryngol. Basel, Karger, 1992, vol 47, pp 32–36

Relationship between Lymphatic and Glandular Tissue in the Larynx

Alžběta Holibková

Department of Anatomy, Medical Faculty, University of Olomouc,
Czechoslovakia

There has been an ever-increasing interest in the study of lymphatic
and glandular tissues in connection with the clinical aspects such as the
production of secretory immunoglobulins and the role these components
play in virus, bacterial and other diseases.

In our previous studies we proved the existence of a lymphatic barrier
in the larynx, which is analogous to Waldeyer's lymphatic ring [1]. We
were also concerned with the problem of the development and topography
of laryngeal glands [2, 4] and other portions of the respiratory tract. An
attempt has been made in the present study to express graphically the
interrelationship of the time course of glandular tissue development and
future localization of individual laryngeal tonsils.

Material and Methods

We studied the laryngeal lymphatic and glandular tissue in material from 101
embryos and fetuses and 68 subjects of both sexes, ranging in age from the third prenatal
month to 95 years. After macroscopic description, the preparations were dehydrated and
embedded in celloidin-paraffin. Serial sections were cut in the frontal, sagittal or trans-
verse plane and were stained with hematoxylin and eosin, after van Gieson, by Hornows-
ky's method.

Results

Focuses of lymphatic tissue were found which were called by us tonsils
(fig. 1). Tonsilla epiglottica is brought in evidence in the seventh fetal
month and reaches its peak development between 4 and 8 years of life

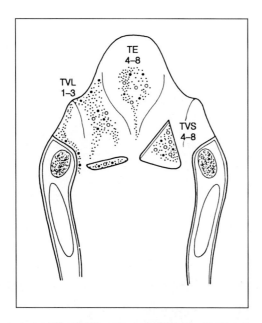

Fig. 1. Distribution of lymphatic tissue in laryngeal mucosa. ● = Primary lymphatic follicles; ○ = secondary lymphatic follicles; TE = tonsilla epiglottica; TVL = tonsilla vestibuli lateralis; TVS = tonsilla ventriculi et sacculi.

(fig. 2). Tonsilla lateralis vestibuli is laid down in the fifth month of intrauterine life, attaining its peak development between 1 and 3 years. Tonsilla ventriculi et sacculi is laid down in the fifth fetal month, attaining its peak development between 4 and 8 years (fig. 3). The glands are laid down in the form of solid epithelial outgrowths between 11 and 16 weeks of the intrauterine life, and in the course of 10–14 days they luminize (fig. 4).

An attempt is made here to represent the development of glandular tissue in relation to the incidence of future tonsils (fig. 5). The y-axis shows the age in prenatal weeks and the x-axis individual groups of laryngeal glands. The first three bars represent groups of epiglottic regions, namely on the dorsal wall (DE), on the lateral wall (LE) and on the ventral wall (VE). Further groups are on the lateral wall of the laryngeal vestibule (LV), in the aryepiglottic folds (PA), in the arytenoid muscle (MA), in the region of the dorsal commissure (CD) and in the region of the ventral commissure (CV), where they occur very rarely and therefore the bar is hatched. Further there is a group of glands in the region of the free side of the ventric-

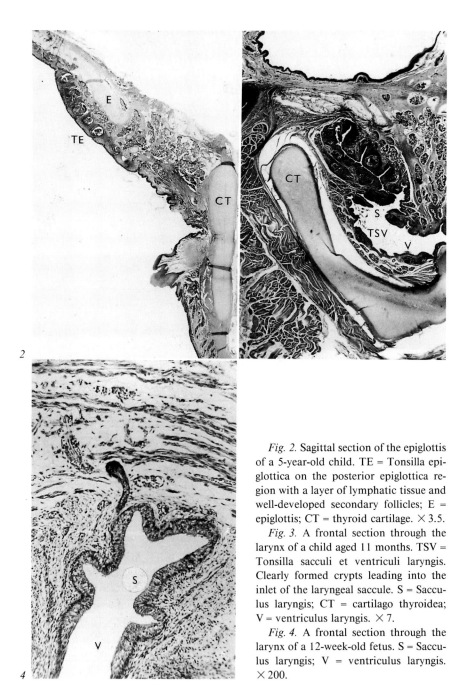

Fig. 2. Sagittal section of the epiglottis of a 5-year-old child. TE = Tonsilla epiglottica on the posterior epiglottica region with a layer of lymphatic tissue and well-developed secondary follicles; E = epiglottis; CT = thyroid cartilage. × 3.5.

Fig. 3. A frontal section through the larynx of a child aged 11 months. TSV = Tonsilla sacculi et ventriculi laryngis. Clearly formed crypts leading into the inlet of the laryngeal saccule. S = Sacculus laryngis; CT = cartilago thyroidea; V = ventriculus laryngis. × 7.

Fig. 4. A frontal section through the larynx of a 12-week-old fetus. S = Sacculus laryngis; V = ventriculus laryngis. × 200.

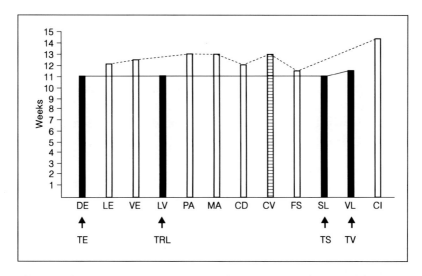

Fig. 5. Relationship between lymphatic and glandular tissue. See text for details and explanation of abbreviations.

ular folds (FS), in the laryngeal saccule (SL) and in the infraglottic cavity (CI). The black bars indicate the anlage of glandular groups at the site of future tonsils. It is evident from figure 5 that at these sites glands make their earlier appearance than in other portions of the larynx, which is suggestive of a close relationship between lymphatic and glandular tissues. These sites are indicated as tonsilla epiglottica (TE), tonsilla recessus lateralis laryngis (TRL), tonsilla sacculi laryngis (TS) and tonsilla ventriculi laryngis (TV).

Discussion

In the period of the maximum development of lymphatic tissue of the larynx, the various tonsils come into contact with each other by means of strips of lymphatic tissue in the aryepiglottic folds, in the region of the anterior and posterior commissure, forming thus a complete laryngeal lymphatic ring at the entrance to the lower respiratory tract, which is comparable to the Waldeyer's tonsillar ring (fig. 1). These anatomical findings are in keeping with the clinical practice as can be seen from the incidence of laryngeal anginas in a relatively old age described by us in collaboration with the Department of Otorhinolaryngology [3]. The graphical representation of the development of individual glandular groups as related to the localization of future tonsils proves the fact that the first to be laid down are the glands at the sites of future tonsils. This close relationship between glandular and lymphatic tissue is not only of morphological but also immunological importance, particularly in the production of secretory immunoglobulins [5].

References

1   Holibková A: Development of the lymphatic tissue of the human larynx. Acta Univ Palacki Olomuc Fac Med 1974;70:101–113.
2   Holibková A: Development and topography of laryngeal glands. Acta Univ Palacki Olomuc Fac Med 1979;90:123–139.
3   Hubáček J, Holibková A: Příspěvek k zánětůům lymfatické tkáně hrtanu (English summary). Česk Otorinol 1979;28:288–291.
4   Holibková A, Výborná E, Hubáček J: Relationship between the development of lymphatic and glandular tissue in the larynx. Acta Univ Palacki Olomuc Fac Med 1989;123:49–54.
5   Kotyza F, Slípka J: Postavení patrových mandlí v imunitním systému člověka (English summary). Česk Otorinol 1988;37:65–72.

Dr. med. Alžběta Holibková, Department of Anatomy, Hněvotínská 3, CS-77515 Olomouc (Czechoslovakia)

Galioto GB (ed): Tonsils: A Clinically Oriented Update.
Adv Otorhinolaryngol. Basel, Karger, 1992, vol 47, pp 37–40

Contacts between Nerves and Lymphocytes in Human Tonsils

J. Lamprecht[a], *M. Hess*[b], *G.E.K. Novotny*[c]

[a] ENT Clinic, RWTH-Aachen, Aachen;
[b] Department of Audiology and Phoniatrics, Free University of Berlin, Berlin, and
[c] Department of Neuroanatomy, Center for Anatomy and Brain Research,
University of Düsseldorf, Düsseldorf, FRG

Recent research has shown innervation of lymphoid tissue in animals [1–3, 5, 6]. Nerves containing various neurotransmitters or neuropeptides [7] have been demonstrated in close contact to immunocompetent cells in organs such as thymus, spleen and lymph nodes of various species. Specific aspects of the innervation of lymph nodes in animals have been reported elsewhere [5, 6]. It has been the aim of our investigation to determine whether the nerves long known to accompany the blood vessels in tonsillar tissues also have contacts to immunocompetent cells. Furthermore, questions as to the distribution of the nerves and their relations to other cells were also addressed.

For our investigations we have employed a reliable staining method for myelinated and unmyelinated nerves in histological sections, combined with immunohistochemical techniques.

Material and Methods

Adenoids and palatine tonsils were obtained from children with chronic infections. Immunohistochemical and silver staining procedures have been published previously [4]. The following antibodies were used: Anti-Leu 3a and Anti-Leu 4 (Becton Dickinson), OKT 3, 4, 8 and OKB (Ortho Diagnostics). The histological sections (double-stained for nerves and lymphocytes) were evaluated using qualitative and semiquantitative methods.

Results

The distribution of nerves in tonsils is inhomogeneous. Large areas devoid of nerves are interspersed with small, intensely innervated areas. In the total extent the connective tissue and parenchyma of the tonsils are only sparsely innervated. Nerves are most frequently found in the connective tissue septa. Nerves accompanying blood vessels must be distinguished from those associated with the vessel wall. The former occasionally send very fine branches into the parenchyma. Single very fine axons, just resolvable under oil immersion optics, may be found in this position in rare instances. It was possible to follow single nerves of less than 1 μm diameter for considerable distances between germinal centers in serial sections. However, terminals that could be identified with any certainty were hardly ever to be found. In the parenchyma there are also nerves accompanying blood vessels. Immunohistochemically stained lymphocyte subpopulations are only occasionally found closely associated with fine nerve fibres. In some instances these nerves possessed varicosities in vicinity of the lymphocytes. At the present stage of our investigations, there is no indication that particular lymphocyte subpopulations are preferentially associated with nerves.

Discussion

Direct contacts between nerves and lymphocytes have been found in lymphatic organs. Earlier immunohistochemical studies on palatine tonsils using fluorescent markers have demonstrated nerves only associated with blood vessels (due to limitations in the effectiveness of fluorescent methods in these tissues) [8]. Silver impregnations have a high signal-to-noise ratio, and has been used for quantitative studies [5, 6].

Nerves are found to be unevenly distributed in the tonsils. They are most frequently present in connective tissue septa together with blood vessels. There are also nerves not innervating blood vessels and giving off very fine branches into the parenchyma. However, so far we have not been able to distinguish any systematic organization. The nerves are inhomogeneously localized to small areas (as in other lymphatic organs). A concentration of nerves within the poles of the tonsils was not observed.

Difficulties were encountered in the attempt to convincingly demonstrate contacts between nerves and lymphocytes, due to the relatively thick sections, which were necessary to be able to follow the course of nerves for any distance, or to be able to recognize nerves in cross section with certainty.

Within the parenchyma, nerves sometimes possessed varicosities. Terminals were only rarely to be demonstrated by means of serial sections. Contacts to lymphocytes at the LM level seemed to be present; in several instances varicosities were seen nearby lymphocytes.

Since electron microscopical studies on rat lymphoid tissues demonstrate the frequent presence of thin cell processes (which cannot be resolved by the light microscope) statements as to the actual presence of nerve contacts to cells must be treated with great caution. However, this does not preclude that functional connections may exist between the nerves and immunocompetent cells with the mediation of the interposed cell. Electron microscopical investigation of these areas on the same section may lead to further information on the relations at the cellular level and possibly give indications as to functional aspects.

In summary, the proximity of lymphocytes to nerves in human tonsils is shown by our double-staining technique of nerves (silver) and lymphocytes (immunohistochemistry). Nerves are mainly confined to connective tissue septa, but occasionally present in the parenchyma. Infrequent varicosities of nerves in close vicinity to lymphocytes can also be demonstrated. Further investigation of possible functional connections requires electron microscopy studies.

References

1   Felten DL, Overhage JM, Felten SY, Schmedtje JF: Noradrenergic sympathetic innervation of lymphoid tissue in the rabbit appendix: further evidence for a link between the nervous and immune systems. Brain Res Bull 1981;7:595–612.
2   Fink T, Weihe E: Multiple neuropeptides in nerves supplying mammalian lymph nodes: messenger candidates for sensory and autonomic neuroimmunomodulation? Neurosci Lett 1988;90:39–44.
3   Giron TG, Crutcher KA, Davis JN: Lymph nodes – A possible site for sympathetic neuronal regulation of immune responses. Ann Neurol 1979;8:520–525.
4   Hess M, Krueger J, Novotny GEK, Thomas C, Lamprecht J: Nachweis von Nerven in Rachen- und Gaumenmandeln – Ein morphologischer Beitrag zur Neuroimmunologie der Tonsillen. Otorhinolaryngol Nova 1991;1:62–66.

5   Novotny GEK, Kliche KO: Innervation of lymph nodes: A combined silver impregnation and electron-microscopic study. Acta Anat 1986;127:243–248.
6   Novotny GEK: Ultrastructural analysis of lymph node innervation in the rat. Acta Anat 1988;133:57–61.
7   Thureson-Klein A, Klein RL, Zhu PC: Exocytosis from large dense-cored vesicles as a mechanism for neuropeptide release in the peripheral and central nervous system. Scanning Electron Microsc 1986;1:179–187.
8   Yamashita T, Kozuki K, Kubo N, Ishibe T, Kumazawa H, Otani K, Kumazawa T: Participation of autonomic nerve in tonsillar focal infection. Acta Otolaryngol (Stockh) 1988(suppl 454):237–240.

Dr. J. Lamprecht, ENT-Clinic, RWTH Aachen, Pauwelsstrasse 30,
D-W–5100 Aachen (FRG)

Galioto GB (ed): Tonsils: A Clinically Oriented Update.
Adv Otorhinolaryngol. Basel, Karger, 1992, vol 47, pp 41–45

Allergic Tonsillitis

A Histopathological Study

Luiza H. Endo, José Vassalo, Silvia R.M.C. Leitão

Department of Otolaryngology and Pathology, Campinas University, São Paulo,
Brazil

Pharyngeal and palatine tonsils undergo alterations in allergic children which become prone to recurrent infection. Daily clinical observations demonstrate that upper airway obstruction (UAO) due to moderate adenoid hypertrophy may be increased in children with allergic rhinitis. Treatment with antihistaminics not only decreases the frequency of infections, but also relieves UAO and surgery may be avoided. X-ray examination shows that adenoid volume decreases after therapy.

Clinicopathological studies have rarely been performed in this area [6]. The authors intended to study surgical specimens of adenoidectomy in order to correlate histological and clinical findings of atopic and nonatopic children.

Material and Methods

Surgical specimens of adenoidectomy performed at our department from January to October 1989, were collected for this retrospective study. 50 cases entered this study.

Surgical specimens were routinely fixed in formalin 10% and embedded in paraffin. Sections (4 μm) were stained with hematoxylin and eosin, Giemsa, toluidine blue (pH 5.0), PAS reaction and Gomori's silver impregnation for reticulin fibers. Slides were histologically evaluated for: chorium edema and presence of eosinophils and mast cells (surface epithelium); crypt epithelium evaluation of lymphatic tissue activity (germinal centers, T zone) fibrosis; acute exsudate. Histological examination was performed without prior knowledge of any clinical information. Patients were divided into three groups according to clinical history and examination, in addition to laboratory results (serum IgE, eosinophil count in nasal mucous): (1) untreated children; (2) allergic children, who had undergone therapy (ketotifen, environmental and alimentary prophylaxis for 3 months), and (3) nonallergic children. Histological data was then correlated with the three groups of patients.

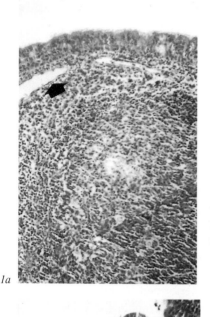

1a

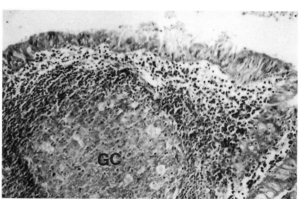

1b

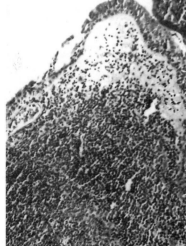

1c

Fig. 1. Histological sections of adenoids. *a* Slight chorion and a dilated vessel (arrow). *b* Moderate chorion edema and an active germinal center (GC). *c* Intense chorion edema. HE. × 100. For details, see text.

Fig. 2. Analysis of the chorium edema.

Fig. 3. Moderate and intense edema in groups 1 and 2.

Results

This study was based on 50 cases divided into three groups: 20 cases of allergic children (group 1), 11 cases of allergic children treated with anti-histamines (group 2) and 19 cases of nonallergic children (group 3). The edema of the chorium was classified as light, moderate and intense (fig. 1a–c). The analysis of the edema of the chorium was made in these

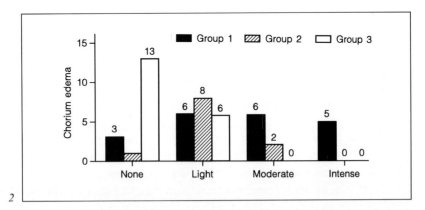

2

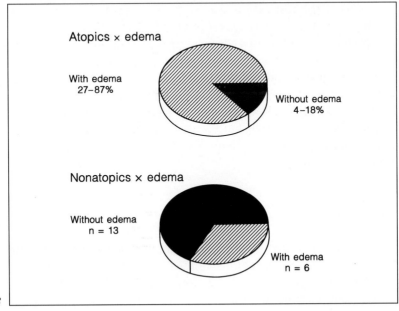

3

different groups (fig. 2). Groups 1 and 2 (atopic patients) showed edema of the chorium in 87.1% and in group 3, in 31.6% (all cases light). Moderate plus intense edema was significantly more frequent in groups 1 and 2 (fig. 3). The eosinophils and mast cells were present in the edema in a few cases in the three groups.

Discussion

The indication of adenoidectomies in allergic children has been very controversial. Some authors say that allergic pathologies may worsen after surgery [1, 2]. On the other hand, some authors assert that there is an improvement in allergic symptoms and little immunological damage [3]. In the literature, we found only one report which studied the interrelation of edema of the chorium with allergic persons [4]. This was the purpose of our study.

The edema was frequently present in the allergic group. We had 20 cases of allergic children (group 1), where the edema was light in 5 cases, moderate and intense in 11 cases and absent in 3 cases. In group 2 (treated allergic children), the edema was present in 10 of 11 cases, but was light. This suggests that the edema in allergic children was responsible for the worsening of the obstruction, due to the increase of size of the adenoid.

In group 3, there was edema in only 6 of 19 patients, and was light. The eosinophils and mast cells were present in a few cases in the three groups. Some authors suggest that the presence of these cells is essential to characterize allergic adenoiditis [4, 5]. On the other hand, other authors were not able to show mast cells in the adenoids of allergic children [6]. Raphael and Kaliner [7] affirm that the pharyngeal tonsil contains significant numbers of mast cells but they had difficulty in isolating these from the surrounding lymphoid tissue and the role of mast cells is not well established in allergy [7].

Conclusion

We concluded that in atopic children, the edema of the chorium was present in 87.1% and the antihistaminic treatment may diminish this edema. Eosinophils and mast cells were present in edema in a few cases in the three groups. Unnecessary surgery may be avoided in children with moderate adenoid hypertrophy and allergic rhinitis presenting UAO by previous administration of antihistaminics in order to diminish adenoid volume. Further studies are necessary to confirm these findings.

References

1   El-Hefny AM: Tonsillectomy and allergic respiratory diseases in children. Acta Allergol 1968;23:312–317.
2   Pialoux P, Laval R: Indictions de l'amydalectomie et de l'adenoïdectomie. Rev Prat 1972;22:82–83.
3   Kjellman NIM, Harder H, Hansson LO, Londwall L: Allergy, otitis media and serum immunoglobulins after adenoidectomy. Acta Paediatr Scand 1978;67:717–723.
4   Studenikin M, Sokolova T: Clinical picture of certain allergic disorders; in Studenikin M, Sokolova T (eds): Allergic Disorders in Children. Moscow, MIR Publishers, 1977, pp 214–233.
5   Loesel LS: Detection of allergic disease in adenoid tissue. Am J Pathol 1984;81:170–175.
6   Tada T, Ishizaka K: Distribution of IgE-forming cells in lymphoid tissue of the human and monkey. J Immunol 1970;104:377–387.
7   Raphael G, Kaliner M: Allergy and the pharyngeal lymphoid tissue. Otolaryngol Clin North Am 1987;20:295–303.

Dr. Luiza H. Endo, Rua Guilherme da Silva, 231/111, Cep. 13.023, Campinas, São Paulo (Brazil)

Galioto GB (ed): Tonsils: A Clinically Oriented Update.
Adv Otorhinolaryngol. Basel, Karger, 1992, vol 47, pp 46–53

Electron Microscope Observations on the Nasopharyngeal Tonsil in Children with Allergic Rhinosinusitis

Todor Karchev, Vesselin Pavlov[1]

Department of Pediatric Otolaryngology, Scientific Institute of
Otorhinolaryngology, Medical Academy, Sofia, Bulgaria

Allergy is being observed at an increasing rate in childhood. According
to Gray [4], till the age of 1 year, the shock organ of allergy is the skin, and
later – till about the age of 6 – the peak of allergic reactions is 'transferred'
to the nose.

Allergic rhinosinusitis is manifested mainly by the symptoms of nasal
obstruction, but practically it is difficult to differentiate the nasal obstruction with allergic genesis from that caused by pathologic hypertrophy of
the nasopharyngeal tonsil. Besides, in some cases allergy and adenoids
contribute substantially to the prevalence of mouth breathing.

It is a long known clinical fact that the lymphoid tissue in the nasopharynx is more or less reconstituted after adenoidectomy in children with
allergic conditions. The reason for this phenomenon is still unclear and the
morphological observations are a path for further investigation.

The ultrastructure alterations in the nasal mucosa after allergic provocation are described by Watanabe and Watanabe [12]. Friedmann and
Bird [3] and Takasaka et al. [10] studied the ultrastructure of the nasal
epithelium in allergic patients. However, no data concerning the ultra-

[1] Thanks are due to Mrs. Ivaneta Dobreva for technical assistance in the processing
of the material for electron microscope observation and to Prof. V.H. Vulchanov for the
help in preparation of the manuscript.

structure of nasopharyngeal tonsil in children with allergic disease have been available in the literature.

In this paper we present our electron microscope observations on the epithelium and lymphoid tissue of the nasopharyngeal tonsil in children with allergic rhinosinusitis.

Material and Methods

Seven children, aged 3–7 years, with case history and physical examination data for nasal obstruction, were included in this study. The extent of hypertrophy of the nasopharyngeal tonsil was defined as obstructive adenoids by means of profile radiogram of the nasopharynx. Allergological tests (performed at the Pediatric Allergological Unit, Medical Academy, Sofia) showed strongly positive reactions to group bacterial antigen. The children suffered periodically with acute inflammation of the upper airways. Adenoidectomy was performed at least 1 month after the last episode of infection and before the onset of desensitizing therapy.

1×1 mm^3 pieces of the surface and the parenchyma of the tonsil were taken immediately after operation and were fixed in 1.6% glutaraldehyde, postfixed in OsO_4, dehydrated in 30–100° alcohol and embedded in Durcopan. Slices were obtained by a Reichert type O_mU_3 ultramicrotome, stained by uranylacetate and lead citrate and examined under a Hitachi HS-7S electron microscope.

As controls we used our previous observations on the ultrastructure of the nasopharyngeal tonsil in children without allergic disease [8].

Results

We found accumulation of eosinophils in tonsillar blood vessels in the children with allergic rhinosinusitis. The eosinophils were directed selectively to the epithelial layer. This caused enlargement of the intraepithelial passages. In children with no allergic disease, the intraepithelial passages, surrounded by precursors of the high cylindrical ciliated cells, were narrow (fig. 1). However, in children with allergic rhinosinusitis, these passages were markedly enlarged and filled with clusters of eosinophils, lymphocytes and erythrocytes (fig. 2, 3). Similar picture was observed in the intraepithelial passages, surrounded by precursors of the M cells (fig. 4).

In some samples eosinophils in degranulation phase were observed (fig. 5), surrounded by lymphocytes and floating in the profuse intercellular liquid, where the granules disappear – a finding which gives us ground to suggest that the granules are quickly dissolved in the liquid.

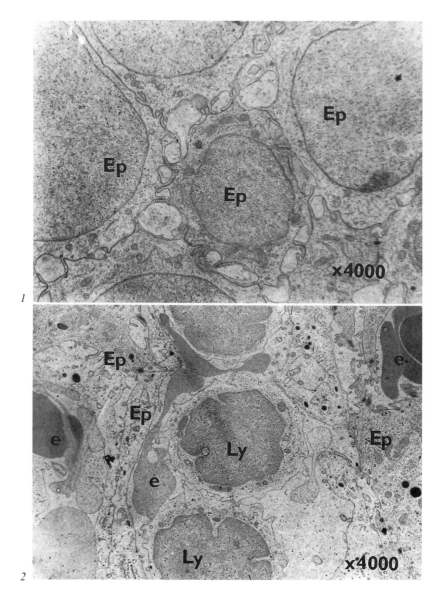

Fig. 1. Precursors of the high cylindrical ciliated cells (Ep).

Fig. 2. Precursors of the high cylindrical ciliated cells (Ep). Ly = Lymphocytes; e = erythrocytes.

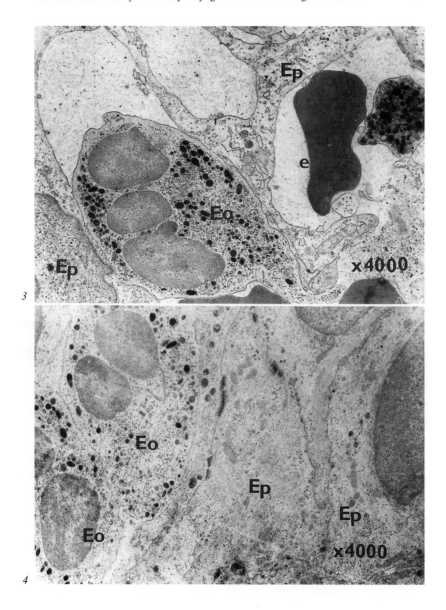

Fig. 3. Precursors of the high cylindrical ciliated cells (Ep). Eo = Eosinophils; e = erythrocytes.

Fig. 4. Precursors of the M cells (Ep). Eo = Eosinophils.

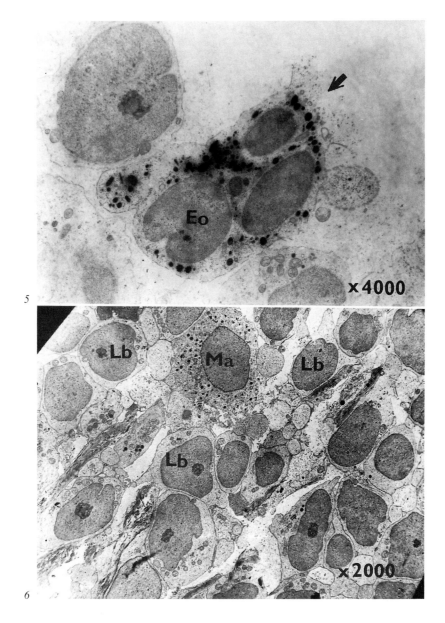

Fig. 5. Eosinophil (Eo): the arrow shows the site of cell membrane disruption.
Fig. 6. Mastocyte (Ma) and lymphoblasts (Lb).

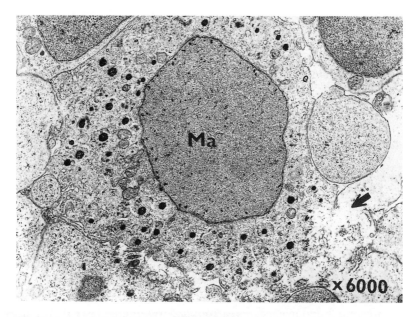

Fig. 7. Mastocyte (Ma): the arrow shows the site of cell membrane disruption and degranulation.

In the lymphoid tissue of nasopharyngeal tonsil in children with allergic rhinosinusitis, eosinophils situated extravasally were very rarely observed. The increased incidence of mastocytes was a characteristic finding. Sometimes mastocytes were surrounded by lymphoblasts, which makes us conclude that mastocytes are probably localized in a germinative center of a lymphoid follicle (fig. 6). A mastocyte in higher magnification is shown in figure 7. A region of disruption of cell membrane with cytoplasmic granules leaving the cell is seen.

Discussion

Businco et al. [1] have demonstrated experimentally that the increase of tissue histamine level is followed by eosinophil infiltration. Honsinger et al. [5], Hübscher [6], and Zeiger et al. [13] consider that eosinophils degrade histamine by means of enzymes, while Wasserman et al. [11] reveal inactivation of slow-reacting substance of anaphylaxis by eosinophil arylsulfatase. Butterworth [2] established that eosinophils phagocytose immune complexes. So it may be accepted that eosinophil accumulation in the adenoids of children with allergic rhinosinusitis is probably due to allergic reaction.

If we believe that eosinophils stand as a morphological marker of histamine concentration, this may mean in our cases that the histamine level in adenoids is highest in the epithelium and probably it is conditioned by the bacterial allergy.

The fact that the histamine producers – mastocytes and basophils – are not encountered in the adenoid epithelium in our preparations, may be explained by the rapid and total destruction of these cells in the epithelial area.

Sydor et al. [9] emphasized that mastocytes may be found in all structures of nasopharyngeal tonsil with the exception of the lymphoid follicles. However, we did not observe mastocytes or basophils in the adenoid epithelium, but found mastocytes surrounded by lymphoblasts, on the basis of which we admit that mastocytes can penetrate the germinative center of the lymphoid follicle. It may be postulated, in accordance with our concept of panautoprotection [7], that mastocytes may be concerned with the immunocompetence of lymphocytes, generated in the respective lymphoid follicles.

In 1984 we introduced the idea that in the normal state, reticulation of the adenoid epithelium occurs in the areas covered by M cells. The findings obtained from the present study show that in allergic conditions the lymphoid cells penetrate also in the intraepithelial passages, surrounded by precursors of the high cylindrical ciliated cells. Normally, in our understanding, these passages can be accessible only for erythrocytes. It remains to investigate how the change in pattern of reticulation, caused by allergy, alters the function of nasopharyngeal tonsil as analyzer of the human immune system.

In conclusion we suggest that the recovery of lymphoid tissue in the nasopharynx after adenoidectomy in children with allergic conditions have to be interpreted immunologically. That is to say the peculiarity of the activity of nasopharyngeal tonsil is in some way necessary for the sensitized organism. Our 20 years' clinical experience allows us to recommend adenoidectomy in allergic children only after objective defining of obstructive adenoids.

References

1   Businco L, Tucci L, di Nardo W, et al: Sodium cromoglycate in allergic diseases. Allergologica 1982;3:3–4.
2   Butterworth AE: The eosinophil and its role in immunity to helminth infection. Curr Top Microbiol Immunol 1977;77:127–168.
3   Friedmann I, Bird ES: Ciliary structure, ciliogenesis, microvilli. Electron microscopy of the mucosa of the upper respiratory tract. Laryngoscope 1971;81:1852–1868.
4   Gray LP: The T's and A's problem: assessment and reassessment. J Laryngol 1977; 91:11–32.
5   Honsinger RW Jr, Silverstein D, Van Arsdel PP Jr: The eosinophil and allergy: Why? J Allergy Clin Immunol 1972;49:142–155.
6   Hübscher T: EDI – an eosinophil-derived inhibitor of histamine release. J Immunol 1975;114:1379–1388.
7   Karchev T: Specialization of tonsils as analyzers of the human immune system. Acta Otolaryngol (Stockh) 1988(suppl 454):23–27.
8   Karchev T, Kabakchiev P: M cells in the epithelium of the nasopharyngeal tonsil. Rhinology 1984;22:201–210.
9   Sydor U, Chodynicki S, Hofman J: Mast cells and histamine level in the pharyngeal tonsil. Otolaryngol Pol 1980;34:461–467.
10 Takasaka T, Sato M, Onoreda A: Atypical cilia of the human nasal mucosa. Ann Otol 1980;89:37–45.
11 Wasserman SI, Goetzl E-J, Austen KF: Inactivation of slow-reacting substance of anaphylaxis by eosinophil aryl sulfatase. J Immunol 1975;114:645–649.
12 Watanabe K, Watanabe I: Changes of nasal epithelial cells and mucus layer after challenge of antigen. Ann Otol 1981;90:204–209.
13 Zeiger RS, Yurdin DL, Colten HR: Histamine metabolism. II Cellular and subcellular localization of the catabolic enzymes, histaminase and histamine methyltransferase in human leukocytes. J Allergy Clin Immunol 1976;58:172–179.

Dr. T. Karchev, Department of Pediatric Otolaryngology, Scientific Institute of Otorhinolaryngology, Medical Academy, BG–1040 Sofia (Bulgaria)

Galioto GB (ed): Tonsils: A Clinically Oriented Update.
Adv Otorhinolaryngol. Basel, Karger, 1992, vol 47, pp 54–58

High Endothelial Venules in the Developing Human Palatine Tonsil

Vladimír Holibka

Department of Anatomy, Medical Faculty, University of Olomouc,
Czechoslovakia

High endothelial venules (HEV) are typical of extrafollicular lymphatic tissue of secondary lymphatic organs. These venules make their appearance in the human palatine tonsil as early as in the 14th gestational week [Holibka, in press]. An attempt has been made in this paper to establish the mode of the movement of the lymphocytes through the venular wall.

Material and Method

Five human fetuses aged 10, 12, 14, 16 and 18 weeks were used for our study. The fixation was made by whole-body perfusion with 3% glutaraldehyde in phosphate buffer (pH 7.2). The region of the palatine tonsil was cut under a dissection microscope into slices of about 1 mm in thickness. These were postfixed in 2% OsO_4 in phosphate buffer, and then dehydrated in ethanol and embedded in Epon. Ultrathin sections were stained with uranyl acetate and lead citrate and examined using a Tesla BS 500 electron microscope.

Results

The migration of lymphocytes through the wall of HEV was seen as early as in the 16th gestational week. Our observations show that in the prenatal period they migrate only through the intercellular spaces, we have never seen the transendothelial movement of the lymphoid cells. The migration begins with the adherence of a circulating lymphocyte to the surface of an endothelial cell by means of the short cytoplasmic projection in the vicinity of the intercellular space (fig. 1a) or away from it (fig. 1b).

The first possibility (a): the cytoplasmic projection of the lymphocyte expands into the cleft between two neighboring endothelial cells (fig. 1a II).

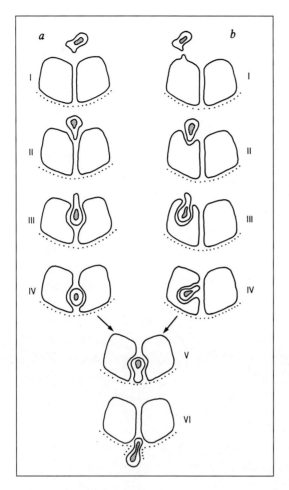

Fig. 1. Schema of the migration of the lymphoid cell. The adherence of the lymphocyte near the intercellular space (*a*) and away from it (*b*).

The desmosomal junctions are disrupted and the projection of the lymphocyte finally fits onto the basal lamina (fig. 1 V, fig. 2).

The second possibility (b): the adherence of lymphoid cell to the endothelial surface away from the intercellular space. In this case the lymphocyte is pressed into the cytoplasm of an endothelial cell from its luminal surface (fig. 1b II, III, fig. 3, 4) and then slides into the intercellular space (fig. 1b IV).

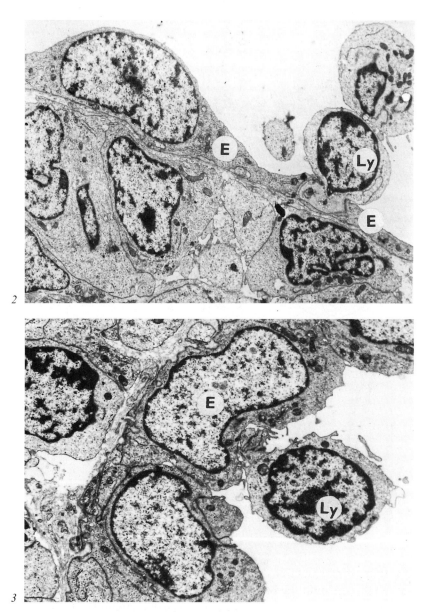

Fig. 2. The projection of a lymphocyte (Ly) lies in the intercellular cleft between two endothelial cells (E). ×1,800.

Fig. 3. The adherence of a lymphocyte (Ly) to the luminal surface of an endothelial cell (E). ×2,550.

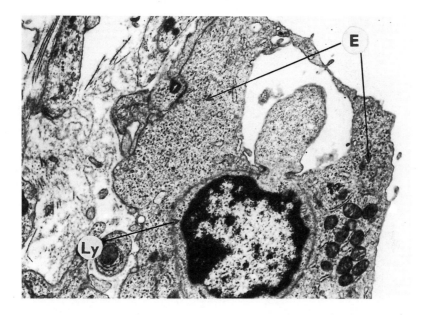

Fig. 4. The lymphocyte (Ly) is pressed deep into the cytoplasm of the endothelial cell (E). × 2,850.

An important moment is the disruption of the basal lamina (fig. 1 VI). The cytoplasm of the lymphocyte contains a great amount of vesicles at the site of contact with the basal membrane. It is possible that these vesicles release enzymes contributing to the disruption of the basal membrane. The migrating cell and also its nucleus elongate. As the opening in the basal lamina is relatively narrow (about 1 μm) a strangulation of the nucleus can be seen in this site (fig. 5). The lymphoid cell then migrates among the lamellae of the subendothelial connective tissue.

Discussion

The development of human palatine tonsil was studied by Gaudecker and Müller-Hermelink [2, 4] from the point of view of development of lymphoid and nonlymphoid cells. HEV are mentioned very briefly. Electron microscopic study of HEV in human prenatal development was made on fetal lymph nodes by Bailey and Weiss [1]. Their results are similar to ours. Unlike some other authors [3], we are of the opinion that true trans-

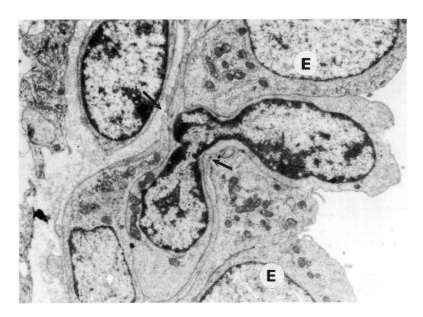

Fig. 5. The nucleus of the lymphocyte elongated and strangulated at the site of the opening in the basal lamina (arrows). E = Endothelial cells. × 3,150.

endothelial movement does not exist. Even when in some sections a lymphocyte is completely surrounded by the cytoplasm of an endothelial cell, it is probably only pressed deep into its cytoplasm.

References

1   Bailey RP, Weiss L: Light and electron microscopic studies of postcapillary venules in development of human fetal lymph nodes. Am J Anat 1975;143:43–58.
2   Gaudecker B, Müller-Hermelink HK: The development of the human tonsilla palatina. Cell Tissue Res 1982;224:579–600.
3   Marchesi VT, Gowans JL: The migration of lymphocytes through the endothelium of venules in lymph nodes: an electron microscope study. Proc R Soc Lond [B] 1964; 159:283–290.
4   Müller-Hermelink HK, Gaudecker B: Ontogenese des lymphatischen Systems beim Menschen. Verh Anat Ges 1980;74:235–259.

Dr. med. Vladimír Holibka, Department of Anatomy,
Hněvotínská 3, CS–775 15 Olomouc (Czechoslovakia)

Galioto GB (ed): Tonsils: A Clinically Oriented Update.
Adv Otorhinolaryngol. Basel, Karger, 1992, vol 47, pp 59–63

Structure of the Palatine Tonsil in European Insectivores

Miroslav Kutal

Department of Anatomy, Medical Faculty, Palacký University Olomouc,
Czechoslovakia

The turn of the century and the thirties saw the boom of the comparative histologico-anatomical studies of the tonsils. The investigators centered their attention mainly on domestic animals of medium and large size, which, however, from the point of view of taxonomy, represented different mammal orders (lagomorphs, carnivora, artiodactyla, perissodactyla) without developmental relationship to the primates. However, to evaluate the development of the tonsils the phylogenetic approach must be applied. The key position of the insectivora order for the evolution of the mammals is well known. They are believed to be ancestors of placental mammals with primates as their early offshoots.

Materials and Methods

Palatine tonsils of 20 common shrews *(Sorex araneus),* 3 common moles *(Talpa europaea)* and 16 hedgehogs *(Erinaceus europaeus)* of both sexes were subjected to the study. The material for light microscopy was processed using standard histological techniques; serial sections at different levels were stained with HE. The samples for SEM were first dehydrated and then dried at critical-point drying, stutter-coated with Au and Pd, and studied using an EM Tesla BS 300.

Results

The shrew palatine tonsils, ovoid in shape and about 1 mm in diameter, are located high up on the lateral pharyngeal walls (isthmus faucium) (fig. 1, 2). The surrounding epithelium on the lingual and palatinal aspects

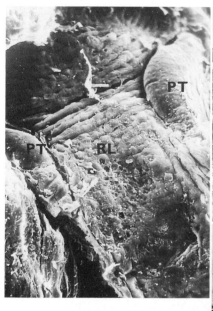

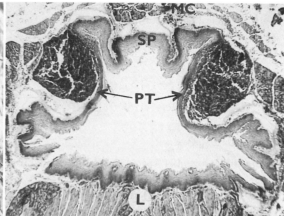

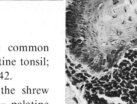

Fig. 1. The fauces of the common shrew *(S. araneus).* PT = Palatine tonsil; RL = radix linguae. SEM. × 142.

Fig. 2. Frontal section of the shrew fauces. SP = Soft palate; PT = palatine tonsil; L = lingua; MC = mucous gland. HE.

Fig. 3. A detail showing the penetration of lymphoid cells through epithelium. HE.

Fig. 4. In lower magnification SEM the shrew palatine tonsil appears as clear-cut ovoid protrusion and epithelial invaginations on lingual (L) and palatinal (P) aspects. SEM. × 205.

Fig. 5. A SEM of the tonsil surface. Note desquamation of the cornified epithelial cells and opening of intraepithelial pathways. × 850.

Fig. 6. Transversal section through the hedgehog palatine tonsil. The crypt (C) branches giving off secondary crypt (SC). HE.

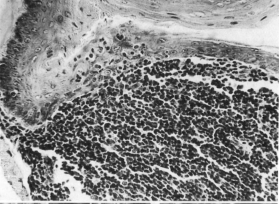

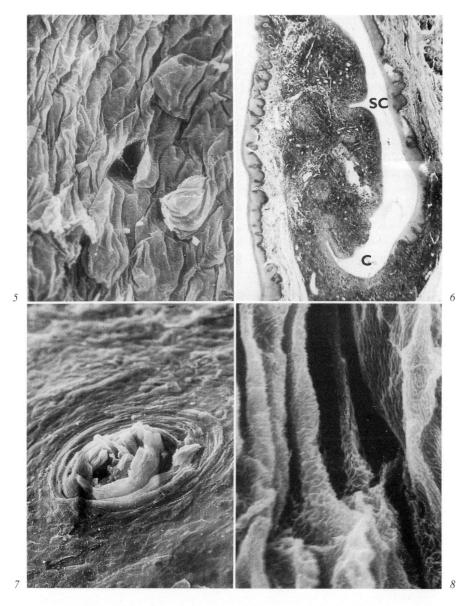

Fig. 7. The opening of the salivary gland on the free surface of the hedgehog palatine tonsil. SEM. × 375.

Fig. 8. The bottom of the crypt: superficial cells of squamous epithelium is of an elongated shape and the labyrinth or mesh-like protrusions can be observed. SEM. × 4,000.

forms deep invaginations. The tonsil is covered with stratified squamous epithelium and is transformed by infiltrating lymphoid cells into reticularized epithelium (fig. 3). In lower magnification SEM (fig. 4), shrew palatine tonsils appear as clear-cut ovoid protrusion and epithelial invaginations on lingual and palatinal aspects. At higher magnifications (fig. 5) the cells of free epithelium show a cobblestone pattern and desquamation of the cornified epithelial cells and openings of intraepithelial pathways. The parenchyma of the shrew palatine tonsil consists of a single lymph node with a germinal center and nonlymphatic cell population.

In moles and hedgehogs the palatine tonsil is monocryptic. In hedgehogs it is 4 mm in length, its greatest width equals 1.5–1.8 mm, in moles 2 × 1 mm. The crypt begins at the anterior pole of the tonsil as a slightly concave arch in the form of a groove, which, at the lower pole of the tonsil, widens and flattens. A transversal section through the hedgehog palatine tonsil shows the distribution of lymphatic tissue (fig. 6). It is localized medial and lateral to the single crypt running longitudinally. Medial to the crypt is the smaller portion of lymphatic tissue, lateral to it is a larger accumulation, which forms visible protrusion above the surrounding epithelium. The medial wall of the crypt is covered with stratified squamous epithelium, which, at the bottom of the crypt, undergoes reticularization. The palatine tonsil is embedded in mucous glands, in some places contact with glandular tissue can be seen. Glandular ducts go through the main mass of tonsils to open on the free surface of the tonsil (fig. 7). The epithelium on the bottom of the crypt is of an elongated shape, forming thus a kind of fold. At higher magnifications the labyrinth or mesh-like protrusions can be observed on cellular surfaces, reminiscent of microridge cells (fig. 8). Palatine tonsils of moles and hedgehogs show many typical secondary lymphatic follicles with germinal centers.

Discussion

The palatine tonsils represent a typical mammalian structure, however, they are lacking in rodents (mice, rat, guinea pig). The human palatine tonsil, as described by others [1–4], is very similar to the primitive insectivora tonsil, which corresponds to the lower developmental stage. Our results are in keeping with those of Kimura and Tohya [4], who described the primitive tonsilar structure in suncus *(Suncus murinus).*

References

1 Howie AJ: Scanning and transmission electron microscopy of the epithelium of human palatine tonsils. J Pathol 1980;130:91–98.
2 Von Gaudecker B, Müller-Hermelink HK: The development of the human tonsilla palatina. Cell Tissue Res 1982;224:579–600.
3 Favre A, Paoli D, Poletti M, Marzoli A, Pesce G, Giampalmo A, Rossi F: The human palatine tonsil studied from surgical specimens at all ages and in various pathological conditions. Z Mikrosk Anat Forsch 1986;100:7–33.
4 Kimura M, Tohya K: Scanning, transmission and immunoelectron microscopical studies of the tonsil-like lymphoid organ of normal and horseradish-peroxidase-injected laboratory suncuses. Acta Anat 1989;136:177–184.

Dr. Miroslav Kutal, Department of Anatomy, Medical Faculty, Hněvotínská 3, CS–775 15 Olomouc (Czechoslovakia)

Immunology and Immunopathology

Galioto GB (ed): Tonsils: A Clinically Oriented Update.
Adv Otorhinolaryngol. Basel, Karger, 1992, vol 47, pp 64–75

Immunology and Immunopathology of Tonsils[1]

Per Brandtzaeg, Trond S. Halstensen

Laboratory for Immunohistochemistry and Immunopathology (LIIPAT),
Institute of Pathology, University of Oslo, The National Hospital, Rikshospitalet,
Oslo, Norway

The lymphoepithelial structures of Waldeyer's ring are well designed for direct transport of foreign material from the exterior to the lymphoid tissue via epithelial crypts. Their initial immunological development does not depend on exogenous antigens as primary B-cell follicles are present in the tonsils as early as at 16 weeks' gestation [1]. However, activation of the tonsillar B-cell system, as evidenced by germinal centre formation, does not take place until after birth, and extrafollicular plasma cells are seen about 2 weeks postnatally [2].

The tonsils and other parts of Waldeyer's ring are strategically located to perform regional immune functions because these structures are exposed to both airborne and alimentary antigens. Their putative immunological role has been debated for many decades, but no consensus has been reached. An extensive account of this topic was recently published [3]. The present short review will mainly focus on the mechanisms involved in tonsillar B-cell activation and possible adverse effects of recurrent tonsillitis on regional antibody defence.

Tonsils May Provide Activated B Cells for the Secretory Immune System

The mucosa of the upper respiratory tract is protected by a secretory antibody system which depends on complex regional and local immune regulation [4]. B cells with a potential for J-chain expression are pri-

[1] Supported by grants from the Norwegian Cancer Society and the Norwegian Research Council for Science and the Humanities.

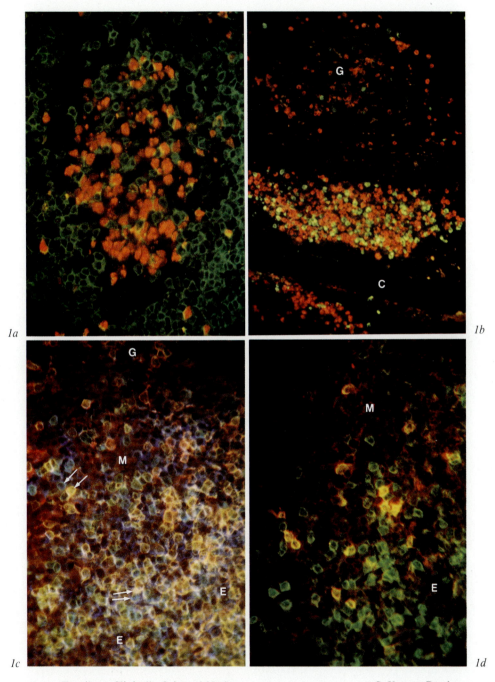

1a

1b

1c

1d

Tonsils: A Clinically Oriented Update

S. Karger, Basel

Fig. 1.

a Two-colour immunofluorescence staining with anti-CD3 (T cells, green) and monoclonal antibody Ki-67 (proliferating cells, red) in tonsillar germinal centre. Note that positivity for Ki-67 is restricted to nuclei of non-T cells (presumably centroblasts and centrocytes derived from activated B cells). ×280.

b Two-colour immunofluorescence staining for IgG (red) and IgA (green) in section of tonsil. Note many cells with cytoplasmic IgG (and some with IgA) in large germinal centre (G). Dense accumulation of positive plasma cells is seen adjacent to crypt (C). ×115.

c Three-colour staining for CD3 (green), CD45RA (dark blue), and CD45R0 (red) in section of tonsil including parts of germinal centre (G), mantle zone (M), and extrafollicular area (E). Note many purely RA+ cells (= B cells) in M, whereas G contains a few memory T cells (CD3+CD45R0+, yellow). Both naive (CD3+CD45RA+, light bluish) and memory T cells are found intermingled in M and E (one of each phenotype arrowed in both compartments). ×280.

d Two-colour staining for CD3 (T cells, green) and CD25 (IL-2R, red) in section of tonsil including parts of mantle zone (M) and extrafollicular area (E). Some T cells expressing CD25 activation marker (yellow) are found in both compartments. Note that many follicular B cells are weakly CD25-positive (faint purely red). ×280.

marily activated in organized mucosa-associated lymphoid tissue (MALT) and migrate thereafter through lymph and blood to glandular sites to become terminally differentiated as immunoglobulin (Ig)-producing plasma cells [5, 6]. Most mucosal plasma cells produce dimers and larger polymers of IgA (poly-IgA), and gut-associated lymphoid tissue (GALT) with the predominating Peyer's patches (PP) are the best recognized precursor source of these local immunocytes [7]. Their product of J-chain-containing poly-IgA is selectively transported through serous glandular cells by a specific epithelial receptor protein called the secretory component (SC) or poly-Ig receptor. J-chain-containing pentameric IgM is also subjected to SC-mediated epithelial transport [5]. The secretory Igs (SIgA and SIgM) perform immune exclusion by inhibiting uptake of soluble antigens and by blocking epithelial colonization of microorganisms [4, 8].

Early animal experiments showed that although activated IgA immunocyte precursors originating from lymph nodes draining bronchus-associated lymphoid tissue (BALT) to a minor extent might migrate to the intestinal mucosa, most of them ended up in the respiratory tract [9]. Because BALT is apparently absent from normal human lungs [10], the tonsils are of particular interest as precursor sources for mucosal Ig-producing cell populations in humans. Both the pharyngeal (adenoid) and palatine tonsils are indeed well equipped for antigen uptake, processing, and presentation [3]; and some of the lymphoid follicles of the adenoids actually form around the ducts of small salivary glands [11]. The tonsillar follicles are strikingly activated even in the normal state [3] as demonstrated by germinal centres containing B cells with a high proliferative rate (fig. 1a) and a marked tendency to undergo terminal differentiation into Ig-producing immunocytes (fig. 1b).

The observed disparity between the gut mucosa and secretory sites of the upper digestive and respiratory tracts as to occurrence of IgD immunocytes and subclass distribution of IgA immunocytes, has led us to propose that a dichotomy exists in the human mucosal immune system [12–14]; the gut mucosa probably receives most of its activated B cells from GALT, whereas the upper mucosal region of the body appears to be seeded mainly by B cells from tonsils (and BALT?) (fig. 2). A similar dichotomy of the secretory immune system has been suggested by B-cell homing studies in the rat [15–17]. Also, it is of great interest that activated human tonsillar B cells migrate to the lung, but not gut mucosa, when transferred into mice with severe combined immunodeficiency [18].

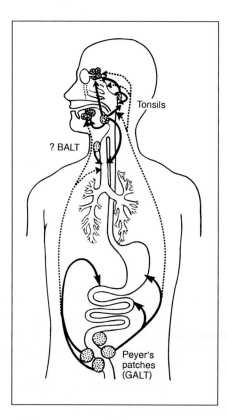

Fig. 2. Putative dichotomy in the human mucosal immune system. Solid arrows indicate major migration routes of B cells stimulated in various lymphoepithelial structures (tonsils, BALT and GALT), whereas broken arrows indicate less consistent routes. Note that BALT does probably not exist in normal human lungs.

Tonsillar T Cells Have Properties Necessary for the Induction of B Cells

The reticular tonsillar crypt epithelium contains macrophages and dendritic cells which can transport antigen to the extrafollicular T-cell areas and to the B-cell follicles. Interdigitating antigen-presenting cells (APC) are present in the extrafollicular areas, often closely surrounded by T lymphocytes which are mainly of the CD4+ ('helper') phenotype [3]. These consist of both naive (CD45RA+) and memory (CD45R0+) subsets (fig. 1c), and some express interleukin-2 receptor (IL-2R or CD25) as a sign of recent activation (fig. 1d). Tonsils therefore appear able to mount both primary and secondary T-cell responses. As there is a close spatial relationship between naive and memory T cells both in the extrafollicular areas and mantle zones (fig. 1c), synergy most likely occurs because of the differ-

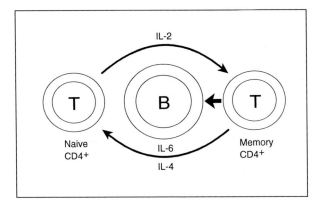

Fig. 3. Synergy may occur when juxtaposed CD4+ naive and memory T cells are stimulated in a microenvironment where both primary and secondary antigens are present. Such synergy will promote local activation of B cells.

ent lymphokine profiles of these two subsets (fig. 3). Importantly, CD4+ memory T cells (a) express adhesion molecules necessary for migration to sites outside the tonsils, such as the secretory tissues; (b) they have less stringent activation requirements than naive T cells, and (c) they provide most of the help required for activation and differentiation of B cells [19, 20].

T cells are also found within the germinal centres (fig. 1a). This subset is almost exclusively of the CD4+CD45R0+ helper memory phenotype (fig. 1c). Some T cells expressing IL-2R are also found in relation to the lymphoid follicles (fig. 1d). A large fraction of the intrafollicular T cells are positive for Leu-7 (CD57), express the early activation marker CD69, and show a particular lymphokine profile [21]. Interestingly, animal experiments have suggested that memory T cells are necessary to promote somatic V-gene mutations leading to the production of high-avidity antibodies in both naive and primed B-cell populations [22].

Role of Tonsillar Lymphoid Follicles in B-Cell Induction

The tonsillar lymphoid follicles are very active B-cell proliferation and differentiation sites and most of the follicles show germinal centres shortly after birth. The follicular dendritic cells (FDC) of germinal centres are

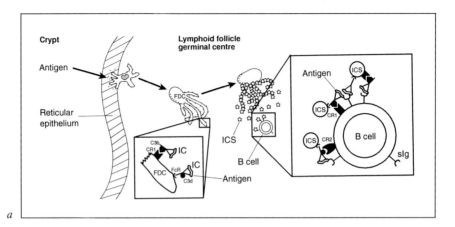

Fig. 4. Schematic depiction of various important events leading to proliferation and differentiation of B cells in tonsillar germinal centre. *a* Antigen is transported from crypt to follicular dendritic cell (FDC) and iccosome (ICS) formation is subsequently induced. Antigen is retained on FCC and ICS in immune complex (IC) bound to surface membrane by complement and Fc receptors (CR1, CR2, and FcR) which also bind ICS to B cell, cooperating with antigen-specific surface immunoglobulin (sIg). Cross-linking of these membrane structures leads to activation of B cells. *b* B cell is also stimulated by receiving help from antigen-specific T cell to which it presents processed antigen in the context of HLA class II determinants. Resulting memory B cells may either emigrate from the tonsils or differentiate locally to plasma cells. TCR = T-cell receptor for antigen.

probably the most important APC for B cells [23], and a variety of adhesion molecules appear to be involved in the interactions taking place between these two cell types [24]. The FDC retain large amounts of antigen in complement-containing immune complexes, mainly involving antibodies of the IgM and IgG classes [25]. This retention is mediated by C3b receptors (CR1, CR2, CR3) and probably also by Ig Fc receptors (fig. 4a). Terminal complement complex (TCC) occurs on the FDC [26], although this generally causes no apparent harm to the germinal centres. Perhaps inhibition of C9 polymerization by associated S-protein (vitronectin) [26] and CD59 [27] renders TCC nonlytic. The latter protein (also called homologous restriction factor or HRF) restricts homologous complement lysis efficiently and its expression on FDC parallels the deposition of TCC [Halstensen et al., unpubl. observations].

Complement activation in germinal centres may, nevertheless, generate inflammatory mediators that cause oedema apparently facilitating iccosome (ICS) dispersion [28]. ICSs, or 'immune complex-coated bodies', are produced by FDC and become attached to B cells [29]. Antigens bound on ICSs are thereafter taken up by B cells in a receptor-specific manner, degraded, and finally presented to T cells in the context of HLA class II molecules [30]. The CD4+CD450+ helper memory cells occurring in the germinal centres will in this way become stimulated and then promote B-cell proliferation and differentiation in an antigen-specific way by topical release of lymphokines (fig. 4b).

Tonsillar B-Cell Differentiation May Be Influenced by the Regional Microbiota

In B-cell ontogeny, surface IgM (sIgM) is first expressed as a receptor for antigen whereas sIgD appears later and predominates on resting B lymphocytes in adults. After being cross-linked, both sIgM and sIgD transmit activation signals to the interior of the B cell by means of an assemblage of receptor-associated accessory molecules [31]. Apparently, sIgM and sIgD can deliver qualitatively different signals to immature B cells, the former isotype inducing growth inhibition and the latter activation [32].

Most strains of *Haemophilus influenzae* and *Moraxella (Branhamella) catarrhalis,* which are frequently colonizing the upper respiratory tract, produce an IgD-binding factor (protein D) and may therefore exert great impact on B-cell activation in the tonsils by cross-linking sIgD and HLA

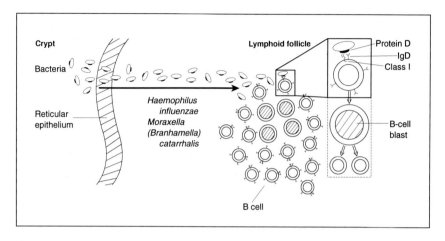

Fig. 5. Putative scheme for the stimulatory effect of bacteria bearing protein D on tonsillar B cells. When HLA class I molecule and surface IgD are cross-linked by protein D, the B cell will proliferate in a polyclonal manner.

class I molecules [33–35]. B lymphocytes of the follicular mantle zones usually express IgD abundantly on their surface [3], and may hence be stimulated to proliferate and differentiate in a polyclonal (antigen-independent) manner by protein D-expressing bacteria (fig. 5). Perhaps this contributes to the fact that there are relatively many IgD- and particularly IgA1-producing cells in the upper digestive and respiratory tracts, in striking contrast to the distal gut where IgA2 production predominates [3, 36]. One might speculate that cross-linking of sIgD favours a sequential differentiation pathway, mainly terminating with IgA1 production (fig. 6), whereas direct switching from IgM to IgA2 predominates in GALT [13].

The preferential production of IgA1 in sinonasal [36] and bronchial [37] mucosae is intriguing in view of the frequent synthesis of IgA1-specific proteases by *H. influenzae, Streptococcus pneumoniae* and *Neisseria meningitidis,* which are prone to produce invasive disease of the upper respiratory tract [38]. A relationship of this proneness to an enzymatically induced deterioration of secretory immunity has been proposed [39]. Also, patients with allergy have increased amounts of IgA1 split products in their nasopharyngeal secretions [40].

Several bacteria of the nasopharyngeal flora thus appear able to evade the protective effects of local SIgA antibodies by a combination of driving the B-cell differentiation towards IgA1 and then cleaving this product by

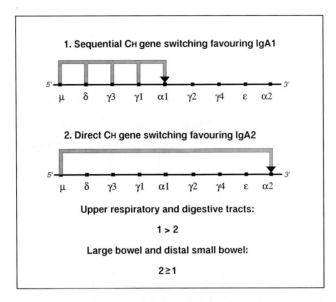

1. Sequential CH gene switching favouring IgA1

5'   μ   δ   γ3   γ1   α1   γ2   γ4   ε   α2   3'

2. Direct CH gene switching favouring IgA2

5'   μ   δ   γ3   γ1   α1   γ2   γ4   ε   α2   3'

Upper respiratory and digestive tracts:

1 > 2

Large bowel and distal small bowel:

2 ≥ 1

Fig. 6. Putative B-cell switching pathways leading to preferential production of IgA1 or IgA2 after activation of the respective C_H genes encoding the constant regions of the Ig heavy chains in various mucosal tissues. Modified from Brandtzaeg et al. [13].

specific proteases. Stimulation of resistant IgA2 antibodies by enteric vaccination to enhance the immunobarrier of the upper respiratory tract is therefore an interesting theoretical possibility, which perhaps may be clinically practical in the future [41]; precursors of poly-IgA-producing plasma cells are indeed able to migrate from human ileal PP to secretory sites of the upper digestive and respiratory tracts [6]. However, *Pseudomonas aeruginosa*, the major pathogen in patients with cystic fibrosis, produces an elastase that is able to cleave both IgA1 and IgA2 [42].

In patients with selective IgA deficiency, SIgA is lacking but often satisfactorily replaced by protective SIgM. In other IgA-deficient patients, however, immunoregulatory 'compensation' gives rise to a large number of IgD-producing cells in respiratory mucosae [43]. IgD cannot act as a secretory antibody and these patients are prone to have recurrent infections. There are thus large individual variations in the regional secretory immune system, which in the future hopefully may be subjected to regulatory manipulation, perhaps by a combination of enteric and pharyngeal immunization.

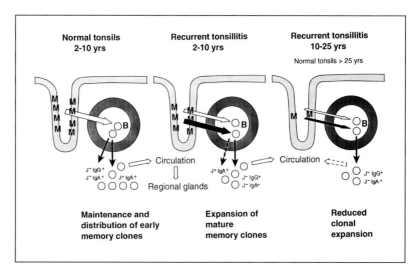

Fig. 7. Hypothetical scheme for age- and disease-associated changes of immunological functions of palatine tonsils. Tissue elements of particular interest are: M cells (M), whose number may decrease in the reticular parts of the crypt epithelium; J-chain-positive IgA-producing (J+IgA+) B cells, and J-chain-negative IgG-producing (J–IgG+) B cells. In addition to being retained in the extrafollicular compartment for terminal differentiation to plasma cells, the B cells may become disseminated to the general circulation. Differentiation to the J+IgA+ phenotype depends on expansion of early memory clones, and may result in homing of poly-IgA precursor cells to regional glands. Differentiation to the J–IgG+ phenotype is favoured by expansion of mature memory clones. The latter development may be related to reduced antigen presentation by M cells (graded open large arrows) and enhanced direct passage of foreign material through crypt epithelium (graded filled large arrows) along with changed T-cell functions. At higher ages, decreased entrance of antigenic material into the tonsils results in reduced expansion of both early and mature memory B-cell clones. Modified from Brandtzaeg [3, 8].

Putative Adverse Effect of Recurrent Tonsillitis on the Immunological Role of Tonsils

The capacity of palatine tonsils for generation of J-chain-expressing B cells is significantly reduced in children afflicted with recurrent tonsillitis [44]. The reason for this is unknown, but it may depend on a change of lymphokine profiles produced by the engaged APC and T-cell subsets. A putative consequence is reduced maintenance of those early memory B-cell clones that may contribute to secretory immunity of the upper digestive and respiratory tracts (fig. 7). Nevertheless, the tonsils retain considerable immunological activity despite repeated inflammatory episodes and increasing age [3]. The putative role of Waldeyer's lymphoid ring in reinforcing immunity of the whole nasopharyngeal region should therefore be considered before tonsillectomy is performed, particularly in early childhood. Also, generalized lack of IgA production, or some other type of immunodeficiency, should be taken into account as a possible cause of infectious disease in the upper respiratory tract. Conversely, tonsillar hyperproduction of poly-IgA in recurrent tonsillitis has been associated with IgA nephropathy [45], but the clinical effect of tonsillectomy in such patients is still being debated [46].

References

1   Von Gaudecker B, Müller-Hermelink HK: The development of the human tonsilla palatina. Cell Tissue Res 1982;224:579–600.
2   Davis DJ: On plasma cells in the tonsils. J Infect Dis 1912;10:142–147.
3   Brandtzaeg P: Immune functions and immunopathology of palatine and nasopharyngeal tonsils; in Bernstein JM, Ogra PL (eds): Immunology of the Ear. New York, Raven Press, 1987, pp 63–106.
4   Brandtzaeg P: Mucosal immunology – with special reference to specific immune defence of the upper respiratory tract. ORL 1988;50:225–235.
5   Brandtzaeg P: Role of J chain and secretory component in receptor-mediated glandular and hepatic transport of immunoglobulins in man. Scand J Immunol 1985;22: 111–146.
6   Mestecky J: The common mucosal immune system and current strategies for induction of immune response in external secretions. J Clin Immunol 1987;7:265–276.
7   Brandtzaeg P, Bjerke K: Immunomorphological characteristics of human Peyer's patches. Digestion 1990;46(suppl 2):262–273.
8   Brandtzaeg P: Immune functions of nasal mucosa and tonsils in health and disease: in Bienenstock J (ed): Immunology of the Lung and Upper Respiratory Tract. New York, McGraw-Hill, 1984, pp 28–95.
9   McDermott MR, Bienenstock J: Evidence for a common mucosal immunologic system. I. Migration of B immunoblasts into intestinal, respiratory, and genital tissues. J Immunol 1979;122:1892–1898.
10 Pabst R, Gehrke I: Is the bronchus-associated lymphoid tissue (BALT) an integral structure of the lung in normal mammals, including humans? Am J Respir Cell Mol Biol 1990;3:131–135.
11 Slípka J: Development of the pharyngeal tonsil with reference to commencement of its immunocompetence. Folia Morphol 1983;31:102–105.
12 Brandtzaeg P, Gjeruldsen ST, Korsrud F, Baklien K, Berdal P, Ek J: The human secretory immune system shows striking heterogeneity with regard to involvement of J chain-positive IgD immunocytes. J Immunol 1979;122:503–510.

13   Brandtzaeg P, Kett K, Rognum TO, Söderström R, Björkander J, Söderström T, Petruson B, Hanson LÅ: Distribution of mucosal IgA and IgG subclass-producing immunocytes and alterations in various disorders. Monogr Allergy. Basel, Karger, 1986, vol 20, pp 179–194.

14   Kett K, Brandtzaeg P, Radl J. Haaijman JJ: Different subclass distribution of IgA-producing cells in human lymphoid organs and various secretory tissues. J Immunol 1986;136:3631–3635.

15   Parmely MJ: Kinetics of mammary and intestinal IgA-producing cells in the lactating rat. J Reprod Immunol 1985;8:89–93.

16   Van der Brugge-Gammelkoorn GJ, Claassen E, Sminia T: Anti-TPN-forming cells in bronchus-associated lymphoid tissue (BALT) and paratracheal lymph node (PTLN) of the rat intratracheal priming and boosting with TNP-KLH. Immunology 1986;57: 405–409.

17   Sminia T, Brugge-Gamelkorn GJ, Jeurissen SHM: Structure and function of bronchus-associated lymphoid tissue (BALT). Crit Rev Immunol 1989;9:119–150.

18   Nadal D, Albini B, Chen C, Schläpfer E, Bernstein JM, Ogra PL: Distribution and engraftment patterns of human tonsillar mononuclear cells and immunoglobulin secreting cells in mice with severe combined immunodeficiency. Role of the Epstein-Barr virus. Int Arch Allergy Appl Immunol 1991;95:341–351.

19   Akbar AN, Salmon M, Janossy G: The synergy between naive and memory T cells during activation. Immunol Today 1991;12:184–188.

20   Mackay CR: T-cell memory: the connection between function, phenotype and migration pathways. Immunol Today 1991;12:189–192.

21   Bowen MB, Butch AW, Parvin CA, Levine A, Nahm MH: Germinal center T cells are distinct helper-inducer T cells. Hum Immunol 1991;31:67–75.

22   Francus T, Francus Y, Siskind GW: Memory T cells enhance the expression of high-avidity naive B cells. Cell Immunol 1991;134:520–527.

23   Heinen E, Cormann N, Kinet-Denoël C: The lymph follicle: a hard nut to crack. Immunol Today 1988;9:240–243.

24   Koopman G, Parmentier HK, Schuurman H.-J, Newman W, Meijer CJLM, Pals ST: Adhesion of human B cells to follicular dendritic cells involves both the lymphocyte function-associated antigen 1/intercellular adhesion molecule 1 and very late antigen 4/vascular cell adhesion molecule 1 pathways. J Exp Med 1991;173:1297–1304.

25   Parmentier HK, van der Linden JA, Krijnen J, van Wichen DF, Rademakers LHPM, Bloem AC, Schuurman H-J: Human follicular dendritic cells: isolation and characteristics in situ and in suspension. Scand J Immunol 1991;33:441–452.

26   Halstensen TS, Mollnes TE, Brandtzaeg P: Terminal complement complex (TCC) and S-protein (vitronectin) on follicular dendritic cells in human lymphoid tissues. Immunology 1988;65:193–197.

27   Lachmann PJ: The control of homologous lysis. Immunol Today 1991;12:312–315.

28   Tew JG, Kosco MH, Szakal AK: The alternative antigen pathway. Immunol Today 1989;10:229–232.

29   Kosco MH: Antigen presentation to B cells. Curr Opin Immunol 1991;3:336–339.

30   Möller G, Alarcón-Riquelme M, Clinchy B, Gontijo CM, Höidén I: The immunoglobulin receptors on B cells bind antigen, focus activation signals to them and initiate antigen presentation. Scand J Immunol 1991;33:111–116.

31   Reth M, Hombach J, Wienands J, Campbell KS, Chien N, Justement LB, Cambier
      JC: The B-cell antigen receptor complex. Immunol Today 1991;12:196–201.
32   Alés-Martínez JE, Cuende E, Martínez AC, Parkhouse RME, Pezzi L, Scott DW:
      Signalling in B cells. Immunol Today 1991;12:201–205.
33   Forsgren A, Penta A, Schlossman SF, Tedder TF: *Branhamella catarrhalis* activates
      human B lymphocytes following interactions with surface IgD and class I major
      histocompatibility complex antigens. Cell Immunol 1988;112:78–88.
34   Ruan M, Akkoyunlu M, Grubb A, Forsgren A: Protein D of *Haemophilus influen-
      zae.* A novel bacterial surface protein with affinity for human IgD. J Immunol 1990;
      145:3379–3384.
35   Janson H, Hedén L-O, Grubb A, Ruan M, Forsgren A: Protein D, an immunoglob-
      ulin D-binding protein of *Haemophilus influenzae:* cloning, nucleotide sequence,
      and expression in *Escherichia coli.* Infect Immun 1991;59:119–125.
36   Kett K, Brandtzaeg P, Radl J, Haaijman JJ: Different subclass distribution of IgA-
      producing cells in human lymphoid organs and various secretory tissues. J Immunol
      1986;136:3631–3635.
37   Burnett D, Crocker J, Stockley RA: Cell containing IgA subclass in bronchi of sub-
      jects with and without chronic obstructive lung disease. J Clin Pathol 1987;40:1217–
      1220.
38   Kilian M, Reinholdt J: Interference with IgA defence mechanisms by extracellular
      bacterial enzymes; in Easmon CSF, Jeljaszewicz J (eds): Medical Microbiology. Lon-
      don, Academic Press, 1986, vol 5, pp 173–208.
39   Kilian M, Mestecky J, Russell MW: Defense mechanisms involving Fc-dependent
      functions of immunoglobulin A and their subversion by bacterial immunoglobulin A
      proteases. Microbiol Rev 1988;52:296–303.
40   Sørensen CH, Kilian M: Bacterium-induced cleavage of IgA in nasopharyngeal
      secretions from atopic children. Acta Pathol Microbiol Immunol Scand [C] 1984;92:
      85–87.
41   McGhee JR, Mestecky J: In defense of mucosal surfaces. Development of novel
      vaccines for IgA responses protective at the portals of entry of microbial pathogens.
      Infect Dis Clin North Am 1990;4:315–341.
42   Heck LW, Alarcon PG, Kulhavy RM, Morihara K, Russell MW, Mestecky JF: Deg-
      radation of IgA proteins by *Pseudomonas aeruginosa* elastase. J Immunol 1990;144:
      2253–2257.
43   Brandtzaeg P, Karlsson G, Hansson G, Petruson B, Bjørkander J, Hanson LÅ: The
      clinical condition of IgA-deficient patients is related to the proportion of IgD- and
      IgM-producing cells in their nasal mucosa. Clin Exp Immunol 1987;67:626–636.
44   Korsrud FR, Brandtzaeg P: Influence of tonsillar disease on the expression of J-
      chain by immunoglobulin-producing cells in human palatine and nasopharyngeal
      tonsils. Scand J Immunol 1981;13:281–287.
45   Nagy J, Brandtzaeg P: Tonsillar distribution of IgA and IgG immunocytes and pro-
      duction of IgA subclasses and J chain in tonsillitis vary with the presence or absence
      of IgA nephropathy. Scand J Immunol 1988;27:393–399.
46   Béné MC, Hurault De Ligny B, Kessler M, Faure GC: Confirmation of tonsillar
      anomalies in IgA nephropathy: a multicenter study. Nephron 1991;58:425–428.

Dr. P. Brandtzaeg, LIIPAT, Institute of Pathology, Rikshospitalet,
N–0027 Oslo (Norway)

Galioto GB (ed): Tonsils: A Clinically Oriented Update.
Adv Otorhinolaryngol. Basel, Karger, 1992, vol 47, pp 76–79

Tonsils: The Gatekeeper of Mucosal Immunity?

David Nadal[a], *Pearay L. Ogra*[b]

[a] Department of Pediatrics, Division of Immunology/Hematology, University of
Zürich, Switzerland, and [b] Department of Pediatrics, University of Texas
Medical Branch at Galveston, Tex., USA

Tonsils are located at the entrance to both the respiratory tract and the
intestinal tract. Do tonsils function as gatekeeper of the mucosal immune
system?

Here we summarize recent experiments from our laboratories [1–3]
using mice with severe combined immune deficiency (SCID) reconstituted
with human tonsillar mononuclear cells (hu-TMC). The aim was to study
immunobiological aspects of tonsillar cells in vivo.

Distribution and Engraftment of hu-TMC in SCID Mice

Mosier et al. [4] reported in 1988 the successful adoptive transfer of
human peripheral blood lymphocytes (hu-PBL) into SCID mice. In analo-
gy, we injected C.B-17 SCID mice intraperitoneally with hu-TMC (50 ×
10^6/mouse) [1]. The hu-TMC-SCID mice were subsequently tested for the
appearance and distribution of human lymphocytes tagged with the
supravital DNA stain H33342, for human immunoglobulin-secreting cells
(hu-ISC) in various systemic and mucosal immunocompetent tissues, and
for the production of human immunoglobulin [1].

After injection of hu-TMC and over a 4-week observation period,
H33342-stained cells were present in large numbers in the omentum, peri-
toneal washing, and in the peripheral blood of the SCID mice. Human
TMC were detected in liver and spleen starting with day 7, in lung and
bone marrow starting with 2 weeks after injection. Stained cells were not
observed in the intestines [1].

Table 1. Human immunoglobulin levels in serum of hu-TMC-SCID mice

Isotype	Weeks after intraperitoneal transfer of hu-TMC		
	2	4	5–7
G	280.8	590.9	1,093.1
A	1.5	5.9	9.0
M	3.2	28.9	95.6

Adapted from Nadal et al. [1]; values represent the means from the levels in 13 animals and are expressed as µg/ml.

Five to seven weeks after administration of hu-TMC, IgG and IgM hu-ISC were detected by means of an enzyme-linked immunospot (ELISPOT) [5] assay with comparable frequency in all murine tissues investigated, except in the intestine. IgA hu-ISC were found in fewer animals. The engraftment of hu-TMC was in the lung quantitatively more extensive than in systemic tissues [1], a feature not seen in hu-PBL-SCID mice [6].

The hu-TMC-SCID mice exhibited serum levels of human immunoglobulins of the isotypes G, A and M increasing with time after cell transfer (table 1).

Reactivity of hu-TMC-SCID Mice to Respiratory Syncytial Virus

In subsequent experiments [2], we tested the reactivity of hu-TMC to respiratory syncytial virus (RSV) within the SCID mice. RSV was chosen as antigen because it is a pathogen restricted to respiratory mucosa. Hu-TMC-SCID mice were challenged intraperitoneally with inactivated RSV or sham immunized 4–5 weeks after reconstitution. Two weeks later, synthesis and distribution characteristics of human antibody to RSV in various murine tissues were studied using an ELISPOT assay [2].

No specific antibody was observed in sham-immunized hu-TMC-SCID mice. In contrast, following intraperitoneal immunization with inactivated RSV, animals engrafted with hu-TMC exhibited the appearance of specific human antibody-secreting cells (hu-ASC). Hu-TMC-engrafted mice showed RSV-specific IgM and, in lower numbers, IgG hu-ASC in

Galioto GB (ed): Tonsils: A Clinically Oriented Update.
Adv Otorhinolaryngol. Basel, Karger, 1992, vol 47, pp 80–90

Antigen-Presenting Cells in the Nasopharyngeal Tonsil

A Quantitative Immunohistochemical Study

Joel M. Bernstein[a], *Sandy Sendor*[b], *Jean Wactawski-Wende*[c]

[a] Departments of Otolaryngology and Pediatrics, State University of New York at Buffalo and Division of Infectious Diseases, Children's Hospital of Buffalo, N.Y.;
[b] Department of Pathology, Children's Hospital of Buffalo, N.Y., and
[c] Department of Gynecology and Obstetrics, State University of New York at Buffalo, N.Y., USA

The nasopharyngeal tonsil, or adenoid, is a lymphoepithelial organ situated in a critical anatomical position in the roof of the nasopharynx. The adenoid directly communicates with the nasopharyngeal orifice of the eustachian tube; the only entrance to the tympanic cavity and middle ear cleft. Furthermore, the nasopharyngeal tonsil is closely associated with the ostia of the paranasal sinuses, particularly the ethmoid and sphenoid sinuses. The adenoid possesses a mucus membrane which has many ciliated cells which synthesize secretory component and, therefore, represents a part of the local immune system of the upper aerodigestive tract [1].

A balance between the microbial colonization of the nasopharyngeal tonsil and the local immune mechanisms available in the nasopharynx would be of importance in the maintenance of the health and well-being of children in whom otitis media and sinusitis represent, by far, the two most common infectious diseases or inflammatory conditions of the upper respiratory tract. It is, therefore, of particular importance to understand the local immune mechanisms available in the nasopharyngeal tonsil and to be able to either control or modify them to maintain the normal health of this important immunological lymphoepithelial organ.

Available studies [2–4] suggest that a local immune system exists in the nasopharyngeal tonsil and plays a critical role in adherence, colonization and spread of bacteria and viruses to the middle ear and paranasal sinuses, and this local immune system of the nasopharyngeal tonsil may modulate and prevent these potential events.

There have been few reports on antigen-presenting cells (APC) in the nasopharyngeal tonsil. APC have come to the attention of immunologists and immunopathologists in recent years, as it has been recognized that they play a central role in antigen presentation in both the germinal centers as well as in the extrafollicular zones [5].

Inasmuch as these cells are responsible for the proper signaling of T cells and B cells in the nasopharyngeal tonsil as well as the palatine tonsil, it is important to know the distribution of these cells in these lymphoepithelial organs as well as to determine whether or not they may become altered or decreased as a result of aging or inflammation. For example, it is now well documented that in the aging mouse the antigen-retaining reticulum (ARR) in the germinal center of lymph nodes is significantly decreased, or almost absent [6]. The purpose of this study, therefore, was to determine the relationship of age, otitis media, tonsillitis, and NTHI, a major pathogen in acute otitis media and acute sinusitis and the APC in various compartments of the nasopharyngeal tonsil.

Materials and Methods

Twenty freshly dissected adenoids and six tonsils from 21 patients undergoing adenoidectomy, or tonsillectomy and adenoidectomy, were used in this study. The age range for the adenoids was 2–17 years and for the tonsils 5–46 years of age. The tissues were

Table 1. Demographics of patients in study

Tissue	Adenoids	20	
	Tonsils	6	
Age, months	Range	21–198	
	Mean	54	
Sex	Male	15	
	Female	6	
		Yes	No
Tonsillitis		10	11
Otitis media		14	7
Bacteriology	NTHI	8	13
	S. pneumoniae	1	20
	M. catarrhalis	1	20

Table 2. Monoclonal antibodies used in this study

Monoclonal antibody	Immunogen	Clone	Specificity	Reactivity
1. Anti-human C3b receptor (Mouse IgG) (Dako-C3bR)	C3b receptor-enriched precipitates from tonsil cell membranes	To 5	Determines single glycoprotein chain with MW of 220 kD. Inh. binding of C3b to receptor of B cells, red cells, neut. mono, MΦ (CD 35 antigen)	Most strongly labelled elements in B cell follicles are follicular dendritic cells. Mantle cell B cells to a lesser extent
2. Anti-human macrophage (Dako-CD68) (Mouse IgG) (dil. 1:50–1:00)	Subcellular fraction of human aveolar macrophages	KP1	Detects a glycoprotein with a MW of 110 kD. Similar molecule is recognized by EBM11 Y1/P2A Y2/131 Kr-M6	Macrophages in a wide variety of human tissues; reacts also with plasmacytoid T cells
3. Monoclonal Ab Dako-MAC 387 Mouse IgG (dil. 1:100)	Purified peripheral blood monocyte components	MAC 387	Human cytoplasmic antigen expressed in granulocytes, blood monocytes, and tissue histiocytes. (1 alpha unit MW 12 kD) (1 beta unit MW 14 kD)	Monocytes/ histocytes but not in GC. Also labels sq. epithelium in skin and tonsils
4. Rabbit anti-cow S-100 (dil. 1:10)	S-100 protein isolated from cow brain		Cross-reacts with human S-100 A and B	Langerhans' cells of skin. Interdigitating reticular cells of lymphoid tissue

transported at 4 °C in physiological saline solution and submitted for immunohistochemical analysis.

The demographics of this study are summarized in table 1. 15 male and 6 female subjects, were used in this study. Middle ear fluid was present in 14 of the 21 patients and the adenoids were taken from 10 children who had a history of tonsillitis or who had undergone tonsillectomy at the time of adenoidectomy. The bacteriological flora of the adenoid was analyzed in every case; in 8 children NTHI was present, however, in only 1 child was *Streptococcus pneumoniae* present and *Moraxella catarrhalis* was present in 2 children. The average age of the patients in the study was 54 months.

Preparation of Tissue Sections
Human adenoid and tonsil tissue were fixed in 10% buffered formalin (pH 7.2) for 5–7 h, processed through a graded series of alcohols and xylene, and embedded in paraffin. Tissue sections were cut at 4 µm and placed in poly-*L*-lysine coated slides to prevent

Table 3. Reactivity of monoclonal antibodies

	MΦ	IDC (T-cell areas)	FDC (follicle + mantle zone areas)
C3bR	−	−	+ +
CD68	+ +	±	−
MAC 387	+ +	−	−
S-100	±	+ +	±

loss during staining. The sections were deparaffinized, rehydrated, and stained with either a mouse alkaline phosphatase, anti-alkaline phosphatase (APAAP) [7] (Dako APAAP Kit, System 40, Carpinteria, Calif., USA) or rabbit III *Strep-Avidin* HRP (Biomeda Corp., Foster City, Calif., USA) commercially available immunohistochemical detection methods using the protocol specified by the manufacturer.

All monoclonal antibodies (C3b, MAC 387, and CD68) were preceded with proteolytic digestion with protease Type XXVII (Sigma Co., St. Louis, Mo., USA) to enhance the staining reaction. Primary antibody dilutions were prepared as follows: C3b receptor 1:200 MAC 387, myeloid-histiocyte antigen 1:100, macrophage CD68 1:50, and S-100 protein 1:200.

The antibodies used in this study are summarized in table 2. The reactivity of both the monoclonal and polyclonal antibodies are summarized in table 3. Briefly, MAC 387 and CD68 are monoclonal antibodies that react with epitopes in the cytoplasm of the monocyte/macrophage cells. S-100 is a protein which is present in interdigitating cells in the T regions of lymph nodes as well as tonsils and adenoids [11]. The antibody directed against S-100 is a rabbit-anti-cow polyclonal antibody. The antibody directed against the C3b receptor is quite specific for the dendritic processes of follicular dendritic cells (FDC) in the germinal centers of the nasopharyngeal tonsil. Using this monoclonal antibody, staining of B cells in the follicle was either very light or absent.

Method for Counting Cells

Cells were counted with a light microscope (American Optical) with a micrometer disc (American Optical) inserted in the ocular. The grid was 1.0 mm^2 with 10 mm^2 divisions. Calibrations were made with a stage micrometer (American Optical) to confirm that one grid equals 0.25 mm^2 at 40 × magnification. Total cell counts were made by counting cells in five squares (center and four corners when possible) at 40 × and multiplying their total by 20. This was performed at four different locations on the slide to obtain total cells/mm^2. Positive cell counts were made for all areas except crypt epithelium by counting all stained slides in one grid at 40 ×. Four different areas were counted and totalled to obtain positive cells/mm^2. Crypt epithelium was defined as four layers of cells below the surface epithelium. Total crypt epithelial counts were made by counting positive cells in five different squares and multiplying them by 20. This was also done at four locations to calculate total positive cells/mm^2. Percent positive was calculated by dividing total positive cells in each area by total cells in that area and multiplying by 100.

Table 4. Average percentage of APC in compartments of nasopharyngeal tonsil

Antibody	MAC 387		CD68	S-100	C3b
Crypt epithelium	6.1 ± 5.7	$\leftarrow p < 0.01 \rightarrow$	0.39 ± 1.13	0.47 ± 0.86	0.01 ± 0.01
Extrafollicular zone	5.4 ± 2.3		4.4 ± 3.6	2.4 ± 1.5	0.01 ± 0.02
Mantle zone	0.17 ± 0.19		0.99 ± 2.4	0.05 ± 0.08	11.0 ± 7.8
Germinal center	0.66 ± 1.2	$\leftarrow p < 0.01 \rightarrow$	2.5 ± 1.3	0.09 ± 0.24	42.0 ± 6.1

C3b staining was difficult to accurately count because cell staining was not clearly defined. For counting purposes, positive staining was defined as staining in some portion of the cell. Total positive staining is most likely somewhat high due to positive processes communicating with other dendritic cells – so-called antigen-retaining reticulum.

Statistics

All data for the monoclonal antibodies in the four different areas of the nasopharyngeal tonsil, as well as the variables of age, sex, presence or absence of tonsillitis, presence or absence or otitis media, and presence or absence of NTHI in the nasopharyngeal microflora, were entered into the Statistical Package for the Social Sciences (SPSS-PC). Statistical significance using the Student t test in this program was defined as $p < 0.05$.

Results

The quantitative distribution of APC in the nasopharyngeal tonsils is summarized in table 4. MAC 387 stained tissue macrophages primarily in the crypt epithelium (fig. 1) as well as in the extrafollicular zone (fig. 2). MAC 387 cells were rarely seen in the mantle zone or germinal center.

CD68 was rarely present in the crypt epithelium, unlike MAC 387, but was present in the extrafollicular zone and germinal centers (fig. 3, 4). The differences for these two tissue macrophages in these two different areas of the nasopharyngeal tonsil were statistically significant (table 4).

S-100 was seen primarily in the extrafollicular zone and was occasionally present in the crypt epithelium, mantle zone, and germinal centers (fig. 5).

C3b is found on active immune complexes, which appeared to be present on FDC. The monoclonal antibody recognizing C3B was exclusively present in the germinal centers and mantle zones (fig. 6, 7). C3b was virtually absent in the crypt epithelium and in the extrafollicular zones. Again, it should be emphasized that counting of FDC by the light microscope is extremely difficult because the ARR appears to intertwine from dendritic process to dendritic process of different cells and, therefore, it is difficult to count these cells accurately. However, an attempt was made to identify these cells in the count inasmuch as this cell takes up the mono-clonal stain much more avidly than the B cells in the follicle. Furthermore, the B-cell nucleus is round, whereas the dendritic cell nucleus cell is extremely irregular. However, it is most likely that other techniques will be necessary for more accurate determination of the actual numbers of FDC or the area of FDC in the germinal center. These cells, however, appeared to be very prominent in the follicle and this appears to be in contrast to the data that has been described in the murine model where only 1–2% of the germinal center is supposed to possess FDC [8].

The relationship of age, sex, otitis media, tonsillitis, and bacteriology, particularly NTHI, and the quantitative distribution of APC in the naso-pharyngeal tonsil was performed using the SPSS-PC Statistical Package. Several interesting findings were obtained. There were significantly more S-100 cells in the extrafollicular zone of children over the age of 5 as compared to those younger than 5 (p = 0.05). This was the only significant finding with the age variable. The presence of NTHI in the microflora did not appear to have any effect on the distribution of the APC in any com-partment of the nasopharyngeal tonsil. The presence of tonsillitis also had an effect on the distribution of S-100 cells in the extrafollicular zone. In this case, there appeared to be almost twice as many interdigitating cells in the extrafollicular zone in patients with tonsillitis as compared with patients who did not have this condition. There appeared to be no signif-icant differences in the distribution of APC in the nasopharyngeal tonsil in regard to sex. Finally, a nearly (p = 0.063) significant decrease in interdi-gitating cells as represented by S-100 staining in the extrafollicular zone was present in children with otitis media as compared to those who did not have middle ear fluid at the time of adenoidectomy.

Thus, in summary, the interdigitating cell was the cell that appeared to have a significant relationship to the variables studied. There was an increase of number of these cells in the adenoid in patients with tonsillitis; a decrease of this cell in patients with otitis media, and an increase of this cell in children over the age of 5 as compared to those children below the age of 5.

Finally, when tonsils as a group were compared to adenoids there was a significant increase in MAC 387 in the extrafollicular zone of adenoids (p = 0.017).

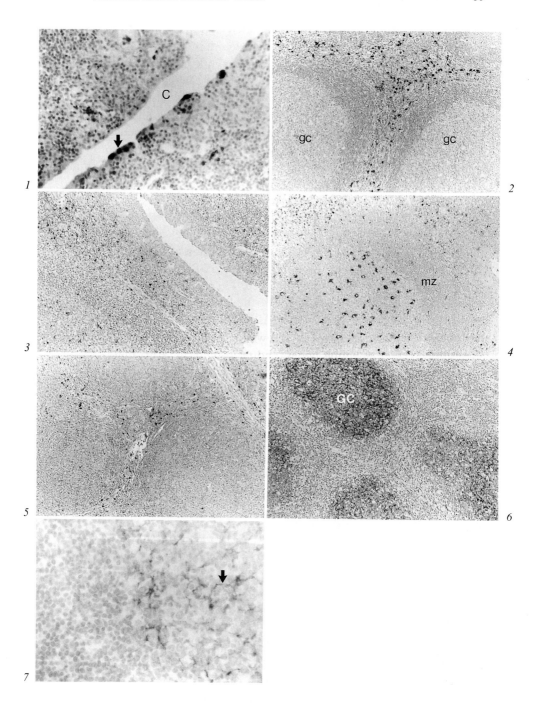

Discussion

APC are clearly needed for proper presentation of antigen to immunocompetent cells. In the absence of APC, as has been suggested in the aging mouse, immunological recognition does not occur and appropriate maturation of B cells into both memory cells as well as into immunoglobulin-secreting cells does not occur [9].

Dendritic cells are a system of APC that function to initiate several immune responses, such as the sensitization of MHC-restricted T cells, the rejection of organ transplants, the formation of T-dependent antibodies, and the presentation of antigen to B cells in the germinal centers of lymph nodes and the tonsils and adenoids.

This study suggests that macrophage, as represented by cells which stain with MAC 387 and CD68, may appear in the crypts of the nasopharyngeal tonsil, but MAC 387 is significantly more common. In contrast to this, CD68 is found in significantly higher numbers in the germinal center compared to MAC 387. Although this study does not permit absolute identification of CD68 cells, it is suggested that CD68 might stain tingible macrophages, which are known as cells which phagocytize effete B cells in the germinal center of lymph nodes, and probably also in the tonsils and adenoids. This concept has also been suggested by Pulford et al. [10].

The extrafollicular zone possesses both MAC 387 and CD68 cells, but it is in this region that S-100 cells are primarily present, and these are specific for interdigitating cells [11]. Thus, the interfollicular area pos-

---

Fig. 1. Immunohistochemical staining using MAC 387 shows staining of macrophages (arrow) in the crypt of the nasopharyngeal tonsil. C = Crypt. APAAP. × 10.

Fig. 2. Immunohistochemical staining of MAC 387 in the extrafollicular zone of the nasopharyngeal tonsil. gc = Germinal center. APAAP. × 4.

Fig. 3. Immunohistochemical localization of CD68 cells in the extrafollicular zone of the nasopharyngeal tonsil. There is a paucity of these cells in the crypt epithelium. APAAP. × 4.

Fig. 4. Immunohistochemical localization of CD68 cells in the germinal center of the nasopharyngeal tonsil. mz = Mantle zone. APAAP. × 4.

Fig. 5. Immunohistochemical localization of cells staining with S-100 in the extrafollicular zone of the nasopharyngeal tonsil. APAAP. × 4.

Fig. 6. Immunohistochemical localization of C3B receptor on the FDC of the nasopharyngeal germinal center. GC = Germinal center. APAAP. × 4.

Fig. 7. High-powered photomicrograph of C3B labeling of the dendritic processes of FDC showing the ARR (arrow). APAAP. × 20.

sesses at least three different types of APC which most likely play a role in antigen presentation to T cells. The multiple signals that are necessary for T cells to recognize antigen on the surface of both macrophage and dendritic cells has been discussed in detail by Geppert et al. [12].

This present study also shows that FDC are present in the germinal centers of the nasopharyngeal adenoid. Tew et al. [13] have demonstrated an alternative antigen presentation pathway in the murine model. The alternative antigen pathway consists of immune complexes present on the dendritic processes of FDC. These complexes are delivered to antigen-specific B cells in the germinal centers, which then process and present antigen to T cells. B cells obtain immunogen from FDC in the form of immune complex-coated bodies or iccosomes and antigen-specific B cells appear to find these newly discovered iccosomes especially palatable. Whether or not this alternative antigen pathway takes place in the human nasopharyngeal tonsil is not as yet known, but it is very likely that it may take place, and thus, the FDC may be a cell for the presentation of immune complexed antigen to be delivered to germinal center B cells. B cells would then ultimately be committed to either memory B cells or mature into immunoglobulin-secreting plasma cells.

It has also been shown by this same group that aging mice have defective ARR and defective follicle development. Therefore, it was of particular interest to determine whether or not older children or children with recurrent tonsillitis and/or otitis media, that is, children who most likely have a pathological microflora in their nasopharyngeal tonsils, might be subject to defective FDC. The numbers of cases in this study are relatively small, and furthermore, the counting of APC in the follicle is exceedingly difficult. Therefore, whether or not there are defective antigen-trapping mechanisms or defective FDC in the nasopharyngeal adenoid in recurrent inflammation cannot be stated at this time. Further studies will need to be performed to determine whether or not this can occur, particularly using the techniques of image analysis and/or immunoelectron microscopy.

One of the purposes of this study was to compare several different variables and the distribution of the APC. Although the numbers are relatively small, there are several trends that may be of some interest and which will need to be further evaluated when more data is available. The presence of tonsillitis, the presence of fluid and the older the child is, may have an effect on the distribution of S-100 cells in the extrafollicular zone. There did not appear to be any other significant findings in regard to the variables studied. Only one significant difference in the distribution of

APC between the tonsils and adenoids was found. MAC 387 was more than twice as common in the extrafollicular zone in the nasopharyngeal tonsil compared to the palatine tonsil. Finally, inasmuch as NTHI is becoming the most common cause of both acute otitis media and is the most common organism present in chronic middle ear effusions, we sought to determine a potential relationship between the presence of NTHI in the adenoidal microflora and the distribution of APC. There was no significant difference in the distribution of the APC in any compartment of the adenoid and the presence or absence of NTHI.

Conclusion

APC consisting of macrophages, interdigitating cells and FDC are distributed in specific areas of the nasopharyngeal tonsil. Whereas MAC 387 cells appear to predominate in the crypts and extrafollicular zone, CD68 cells predominate in the extrafollicular zone and follicle and are extremely rare in the crypt. It is, therefore, cautiously suggested that these latter cells in the follicle could represent phagocytizing macrophage – so-called tingible body macrophages.

C3b was identified in the germinal center of the nasopharyngeal tonsil and appeared to be located on the dendritic processes of the FDC, suggesting that immune complexes are retained on the dendritic processes of these APC. C3b did not appear to be present in any other region of the nasopharyngeal tonsil. The presence of MAC 387 in the extrafollicular zone was the only significant difference in the APC between the tonsils and adenoids. The relationship between tonsillitis, age, otitis media, and the distribution of S-100 in the extrafollicular zone appears interesting and may be of some biological significance, but the numbers in this study are too small to make any meaningful conclusion. Further studies using image analysis and immunoelectron microscopy will be needed to study these cells in the future.

Immunological studies of this type may help us to determine the immunological reactivity of the nasopharyngeal tonsil as it relates to the development of both arms of the immune system, namely cell-mediated immunity and humoral immunity. Ultimately, this information may help the otolaryngologist and clinical immunologist understand the events that control colonization, replication and migration of pathogenic bacteria into the eustachian tube and sinus ostia – the critical events that lead to otitis media and sinusitis.

References

1   Brandtzaeg P: Immune functions and immunopathology of palatine and nasopha-
    ryngeal tonsils; in Bernstein JM, Ogra PL (eds): Immunology of the Ear. New York,
    Raven Press, 1987, pp 63–106.
2   Bernstein JM, Loos B, Dryja D, Dickinson D: Analysis of total genome restriction
    fragments of paired nasopharyngeal and middle ear isolates. Otolaryngol Head Neck
    Surg 1989;110:206–209.
3   Faden H, Bernstein JM, Stanievich J, Hong JJ: Otitis media in children. I. The
    systemic immune response to nontypable *Haemophilus influenzae.* J Infect Dis
    1989;160:999–1004.
4   Kurono Y, Fujiyoshi T, Mogi G: Secretory IgA and bacterial adherence to nasal
    mucosal cells. Ann Otol Rhinol Laryngol 1989;98:273–277.
5   Tew JG, Thorbecke J, Steinman R: Dendritic cells in the immune response: Char-
    acteristics and recommended nomenclature (A report from the Reticuloendothelial
    Society on Nomenclature). J Reticuloendothel Soc 1982;31:371–380.
6   Szakal AK, Taylor JK, Smith JP, Kosco MH, et al: Kinetics of germinal center
    development in lymph nodes of young and aging mice. Anat Rec 1990;227:475–
    485.
7   Cordell JL, Falini B, Erber WN: Immunoenzymatic labeling of monoclonal anti-
    bodies using immune complexes of alkaline phosphatase and monoclonal-alkaline
    phosphatase (APAAP complexes). J Histochem Cytochem 1984;32:219–229.
8   Szakal AK, Taylor JK, Smith JP, Kosco MH, et al: Morphometry and kinetics of
    antigen transport and developing antigen-retaining reticulum of follicular dendritic
    cells in lymph nodes of aging immune mice. Aging Immunol Infect Dis 1988;1:
    7–21.
9   Tew JG, Kosco MH, Szakal AK: An alternative antigen pathway. Immunol Today
    1989;10:229–231.
10 Pulford KA, Rigney EM, Micklem KJ, Jones M, et al: KP1: A new monoclonal
    antibody that detects a monocyte/macrophage associated antigen in routinely pro-
    cessed tissue sections. J Clin Pathol 1989;42:414–421.
11 Nakajima T, Watanabe S, Sato Y, Kamey T, et al: An immunoperoxidase study of
    S-100 protein distribution in normal and neoplastic tissues. Am J Surg Pathol 1982;
    6:715–727.
12 Geppert TD, Davis LS, Gur H, Wacholtz MC, Lipsky PE: Accessory cell signals
    involved in T-cell activation. Immunol Rev 1990;117:5–58.
13 Tew JG, Kosco MH, Burton G, Szakal AK: FDC as accessory cells. Immunol Rev
    1990;117:185–211.

Joel M. Bernstein, MD, PhD, 15 South Forest Rd.,
Williamsville, NY 14221 (USA)

Galioto GB (ed): Tonsils: A Clinically Oriented Update.
Adv Otorhinolaryngol. Basel, Karger, 1992, vol 47, pp 91–96

HLA-DR Antigen Expression in Tonsillar Epithelium

Takaaki Kimura

Otorhinolaryngological Department, Wakayama Medical College,
Wakayama City, Japan

HLA-DR antigen, a class II major histocompatibility complex (MHC) in man, is closely involved in cellular immune responses. Recently, the appearance of HLA-DR antigen in epithelial cells has been interpreted as an early sign of the development of autoimmunity [1, 2]. Promoted by Brandtzaeg [3], who showed the appearance of HLA-DR antigens in the tonsillar epithelium, we reported previously the relationship between HLA-DR positivity and three different diseases [4].

Material and Methods

Twenty-six surgically removed tonsillar specimens were used. The patients consisted of 10 with hypertrophic tonsil, 7 with recurrent tonsillitis, and 10 with tonsils with palmoplantar pustulosis (PPP). These specimens were fixed to make acetone-fixed frozen sections, and stained by fluorescent staining using anti-HLA-DR monoclonal antibody (Becton-Dickinson) as the primary antibody and goat anti-mouse immunoglobulin (DAKO) as the secondary antibody. To evaluate the specimens for HLA-DR positivity, we calculated the rate of HLA-DR-positive area to total epithelial area by an image-analyzing computer program [5], and thus compared the three tonsillar diseases. We used an electron microscope as well as a light microscope. Moreover, we stained the frozen tonsillar sections by avidin-biotin-peroxidase staining using the following monoclonal antibodies as the primary antibody: CD 3 (pan T); CD4 (helper/inducer T); CD8 (suppressor/cytotoxic T); CD22 (pan B), and CD25 (activated T). We counted the lymphocytes infiltrating the tonsillar epithelium, and investigated the relationship between HLA-DR positivity and the degree of lymphocyte infiltration in the tonsillar epithelium. The HLA-DR expression on the epithelium was conveniently classified into four types (fig. 1), namely: type I: negative to HLA-DR; type II: positive to only the basal layer; type III: intermediate between types II and VI; type VI: all the layers are positive to HLA-DR.

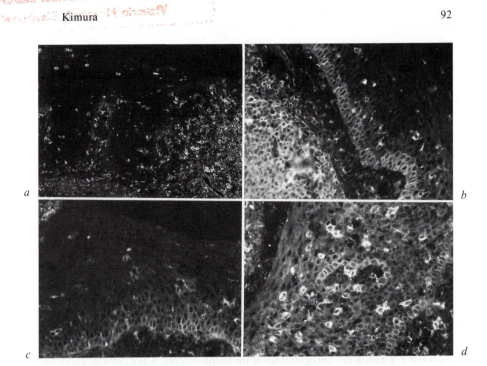

Fig. 1. Immunofluorescent staining of the tonsillar epithelium using anti-HLA-DR antibody. *a* Type I: the epithelium was completely negative for HLA-DR. *b* Type II: only the single basal layer was positive. *c* Type III: an intermediate pattern between types II and VI. *d* Type VI: all the layers were positive for HLA-DR.

Results

HLA-DR antigen was detected on the tonsillar epithelium electron microscopically as well as light microscopically (fig. 1, 2). The immunofluorescent staining resulted in four different patterns of HLA-DR expression mentioned in the Material and Methods. The site on which the HLA-DR antigen was mainly positive was the cytoplasm of epithelial keratinocytes in the immunofluorescent study, and the cellular surface under an electron microscope. When the image-analyzing program was used, the positive reaction of HLA-DR antigen was stronger in hypertrophic tonsil and focus tonsil than in recurrent tonsillitis (fig. 3). For the infiltrating lymphocytes, CD4- and CD8-positive cells, unlike CD3- and

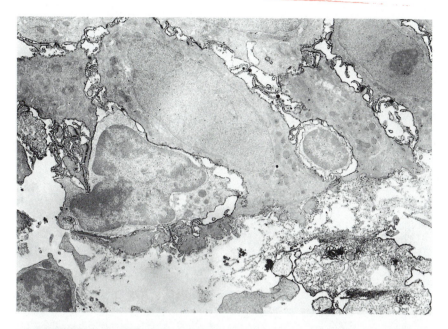

Fig. 2. Electron microscopic image of the tonsillar epithelium stained by anti-HLA-DR antibody.

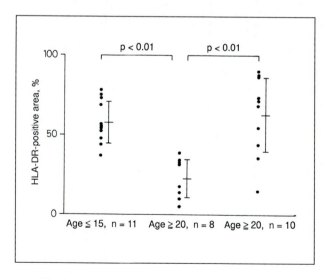

Fig. 3. HLA-DR antigen expression in several tonsillar diseases.

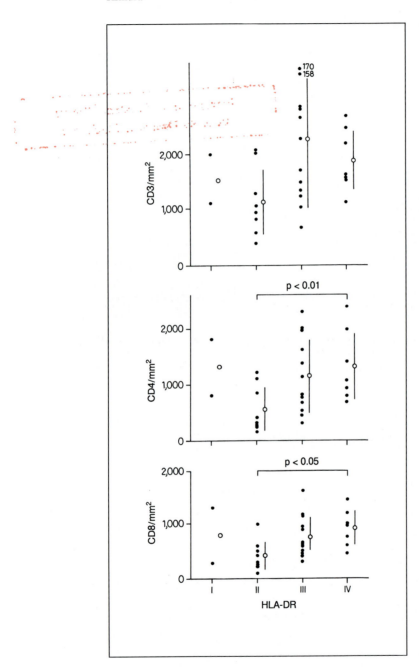

Fig. 4. Relationship between HLA-DR positivity and infiltrating lymphocytes.

CD22-positive cells which seemed to be independent of HLA-DR positivity, tended to increase with the increasing positivity of HLA-DR antigen (fig. 4).

Discussion

The pathogenesis of PPP is not clear, but some contribution of the tonsil is suspected when the efficacy of tonsillectomy is taken into account [6]. A comparison between recurrent tonsillitis and focus tonsil, whose patients are over 20 years of age, shows that the appearance of HLA-DR antigen is stronger in the latter, partly because HLA-DR positivity is thought to have some effects on the PPP etiology. In an early stage of palmar or plantar pustules, T-lymphocyte infiltration in epidermis is a major pathological finding [7]. Taking account of the previous reports [8] that lymphocytes are likely to infiltrate HLA-DR-positive epidermal keratinocytes, in our study, CD4- and CD8-positive cells tended to infiltrate strongly HLA-DR highly positive epithelial area. Opposed to the general concept that is related to humoral immunity, we suspected, from the study, an important role of T lymphocyte and HLA-DR antigen in its onset, and supposed that the tonsillar T lymphocytes stimulated by tonsillar epithelial keratinocytes injure the palmar and plantar skin. Though convincing data are not available, excluding PPP, HLA-DR positivity must have a close relationship to aging. It is assumed that the predominant proliferation of lymphatic organs in childhood has some effects on the upper respiratory tract as expressed by this antigen in the tonsillar epithelium.

References

1   Volc-Platzer B, Groh V, Wolff K: Differential expression of class II alloantigens by keratinocytes in disease. J Invest Dermatol 1987;89:64–68.
2   Hedberg NM, Hunter N: The expression of HLA-DR on keratinocytes in oral lichen planus. J Oral Pathol 1987;16:31–35.
3   Brandtzaeg P: Immune functions of human nasal mucosa and tonsils in health and disease; in Bienenstock J (ed): Immunology of the Lung and Upper Respiratory Tract. New York, McGraw-Hill, 1984, pp 28–95.
4   Kimura T, Fujiwara K, Kuki K, Hayashi Y, Tabata T: HLA-DR antigen expression in tonsillar epithelium. Acta Otolaryngol 1990;110:459–465.

5   Kimura T, Kunimoto M, Tamura S, Fujiwara K, Yokota M, Kuki K, Hayashi Y,
    Tabata T: HLA-DR expression in pharyngeal epithelium and intraepithelially infil-
    trating T-lymphocytes. Stomato-Pharyngol 1990;2:155–160.
6   Ono T, Jono M, Kito M: Evaluation of tonsillectomy as a treatment for pustulosis
    palmaris et plantaris. Acta Otolaryngol 1983(suppl 401):12–16.
7   Kimura T, Kunimoto M, Tamura S, Fujiwara K, Tabata T: Study on the onset of
    tonsil with focal infection (with special reference of palmoplantar pustulosis). Jpn J
    Tonsil 1990;29:133–137.
8   Smolle J, Soyer HP, Juettner FM, Torne R, Stettner H, Kerl H: HLA-DR-positive
    keratinocytes are associated with suppressor lymphocyte epidermotropism. Am J
    Dermatol 1988;10:128–132.

T. Kimura, MD, Otorhinolaryngological Department,
Wakayama Medical College, 7-Bancho 27, Wakayama City (Japan)

Galioto GB (ed): Tonsils: A Clinically Oriented Update.
Adv Otorhinolaryngol. Basel, Karger, 1992, vol 47, pp 97–100

Immunohistological Studies on Immunocompetent Cells in Palatine Tonsil

Akikatsu Kataura, Yasuaki Harabuchi, Hideaki Matsuyama,
Noboru Yamanaka

Department of Otolaryngology, Sapporo Medical College, Sapporo, Japan

The palatine tonsil, a major lymphatic organ, is situated at the beginning of both the respiratory tract and the gastrointestinal tract, and appears to play an important role in the immune defense against bacteria, virus, and the other antigens. On the other hand, it is also the focus for infections such as habitual angina and tonsillar focal infections. The immune response in any lymphatic organ requires multiple interactions among various immunocompetent cells such as T cells, B cells, macrophages, etc. The determination of the distribution of such immunocompetent cells in the palatine tonsil is of much importance to clarify the cellular interactions in tonsil as well as the pathogenesis of tonsillar lesions.

In previous papers [1–3] we have reported data on the immunohistological analyses of the distribution of various immunocompetent cells in palatine tonsils using monoclonal antibodies (MoAb). In this study, we performed quantitative analyses for the lymphoid cells in the tonsils. To identify the distribution of various T-cell subsets on the tonsillar compartments, the double immunoenzymatic labeling technique using alkaline phosphatase and peroxidase was employed. In addition, to analyze the cell suspensions of tonsillar lymphocytes, flow cytometry was performed, and to measure the proportion of various lymphoid cells in the tonsillar compartments, image analysis was done.

Material and Methods

Tonsils were obtained from 96 patients aged from 3 to 66 years who had undergone tonsillectomy for therapeutic purposes – obstructive sleep apnea syndrome (OSA), recurrent tonsillitis (RT), and pustulosis palmaris et plantaris (PPP).

MoAb, which react with T-cell surface antigens (CD4, CD8, CD11, CD25, CD29, CD45RA, and Leu8) and every isotype of immunoglobulin (IgG, IgM, IgA, and IgD), Ki-67 recognizing the antigen appearing during proliferating phases of the cell cycle, OKT9 detecting a transferrin receptor on the proliferating cells, and L29 defining the activated B cells, were employed.

Two-color flow cytometric analysis [4] was performed using an Epics C cytofluorograph (Coulter Electronics Inc., USA) to analyze the suspended tonsillar lymphocytes stained simultaneously with fluorescein isothiocyanate (FITC)-labeled MoAb and phycoerythrin (PE)-labeled MoAb.

The double immunoenzymatic labeling method [5] was used on the tonsillar section. Briefly, the T-cell surface antigen was stained using the alkaline phosphatase-antialkaline phosphatase method. After blocking for remaining antibodies using normal mouse serum, another T-cell antigen was detected by the avidin-biotin-peroxidase method.

The image analysis [6–8] was carried out by an Image Analyzing System, CUE-2 (Olympus Inc., USA). The immunostained section examined by light microscopy was filmed with a TV camera and processed by a personal computer. The image analysis was performed following enhancement and preprocessing on the display, picture stretching and segmentation by thresholding. Then the subarea to be analyzed was selected from the picture. Small objects and binary noise in it were removed. After separating overlapping particles and filling all holes of surface-positive particles, the percentage of positive cells in the subarea was calculated.

Results and Discussion

In two-color flow cytometric analysis, the helper T cells (CD4+Leu8−) were found in about 20% of the tonsillar lymphocytes. Each T-cell subset, the helper-inducer (CD4+CD29+), the suppressor-inducer (CD4+CD45RA+), and the cytotoxic T cells (CD8+CD11−), was seen in 5–9%. However, only 1% of the tonsillar lymphocytes were recognized as suppressor T cells (CD8+CD11+). These data show that tonsil contains more helper T cells and fewer suppressor T cells than peripheral blood does.

In double enzymatic labeling analysis, almost all the CD4-positive cells in the germinal center never expressed Leu8, CD29, and CD45RA. On the other hand, the CD4-positive cells dual expressing such antigens were seen in the interfollicular area. These findings indicate, as shown in figure 1, that aside from the suppressor T-cell subsets, all T-cell subsets, the helper, the helper-inducer, the suppressor-inducer, and the cytotoxic T-cell subsets, are distributed in the interfollicular area; conversely, the vast majority of the T cells in the germinal center are helper T cells which help the activation and differentiation of B-cell lineage.

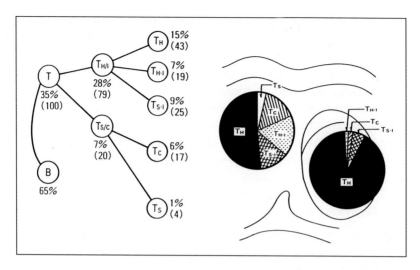

Fig. 1. Distribution of the T-cell subsets in the tonsil.

The data obtained from the image analysis on the stained tonsillar sections showed that every isotope of Ig-positive cells was decreased with aging with significant negative correlation, whereas the amount of the connective tissue fibers stained by Heidenhain's aniline blue in the tonsil increased with age showing significant positive correlation. In the germinal center, aside from the CD25-positive cells defining the activated T cells, each activated lymphoid cell reactive with Ki-67, OKT9, and L29, decreased significantly with aging. In the interfollicular area, CD25 cells showed significant reduction with aging, as well. For T-cell subsets, the CD4-positive cells in the subepithelial area and the CD8-positive cells in the interfollicular area are significantly decreased in older patients. These results suggest a decrease of immune function of the tonsil during aging.

The child patients with RT demonstrated a significant increase of IgG-positive cells and IgD-positive cells in the tonsil and a decrease of CD4-positive cells both in the germinal center and in the interfollicular area, in comparison with the age-matched patients with OSA. The IgE-positive cells distributed in the interfollicular area were significantly increased in patients complicated with nasal allergy.

Aside from IgE, every Ig expression and the Ki67 expression in the tonsillar compartments of the patients with PPP increased as compared with those of the age-matched patients with RT and OSA. In addition, the marked change in proportion of these cells was seen in patients with PPP cured through tonsillectomy in comparison with patients with PPP not cured through tonsillectomy. These data support that PPP is one of the tonsil-related autoimmune diseases.

The data described above show that the image analysis, the double immunoenzymatic labeling method and the two-color flow cytometry, will give us useful information about the roles of the immune response of tonsils and the pathogenesis of various tonsillar lesions.

References

1   Yamanaka N, Sambe S, Harabuchi Y, Kataura A: Immunohistological study of tonsil. Distribution of T cell subsets. Acta Otolaryngol (Stockh) 1983;96:509–516.
2   Harabuchi Y, Yamanaka N, Kataura A: Immunohistological identification of B cell differentiation in human tonsillar follicles by using monoclonal antibodies. Tohoku J Exp Med 1985;147:21–31.
3   Ryan Y, Harabuchi Y, Kataura A: Immunohistological identification of the activated lymphocytes in human palatine tonsil. J Otolaryngol Jpn 1989;92:1958–1963.
4   Harabuchi Y, Koizumi S, Osato T, Yamanaka N, Kataura A: Flow cytometric analysis of Epstein-Barr virus receptor among the different B-cell subpopulations using simultaneous two-color immunofluorescence. Virology 1988;165:278–281.
5   Ryan Y, Harabuchi Y, Kataura A: Double immunoenzymatic and two-color flow cytometric analyses of tonsillar T-cell subsets. J Otolaryngol Jpn 1990;93:1869–1873.
6   Matsuyama H, Yamanaka N: Immunohistological study on immunocompetent cells in palatine tonsil and pharyngeal tonsil. The quantitative study by image analyzer. J Otolaryngol Jpn 1989;92:2064–2078.
7   Matsuyama H, Yamanaka N: Immunohistological study on human palatine tonsils in cases with pustulosis palmaris et plantaris. The quantitative study by image analyzer. J Otolaryngol Jpn 1990;93:6–17.
8   Yamanaka N, Matsuyama H, Harabuchi Y, Kataura A: Distribution of lymphoid cells in tonsillar compartments in relation to infection and age. Acta Otolaryngol (Stockh) 1992;112:128–137.

Akikatsu Kataura, Department of Otolaryngology, Sapporo Medical College, S1 W16, Chuo-Ku, Sapporo City (Japan)

Galioto GB (ed): Tonsils: A Clinically Oriented Update.
Adv Otorhinolaryngol. Basel, Karger, 1992, vol 47, pp 101–106

T-Lymphocyte Role in the Immunological Reactivity of Palatine Tonsil

G. Cortesina[a], *M.T. Carlevato*[a], *M. Bussi*[a], *G. Valente*[b], *M. Sacchi*[a], *G. Palestro*[b]

[a] Istituto di Clinica ORL, II Cattedra, Università di Torino;
[b] Dipartimento di Scienze Biomediche e Oncologia,
Sezione di Anatomia e Patologica, Università di Torino, Italia

Tonsillar T lymphocytes have been studied in detail by characterization of cellular phenotype and evaluation of spatial and functional relationships with other tonsillar and circulating immune cells.

Phenotypically, in paracortical and interfollicular areas, CD3+CD4+ (helper/inducer) T lymphocytes are the most represented cells. CD3+CD8+ (suppressor/cytotoxic) cells are infrequent and they further decrease in a situation of follicular hyperplasia. In the germinal centers, CD3+CD4+ cells seem to have a regulatory role for the tonsillar immune response [1].

The percentage of CD3+ cells expressing TCR-δ is 0.7 ± 0.5% in tonsil, being 12.5 ± 8.1% in spleen, 4 ± 3.1% in peripheral blood, 2.2 ± 1% in lymph nodes, and 1.4 ± 5% in thymus [2]. Tonsil T lymphocytes carrying TCR-δ are mainly positive for BB3 monoclonal antibody (MoAb), specific for the disulfide-linked form of this antigen [3]. In tonsil, TCR-δ1+ cells represent about 3% of the CD3+ cells and they are found mostly under the epithelium, in interfollicular areas, close to the high endothelial venules (HEV). T cells expressing γ/δ antigen are reported to be mature 'resting' cells, playing a suppressor/cytotoxic role.

Recently, distribution of T lymphocytes expressing the different leukocyte common antigen (LCA) polypeptides (CD45+, CD45R+ and CD45/p180 cells) have been studied. T lymphocytes of germinal centers are mostly CD4$^+$CD45/p180$^+$ cells, some of them are also HNK1$^+$ (Leu7$^+$). T lymphocytes of paracortical areas express CD45R or CD45/p180 antigen in the same proportion. 5% of them express both the determinants simultaneously, a possible index of recent activation [4]. It should be noted that expression of CD45, CD45R, and CD45/p180 indicate the activation state of T lymphocytes and not of B lymphocytes of the tonsil [5].

The distribution of the various T-cell subpopulations in tonsil may change with the different physiologic and pathologic conditions of tonsil. For instance, the number of T lymphocytes infiltrating each epithelial unit [6] and of T lymphocytes activated (i.e. expressing CD25) [7] decreases with ageing, demonstrating the ending of the 'educational' phase of tonsillar activity. Similarly, there is a significant correlation between the increase of bacterial load (measured as colony-forming units/g of tonsil) and the increase of CD3$^+$CD4$^+$ lymphocytes [8].

From a functional point of view, many properties of tonsillar T lymphocytes still need a clear interpretation. It has been noted that tonsillar T lymphocytes incorporate less efficiently ^{3}H-TdR than B lymphocytes [9]. In addition, following incubation in presence of IL-4, tonsillar T lymphocytes do not express CD25, while B lymphocytes do [10].

Tonsillar lymphocytes stimulate IgM and IgG production by peripheral blood B lymphocytes preactivated by streptococci antigens. Since in the absence of tonsillar lymphocytes only IgM are produced, it has been postulated that tonsillar T lymphocytes can promote an immunoglobulin switch IgM → IgG through a cognate-like interaction [11].

The proliferative response to IL-4 and mitogens of tonsillar lymphocytes appears to be modulated by expression of CD23 antigen on cell surface, and activated tonsillar cells but not peripheral blood lymphocytes express this antigen [12].

More recently, interesting data regarding the genomic rearrangement for antigen specificity of tonsillar T lymphocytes have been presented. This rearrangement appears to be V γ – (D δ) – J δ and V δ – (D δ) – J γ; in addition, the antigenic specificity seems to be due to chimeric geni as a consequence of translocations, and this mechanism increases the number of possible receptors [13].

The activity of tonsillar T lymphocytes is influenced by the relationship with other tonsillar cells [14] such as macrophages, modulating proliferative response to IL-2 and PHA [15], and follicular dendritic cells, inducing IL-6 and TNF production in tonsillar T and B MLC [16] and T-cell clonal proliferation [17].

Observations in vivo using anti-S100, OKT6 and Leu3a MoAbs have shown that activation of T lymphocytes by antigen-presenting cells takes place at an epithelial level and also in interfollicular areas [18].

Fetal tonsillar T lymphocytes express CD44, a homing antigen which appears to modulate recirculation of both mature T lymphocytes and pro-thymocytes. Migration of prothymocytes into the developing tonsil seems to take place prior to HEV formation, which is followed by lymphocyte colonization [19].

Finally, regarding tonsillar relationship with other structures of MALT, even if cell phenotype of tonsils and adenoids appears to be the same [20], tonsil has been considered the primary structure of MALT for humoral immunity [21]. It may be possible that a similar role is played by tonsil for T-dependent immunity, due to the close relation between B and T lymphocytes. In fact, repeated inoculations of horseradish peroxidase (HRP) into tonsillar crypt induce production of antibodies anti-HRP both in tonsils and regional lymph nodes, followed by glomerular changes [22]. The response to HRP is mainly due to B lymphocytes, which colonize lymph nodes and migrate into peripheral blood; on the other hand, T lymphocytes acquire immunologic memory for HRP.

Personal Data

Material and Methods

Patients. 50 patients, ranging from 3 to 30 years of age, who had undergone tonsillectomy alone or tonsillectomy and adenoidectomy at our institution, were included in this study. On the basis of anamnestic, clinical and laboratory data, they were divided into three groups: (1) 22 patients with hypertrophic tonsillitis; (2) 21 patients with recurrent tonsillitis due to common bacterial agents (as demonstrated by the pharyngeal swab); (3) 7 patients with chronic tonsillitis and focal disease, untreated for the last 3 months.

Cell Isolation. The studies were performed in vitro on tonsillar mononuclear cells (TMNC) isolated from tonsillar tissue obtained at the time of surgery. TMNC were obtained from tonsillar tissue minced in culture medium and treated: (a) with vortex agitation for 15 min; (b) 5 min sedimentation; (c) supernatant aspiration; (d) separation with Ficoll density gradient. Cells were then washed in tissue culture medium.

Phenotypical Study. TMNC were counted and concentrated at 2.5×10^6 cells/ml. MoAbs were employed for characterization of phenotypical lymphocyte subsets. Direct-indirect fluorescence and double staining techniques were employed. The percentage of positive cells was evaluated using a FACScan (fluorescence activated cell sorter). In addition to cell suspensions evaluation, some specimens were comparatively studied on frozen sections, testing the same MoAbs by immunohistochemical techniques (table 1).

Table 1. Phenotypical study: the mean percentages of cells positive for the different MoAbs

	CD3+	CD4+	CD8+	CD19+	HLA-DR+	IL-2R+	CD4/CD8
Hypertrophic tonsillitis	43.113 ±12.6	30.454 ±8.6	15.000 ±6.1	55.204 ±14.1	35.681 ±17.7	15.259 ±8.9	2.626 ±1.8
Recurrent tonsillitis	51.100 ±11.8	38.461 ±11.8	15.609 ±6.7	44.023 ±12.9	32.842 ±8.6	13.057 ±6.4	2.808 ±1.3
Focal diseases	37.857 ±12.1	40.000 ±5.4	18.714 ±7.0	55.071 ±14.0	36.428 ±10.1	12.571 ±9.1	3.060 ±3.0

Results

The mean percentages of cells positive for the different MoAbs are shown in table 1.

The Student t test performed in order to find differences among the three different groups confirmed:

(1) A significant increase of CD3+ cells in the recurrent tonsillitis when compared with hypertrophic and focal ones and a significant increase of CD4+ cells in recurrent and focal tonsillitis (without significant differences between these two groups) vs. hypertrophy.

(2) No significant differences were found among the three pathological groups as far as CD8+, HLA-DR+, and IL-2R+ cells are concerned, although a trend to higher percentages of HLA-DR+ and IL-2R+ cells was observed in hypertrophic tonsillitis.

(3) A trend to higher values of the CD4/CD8 ratio was found in recurrent and focal tonsillitis, but it was not proved statistically.

The studies performed on frozen sections confirmed the findings obtained with the cell suspensions.

References

1   Ge ZH, Lin ZQ, Wang RY: A study of lymphocyte subsets in human normal tonsil and lymph node. Shin Yen Sheng Wu Hsueh Pao 1989;22:75–85.
2   Inghirami G, Zhu BY, Chess L, Knowles DM: Flow cytometric and immunohis-

tochemical characterization of the gamma/delta T-lymphocyte population in normal human lymphoid tissue and peripheral blood. Am J Pathol 1990;136:357–367.

3 Falini B, Flenghi L, Pileri S, Pelicci P, Fagioli M, Martelli MF, Moretta L, Ciccone E: Distribution of T cells bearing different forms of the T cell receptor gamma/delta in normal and pathological human tissues. J Immunol 1989;143:2480–2488.

4 Janossy G, Bofill M, Rowe D, Muir J, Beverley PC: The tissue distribution of T lymphocytes expressing different CD45 polypeptides. Immunology 1989;66:517–525.

5 Zola H, Melo JV, Zowty HN, Nikoloutsopopulos A, Skinner J: The leukocyte-common antigen (CD45) complex and B lymphocyte activation. Hum Immunol 1990; 27:368–377.

6 Harada K: The histopathological study of human palatine tonsils – especially age changes. Nippon Jibiinkoka Gakkai Kaiho 1989;92:1049–1064.

7 Ryan Y, Harabuchi Y, Kataura A: Immunohistological identification of the activated lymphocytes in human palatine tonsil. Nippon Jibiinkoka Gakkai Kaiho 1989;92:1958–1963.

8 Brodsky L, Moore L, Stanievich JF, Ogra PL: The immunology of tonsils in children: the effect of bacterial load on the presence of B- and T-cell subsets. Laryngoscope 1988;98:93–98.

9 Horvath L, Sasvari Szekely M, Spasokukotsakaja T, Antoni F, Staub M: Follicular cells of tonsils metabolise more deoxycytidine than other cell populations. Immunol Lett 1989;22:161–166.

10 Butcher RD, McGarvie GM, Cushley W: Recombinant interleukin-4 promotes expression of the CD25 (Tac) antigen at the plasma membrane of high density human tonsillar B lymphocytes. Immunology 1990;69:57–64.

11 Shinomiya N, Kuratsuji T, Yata J: The role of T cells in immunoglobulin class switching of specific antibody production system in vitro in humans. Cell Immunol 1989;118:239–249.

12 Armitage RJ, Goff LK, Boverley PC: Expression and functional role of CD23 on T cells. Eur J Immunol 1989;19:31–35.

13 Tycko B, Palmer JD, Sklar J: T cell receptor gene transrearrangements: chimeric gamma-delta genes in normal lymphoid tissues. Science 1989;245:1242–1246.

14 King PD, Katz DR: Human tonsillar dendritic cell-induced T cell responses: analysis of molecular mechanisms using monoclonal antibodies. Eur J Immunol 1989;19:581–587.

15 Cai FF: Effect of tonsillar macrophages on several immune functions. Chung Kuo I Hsuch Ko Hsueh Yuan Hsueh Pao 1989;11:125–128.

16 Tsunoda R, Cormann R, Haiaine E, Onozaki K, Coulie P, Akiyama Y, Yoshizaki K, Kinet-Deneel C, Simar LJ, Kojima M: Cytokines produced in lymph follicles. Immunol Lett 1989;22:129–134.

17 Okato S, Magari S, Yamamoto Y, Sakanaka M, Takahashi H: An immunoelectron microscopic study on interactions among dendritic cells, macrophages and lymphocytes in the human palatine tonsil. Arch Istol Cytol 1989;52:231–240.

18 Steinman RM: Dendritic cells: clinical aspects. Res Immunol 1989;140:911–918.

19 Horst E, Meijer CG, Duijvestijn AM, Hartwing N, Van der Harten HJ, Pals ST: The ontogeny of human lymphocyte recirculation: high endothelial cell antigen (HECA-452) and CD44 homing receptor expression in the development of the immune system. Eur J Immunol 1990;20:1483–1489.
20 Matsuyama H, Yamanaka N: Immunological study on immunocompetent cells in palatine tonsil and pharyngeal tonsil – the quantitative study by image analyzer. Nippon Jibiinkoka Gakkai Kaiho 1989;92:2064–2078.
21 Bachert C, Moller P: Die Tonsille als MALT (mucosa-associated lymphoid tissue) der Nasenschleimhaut. Laryngol Rhinol Otol Grenzgeb 1990;69:515–520.
22 Mitani T, Tomoda K, Maeda N, Yamashita T, Kumazawa T: The tonsillar immune system: its response to exogenous antigens. Acta Otolaryngol (Stockh) 1990;(suppl 475):1–14.

Prof. Giorgio Cortesina, Dir. II Clin. ORL, Università di Torino, via Genova 3, I–10126 Torino (Italy)

Galioto GB (ed): Tonsils: A Clinically Oriented Update.
Adv Otorhinolaryngol. Basel, Karger, 1992, vol 47, pp 107–113

Function and Morphology of Macrophages in Palatine Tonsils

Yuzo Yamamoto, Shuichiro Okato, Masanobu Nishiyama,
Hiroaki Takahashi[1]

Department of Otolaryngology, Osaka Medical College, Osaka, Japan

Antigen-presenting cells include monocyte-macrophage cells, dendritic cells and B lymphocytes. When these cells present antigens to T lymphocytes, the expression of MHC class II antigens, that is, HLA-DR antigens, is necessary on their surface membranes. Dendritic cells and B lymphocytes persistently express HLA-DR antigens, whereas monocyte-macrophage cells can express them when the cells are activated by interferon-γ. Therefore, it is speculated that the immunological condition of the palatine tonsils may be represented by the percentage of HLA-DR-positive monocyte-macrophage cells in the total macrophage population.

In our previous study, we demonstrated the distribution and densities of dendritic cells and monocyte-macrophage cells in the palatine tonsils [1]. In the present study, the localization of HLA-DR-positive monocyte-macrophage cells was clarified in three groups of diseased tonsils by the immunohistological method, and the interaction between antigen-presenting cells, such as HLA-DR-positive monocyte-macrophage cells and dendritic cells, and lymphocytes was examined by immunoelectron microscopy. The significance of HLA-DR-positive monocyte-macrophage cells in the palatine tonsil is discussed.

[1] The authors thank Prof. Sumiko Magari of the Department of Anatomy for technical help with immunoelectron microscopy.

Materials

Pieces of palatine tonsils were obtained from 12 tonsillectomized patients, who were classified into three groups according to the clinical diagnosis: (1) tonsillar hypertrophy, 3 patients aged 7–13 years (average 10.0); (2) recurrent tonsillitis, 5 patients aged 8–22 years (average 13.4); (3) tonsils with focal infection, 4 patients aged 18–42 years (average 30.0).

Methods

Light microscopic observation, immunohistochemical study and immunoelectron microscopic studies were performed.

The reagents used in the present study were: rabbit antisera to lysozyme, CD68 (anti-human macrophage KP1) and anti-human myeloid/histiocyte MAC387 for the monocyte-macrophage cell lineage; rabbit antisera to S-100 protein for the dendritic cells (Dakopatts, Japan); anti-HLA-DR antibody (Nichirei and Becton-Dickinson, Japan), biotin-labelled antibody and avidin-biotin-peroxidase complex (ABC) (Vector, Funakoshi, Japan), Dako APAAP kit (Dakopatts):

(1) For light microscopy, the materials were fixed in 10% formalin solution, dehydrated with alcohol and embedded in paraffin. Sections were cut in 3-μm slices and stained with hematoxylin and eosin (HE).

(2) For immunohistochemical studies, paraffin sections and fresh sections were stained by an indirect immunoperoxidase method and a double immunoenzymatic labelling method (ABC method and APAAP method).

(3) Immunohistochemical demonstration of HLA-DR-positive monocyte-macrophage cells: The cells stained with both antilysozyme and anti-HLA-DR antibodies and the cells stained only by antilysozyme antibody were counted in the lymphoepithelial symbiosis area, the interfollicular area and germinal center, and then the percentage of HLA-DR-positive monocyte-macrophage cells among all monocyte-macrophage cells was determined in each tissue compartment.

(4) For immunoelectron microscopy, the unlabelled antibody peroxidase-antiperoxidase (PAP) complex method was used. The procedure was the same as that described in our previous paper [1].

Results

Light Microscopic Immunohistochemical Findings

The distribution and the densities of S-100 protein-positive cells and lysozyme-positive cells were described in our previous paper [1]. The localization of HLA-DR-positive cells and MAC387-positive cells was the same as that in previous reports [2–5]. A double immunoenzymatic labelling stain revealed the cells stained by both antisera to lysozyme and anti-HLA-

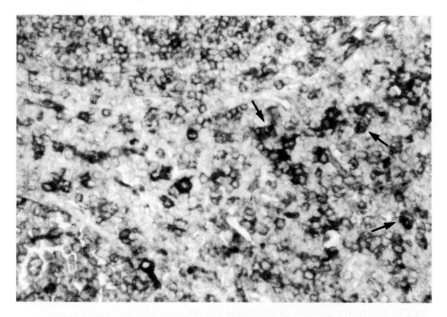

Fig. 1. Double immunoenzymatic labelling stain with antisera to lysozyme and anti-HLA-DR antibody in paraffin section from a patient with recurrent tonsillitis. Lysozyme-positive cells show brown staining in their cytoplasm with the ABC reaction, and HLA-DR-positive cells red staining in their surface membranes with the APAAP reaction. Cells immunostained with both antibodies are seen (arrows). The interfollicular area is shown. × 380.

DR antibody and by both MAC387 antibody and anti-HLA-DR antibody. Those cells were thought to be HLA-DR-positive monocyte-macrophage cells.

Immunohistochemical Demonstration of HLA-DR-Positive Monocyte-Macrophage Cells

A few HLA-DR-positive monocyte-macrophage cells were seen in the lymphoepithelial symbiosis area and the interfollicular area (fig. 1). The germinal centers contained some HLA-DR-positive monocyte-macrophage cells, which were thought to be HLA-DR-positive tingible body macrophages. Close apposition of HLA-DR-positive monocyte-macrophages to HLA-DR-positive lymphocytes was occasionally seen in each tissue compartment. The findings mentioned above were almost the same in the three types of tonsillar diseases. On the basis of the double immunostain-

Table 1. Percentages of HLA-DR-positive monocyte-macrophage cells in total population of monocyte-macrophage cells in different tissue compartments (mean percentage ± SD)

	n	Lymphoepithelial symbiosis area	Interfollicular area	Germinal center		
Tonsillar hypertrophy	3	7.4±1.4	17.8±2.7	42.3±5.0		
Recurrent tonsillitis	5	6.2±2.3 } $p < 0.05$	16.6±2.9	34.5±10.9 } $p < 0.05$	} $p < 0.01$
Tonsil with focal infection	4	4.7±0.6	17.3±2.5	19.0±2.8		

ing with antilysozyme and anti-HLA-DR antibodies, the percentage of HLA-DR-positive monocyte-macrophage cells among all monocyte-macrophage cells was determined in each tissue compartment of the three tonsillar diseases. The results are listed in table 1. In tonsils with focal infection, the percentages of HLA-DR-positive monocyte-macrophage cells in the lymphoepithelial symbiosis area and the lymphoid follicle were lower than in the other groups of diseased tonsils.

Immunoelectron Microscopic Findings

S-100 proteins were observed as granular electron-dense products in the cytoplasm of dendritic cells. Reaction products of lysozyme were seen in phagosomes of monocyte-macrophage cells. These findings were similar to those noted in our previous report [1]. Immunoreactive products of HLA-DR antigens were detected on the surface membranes of lymphocytes, dendritic cells and macrophages. In the subepithelial area, an HLA-DR-positive cell which had phagosomes characteristic of the monocyte-macrophage cell lineage was seen in the cytoplasm. The HLA-DR-positive monocyte-macrophage cell extended long cytoplasmic processes to lymphocytes, surrounded them and was in partial contact with them (fig. 2). HLA-DR-positive dendritic cells and HLA-DR-positive lymphocytes were sometimes in close contact in all compartments of the tonsil.

Discussion

It has long been known that monocyte-macrophages are involved in inflammation, host defense, and reaction against a range of autologous and foreign materials [6]. Recently, it has become clear that they play a key role

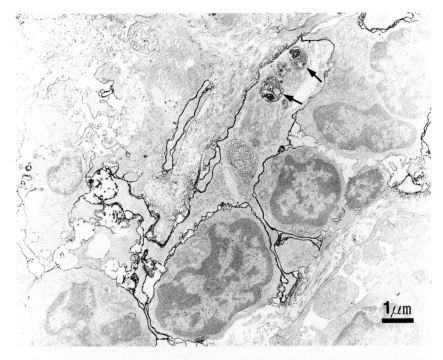

Fig. 2. Immunoelectron micrograph of HLA-DR-positive monocyte-macrophage cell in the subepithelial area. The cell has characteristic phagosomes (arrows) in the cytoplasm, protrudes long cytoplasmic processes to lymphocytes and is in contact with them.

in immunologic reactions. Among their immunologic functions, antigen presentation is of special importance as the first step in the processing of antigens. In the present study, we demonstrated the distribution and densities of HLA-DR-positive monocyte-macrophages in palatine tonsils immunohistochemically and electron microscopically. Moreover, we noted direct contact between HLA-DR-positive monocyte-macrophage cells and lymphocytes, and close apposition of HLA-DR-positive monocyte-macrophage cells to HLA-DR-positive lymphocytes. In our previous studies [1, 7], using the same methods, we investigated interactions between dendritic cells and lymphocytes in palatine tonsils and demonstrated direct contact between the two. These findings strongly suggest that antigen presentation is going on between antigen-presenting cells, such as monocyte-macrophage cells and dendritic cells, and lymphocytes.

In tonsils with focal infection, the percentages of HLA-DR-positive monocyte-macrophage cells in the lymphoepithelial symbiosis area and the lymphoid follicle were lower than those in tonsillar hypertrophy and recurrent tonsillitis. These results may be explained from the viewpoint of both cell-mediated immunity and humoral immunity. With respect to the former, our previous study revealed a decreased number of dendritic cells in the lymphoepithelial symbiosis area in tonsils with focal infection [1]. The present results are closely related to those of the previous study. Accordingly, insufficiency of antigen presentation might suppress the subsequent immune response, resulting in poor development of the germinal centers. With respect to the latter, tonsils with focal infection are in an exhausted state, as described by Kawaguchi et al. [8], or sometimes in a burnt-out state, because antibodies to a certain antigen have been produced for a long time. Consequently, immune competent cells which are involved in the production of antibodies might be decreased in number in tonsils with focal infection.

However, the functions and significance of HLA-DR-positive monocyte-macrophage cells are not yet well understood. Although their involvement in cell-mediated immunity, especially antigen presentation, is obvious, there are still some other possibilities; for example, activation of macrophages by nonimmune stimulation, and the control of the percentage of HLA-DR-positive monocyte-macrophage cells by unknown factors.

In the present study we focused on the immunological aspect of macrophages, especially antigen presentation. Further investigations are necessary to clarify the significance of HLA-DR-positive monocyte-macrophage cells in the palatine tonsils in several conditions.

References

1   Yamamoto Y, Okato H, Takahashi H, Takeda K, Magari S: The distribution and morphology of macrophages in the palatine tonsils. Acta Otolaryngol (Stockh) 1988 (suppl 454):83–95.
2   Van der Valk P, van der Loo EM, Jansen J, Daha MR, Meijer CJLM: Analysis of lymphoid and dendritic cells in human lymph node, tonsil and spleen. Virchows Arch B Cell Pathol 1984;45:169–185.
3   Wood GS, Turner RR, Shiurba RA, Eng L, Warnke RA: Human dendritic cells and macrophages. Am J Pathol 1985;119:73–82.
4   Isaacson PG, Jones DB: Immunohistochemical differentiation between histiocytic and lymphoid neoplasms. Histochem J 1983;15:621–635.

5   Shimoda F, Kawaguchi M, Ishizawa S, Odake H, Koizumi F: Immunohistochemical study of MAC387-positive cells in human palatine tonsils. Jpn J Tonsil 1990;29: 66–69.

6   Unanue ER: Mononuclear phagocyte: Macrophage, antigen-presenting cells, and the phenomena of antigen handling and presentation; in Paul W (ed): Fundamental Immunology. New York, Raven Press, 1989, pp 96–101.

7   Okato S, Magari S, Yamamoto Y, Sakanaka M, Takahashi H: An immuno-electron microscopic study on interactions among dendritic cells, macrophages and lymphocytes in the human palatine tonsil. Arch Histol Cytol 1989;52:231–240.

8   Kawaguchi M, Sakai T, Koizumi F: Histopathological characteristic findings of the palatine tonsils and skin of the soles obtained from patients with pustulosis palmaris et plantaris. Jpn J Tonsil 1991;30:162–167.

Dr. Y. Yamamoto, Department of Otolaryngology, Osaka Medical College, Daigaku-cho, Takatsuki, Osaka 569 (Japan)

Galioto GB (ed): Tonsils: A Clinically Oriented Update.
Adv Otorhinolaryngol. Basel, Karger, 1992, vol 47, pp 114–119

The Role of Integrins in Tonsil

Hiroshi Tsubota, Shinji Ohguro, Akikatsu Kataura

Department of Otolaryngology, Sapporo Medical College, Japan

A palatine tonsil has very unique features in its functions and construction. They have been studied for years by means of immunology or histology independently, but because the functions and structures are not separable, some instruments with which both things can be grasped at the same time have been sought.

In recent years, studies of a series of molecules called cell adhesion molecules (CAM) or integrins have been current. It has been proved that such molecules play crucial roles not only in adhesion of cells and maintaining of structure of tissues but also in cell functions such as signal transductions, recognition of cells, etc. [1, 2]. Therefore, it is expected that they can be very useful tools for the study of the details of biology of a tonsil.

In the present study, we have investigated the distributions of cell adhesion molecules on tonsillar tissues and made a comparison of them between tonsils and other lymphoid organs. Moreover, on the basis of these results, we have tried making a discussion on the roles of integrins in tonsils.

Materials and Methods

All specimens of palatine tonsils, lymph nodes and thymus were surgically removed from the patient at regular operations. Peripheral blood lymphocytes (PBL) were separated from venopunctually obtained blood by Ficoll-Conray gradient density centrifugation. Frozen sections prepared from lymphoid organs were fixed with acetone, then immunohistochemically stained by the ABC method with a series of monoclonal antibodies recognizing various cell adhesion molecules. Dual-color staining utilizing monoclonal antibodies labeled with FITC or phycoerythrin respectively was performed on tonsillar lymphocytes prepared as a form of free cell suspension and PBL. These cells were then analyzed with a flow cytometer (FACScan).

Table 1. Cell adhesion molecules

	Subunit	Ligand
VLA family		
VLA-1	α1β1	LM, collagen
VLA-2	α2β1	collagen
VLA-3	α3β1	FN, LM, collagen
VLA-4	α4β1	FN, VCAM
VLA-5	α5β1	FN
VLA-6	α6β1	LM
β2 family		
LFA-1	αLβ2	ICAM-1 (CD54)
Ig supergene family		
ICAM-1		LFA-1
Extracellular matrix		
Fibronectin (FN)		
Laminin (LM)		
Vitronectin (VN)		
Another subunit of VLA family	αxβ4	

Tonsillar epithelial cells were also prepared in vitro. Briefly, surgically obtained tonsils were minced and washed with phosphate buffer saline, then the cells including chips of epithelium and tonsillar lymphocytes were seeded in a culture flask and maintained in 10% FCS-supplemented RPMI 1640 medium. Expanded epithelial cells were dried and stained by the ABC method with monoclonal antibodies reactive with CAMs.

Results and Discussions

Table 1 lists the CAMs that were examined. First of all, we investigated the distributions of CAMs on tonsillar tissues and other lymphoid organs, peripheral lymph nodes and thymus as a representative central lymphoid organ, then comparisons were made among their CAM expressions.

Distributions of CAMs on Tonsillar Tissues

As shown in figure 1, the subunits of the VLA family were distributed in the tonsillar capsule. There were basal membrane-like expressions lining the innermost part of a capsule except for α2. The observation that α6 and

a   b   c   d

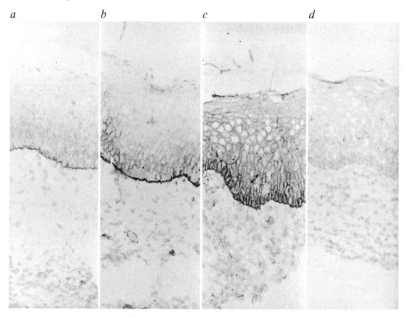

Fig. 1. Immunohistochemical staining of a capsule of a palatine tonsil. Frozen sections were prepared from a surgically obtained palatine tonsil, fixed with acetone, then stained by the ABC method with mouse or rat monoclonal antibodies recognizing a subunit of VLA antigens as indicated in each part of the figure. *a* β4, *b* α6, *c* α3, *d* α2.

β4 had very similar expressions suggested that the heterodimer of α6 here was not generally α6β1 but α6β4, which has been known to be involved in determination of polarity of cells.

Figure 2 indicates the distributions of CAMs in lymphoepithelial symbiosis (LES) that is a unique structure of a palatine tonsil. There were also basal membrane-like expressions of VLAs continuous from a capsule, and that made a definitive border between the inside and outside of LES. This observation supports the hypothesis that LES is developed by massive infiltration of lymphocytes into the formerly established epithelial structure, but not by the random arrangements of lymphocytes and epithelial components.

Each extracellular matrix (ECM) showed a significantly different distribution. Fibronectin seemed to surround a follicle, whereas vitronectin was strongly expressed in a germinal center of a lymphoid follicle. Fibronectin was therefore thought to play a crucial role in sustaining a three-

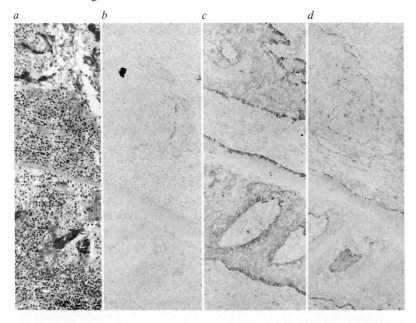

Fig. 2. Standard hematoxylin and eosin staining and immunohistochemical staining of a LES of a palatine tonsil. Specimens were prepared as described in the legend for figure 1. *a* HE, *b* α2, *c* α3, *d* α6.

dimensional structure of a follicle or to do something to support the cells in the interfollicular areas. On the other hand, vitronectin might be important in keeping activated B cells in a germinal center.

It has been reported that α4, which showed a very similar expression pattern to that of vitronectin in a germinal center, is involved in adhesion of activated B cells there in association with VCAM. We also examined LFA-1/ICAM-1 interaction in tonsils. There was the positive relationship between LFA-1 and ICAM-1 distributions not only in a follicle but also in a capsule and LES. We also demonstrated the positive relationship between these two molecules in the thymus. However, it has been reported that LFA-1/ICAM-1 interaction is not involved in the binding of thymocytes to cultured thymic epithelial cells in vitro [3]. So, it should be very interesting to examine how LFA-1/ICAM-1 interaction works in a tonsil [4]. We are now in the middle of such trials and have found that the in vitro expanded tonsillar epithelial cells were ICAM-1 positive.

Comparison between Tonsils and Other Lymphoid Organs on
CAM Expression

It is obvious that a palatine tonsil and a peripheral lymph node share many similarities histologically based upon basic hematoxylin and eosin staining. Both of them are enwrapped by a capsule and have lymphoid follicles as the central components. However, a palatine tonsil lacks afferent ducts and has LES instead.

We examined if such similarities and differences were also proved by distributions of CAMs. α6 expression was picked up first. A palatine tonsil and a peripheral lymph node had an identical pattern as having follicles, but in the capsule region, a basal membrane-like lining by α6 which was very distinctive in a palatine tonsil was not observed. It might be because a tonsillar capsule is a mucous membrane composed of squamous cells, whereas a lymph node capsule is a connective tissue. However, thymus has the significant basal membrane-like distribution of α6 though its lobules are divided by connective tissue.

α6 was also expressed in thymic medulla. The fact that a great part of the thymic medulla is occupied by epithelial components suggests that we compare the roles of α6 molecule in thymus with that of tonsillar epithelial cells, especially a tonsillar capsule. Because β4 is also distributed in thymic medulla in a similar manner to α6, there is probably α6β4 heterodimer expression in a thymus as well as a palatine tonsil.

Comparison between Tonsillar Lymphocytes and Circulating PBL on
ECM Expression

In previous sections, the role of CAMs were investigated as the elements of a solid structure. On the contrary, tonsillar lymphocytes were prepared as free cell suspension in the following experiments and cell surface expressed CAMs were analyzed in comparison with those of circulating PBL.

Tonsillar lymphocytes were fractioned as CD3$^+$ or CD3$^-$ subpopulations for the comparison of percent expression of each CAM in adult and juvenile cases. To start with, an increase of percent expression of several CAMs that seemed to be caused by aging was observed. α5, α6 and ICAM-1 expression on CD3$^+$ cells and α1 expression on CD3$^-$ cells showed such an increase. On tonsillar lymphocytes, α1, α5 and α6 showed higher expression in adult cases than in juvenile cases. On the other hand, compared to tonsillar lymphocytes, PBL had stronger expression of α1 and α4–6.

It is not easy to discuss how such differences are made or what they mean functionally. The changes of CAM expression by aging might be explained as a result of the changes of the whole immune system of an individual by aging. For instance, the changes of the proportion of lymphocyte subsets leads to the changes of the release of cytokines that should affect the CAM expression. One more important thing is that the intensity of CAM expression does not always reflect directly their functions. In general, adhesion activities of integrins are modified by conformational changes caused by various stimuli. Therefore, it is not always true that the cell surface expressed molecules are functional or 'fully' functional. It is also possible that the localization of CAMs on cells are different according to the condition under which these cells are.

In context with the above, the real adhesion activities of CAMs need to be investigated. At present we are planning to examine the adhesion activities of various subsets of tonsillar lymphocytes via CAMs in association with in vitro expanded tonsillar epithelial cells.

Conclusions

To conclude: (1) each adhesion molecule showed a significant distribution on a tonsillar tissue; (2) comparison of the distributions of CAMs on various lymphoid tissues revealed the differences and similarities of them other than histology, and (3) the fact that many CAMs expressed on tonsillar lymphocytes showed the changes by aging might reflect the dynamic changes of the functional aspects of them by individual development.

References

1   Springer TA: Adhesion receptors of the immune system. Nature 1990;346:425–434.
2   Stoolman LM: Adhesion molecules controlling lymphocyte migration. Cell 1989;56:907–910.
3   Singer KH, Denning SM, Whichard LP, Haynes BF: Thymocyte LFA-1 and thymic epithelial cell ICAM-1 molecules mediate binding of activated human thymocytes to thymic epithelial cells. J Immunol 1990;144:2931–2939.
4   Dustin ML, Singer KH, Tuck DT, Springer PA: Adhesion of T lymphoblasts to epidermal keratinocytes is regulated by interferon-gamma and is mediated by intercellular adhesion molecule-1. J Exp Med 1988;167:1323.

Dr. H. Tsubota, Department of Otorhinolaryngology, Sapporo Medical College, S1,W16, Chuo-ku, Sapporo 060 (Japan)

Galioto GB (ed): Tonsils: A Clinically Oriented Update.
Adv Otorhinolaryngol. Basel, Karger, 1992, vol 47, pp 120–123

Immunological and Bacteriological Studies on Mucosa-Associated Lymphatic Tissue in Children with SOM

Britta Rynnel-Dagöö[a], Joachim Forsgren[a], Anders Samuelson[b]

Departments of [a]Otorhinolaryngology and [b]Clinical Bacteriology,
Karolinska Institute, Huddinge University Hospital, Huddinge, Sweden

Some children requiring surgery for hypertrophy of the adenoid may completely lack medical history of otitis media with effusion (OME) or upper respiratory tract infections while others suffer longstanding secretory otitis media, recurrent acute otitis media and nasopharyngitis. The aim of this study was to investigate bacteriological and immunological reflections of this clinically observed difference.

Materials and Methods

Patient Groups

The study group consisted of children admitted for adenoidectomy because of varying degrees of nasal obstruction. Children having had more than one episode of longstanding OME (> 3 months) were placed in the infection group designated 'OME'. Children without any history of middle ear affection or recurrent upper respiratory tract infections were placed in the hypertrophy group designated 'HT'. Thirty-six patients were included, ranging in age from 28 to 139 months, 18 in the OME group and 18 in the HT group. Patients were not included in the study in case of infectious illness or antibiotic treatment during the month prior to the operation.

Bacteriology

Immediately after the operation the adenoid tissue was divided aseptically. Several specimens were deep-frozen in liquid nitrogen and stored at $-70\,°C$. One specimen was homogenized and after dilution, a 0.1-ml sample from each concentration was plated onto 5% sheep blood and chocolate agars. The plates were incubated at $37\,°C$ aerobically or under 5% CO_2 (chocolate) and examined at 24 and 48 h. The bacteria were identified using standard bacteriologic techniques, counted and reported as colony-forming units (CFU)/g adenoid.

Immunology

Sections 6 μm thick were cut on a Leitz 1720 cryostat and mounted on gelatine-coated slides, dried and stored at – 70 °C until use. After acetone fixation and removal of unspecific peroxidase activity with 0.3% peroxide, peroxidase-antiperoxidase (PAP) staining was performed with commercially available monoclonal antibodies. Rabbit anti-mouse immunoglobulin served as secondary antibody and unspecific binding was blocked with normal rabbit serum.

Detection of Pneumococcal C-Polysaccharide; ELISA

A monoclonal antibody [1] directed against the phosphorylcholine residue of the pneumococcal C-polysaccharide (PnC) served as catcher and an affinity-purified poly-clonal anti-PnC rabbit antiserum was used for detection in an ELISA earlier described [2].

Statistical Evaluation

Differences were compared using an unpaired, two-tailed Student's t test and the χ^2 test.

Results

Both clinical groups had similar age distribution, with a mean age of 6 years and a 50-50 ratio between the sexes.

Bacteriology

Haemophilus influenzae, Branhamella catarrhalis, Streptococcus pyogenes and *Streptococcus pneumoniae* were the most common pathogens cultured in both groups, but nonencapsulated *H. influenzae* was found to be the dominant one (> 75% of CFU/g) twice as often in the HT group as in the OME group; 10/18 (56%) compared to 5/18 (28%). Further, *H. influenzae* was found in significantly higher concentrations in the HT group than in the OME group (p < 0.05) shown in table 1. *H. influenzae* was also isolated significantly more often (p < 0.01) from children aged 3–8 years (n = 26) than from children aged 8–12 years (n = 10), and in higher mean concentrations, $7.0 \pm 9.0 \times 10^5$ CFU/g compared with 0.01×10^5 CFU/g (p < 0.05).

Cryostat Sections

Immunohistochemical staining revealed homogenous and intense expression of HLA-DR on the epithelial cells, whereas HLA-DP and HLA-DQ were only seen on scattered cells within the epithelium, the latter being less intense. The pan-T marker CD3 was expressed, apart from in the

Table 1. Quantitative culture of aerobic pathogens in adenoid tissue

	OME (n = 18)	HT (n = 18)	p value[1]
H. influenzae[2]	2.0±3.7	8.2±10	<0.05
S. pneumoniae[2]	0.04±0.1	0.3±0.9	NS
B. catarrhalis[2]	1.7±5.4	0.2±0.4	NS
S. pyogenes[2]	0.01±0.04	0.7±2.0	NS

[1] Unpaired, two-tailed t test.
[2] CFU $\times$ 10^5/g; ± SD.

Table 2. Detection of pneumococcal C-polysaccharide in adenoid tissue

	OME (n = 13)	HT (n = 16)	
Absorbance (mean ± SD)	0.27±0.13	0.30±0.18	NS
Positive tests (>0.25)	9	9	NS
Negative tests (<0.1)	4	7	NS

interfollicular T-cell area, on scattered intraepithelial lymphocytes (IEL) at an approximate rate of 1/20 to 1/100 epithelial cells. IEL only occasionally were CD22+ (B-cell marker). No difference was seen between the two clinical groups. The same finding was also recently reported by van Nieuwkerk et al. [3].

Pneumococcal C-Polysaccharide Detection by ELISA

The background level in the assay was low, 0.04. An absorbance greater than 0.25 is regarded as a positive value in this test and was the finding in 9/13 and in 9/16 of the OME and of the HT groups respectively, i.e. no difference between the clinical groups could be seen (table 2).

Discussion

The adenoid tissue has been suggested as a source of infection contributing to the chronicity of OME [4]. In the present study quantitative culture of aerobic, pathogenic upper respiratory tract bacteria show equal amounts in the adenoid both from children of the OME group and from the HT group. One exception is *H. influenzae* which is more often isolated from the hypertrophic adenoids which is in accordance with studies on palatine tonsils [5]. Despite the low number of cultures positive for *S. pneumoniae,* more than 50% of the homogenized adenoid tissue samples from both groups were found to contain pneumococcal C-polysaccharide. This might imply that varying amounts of bacterial products are harbored within the lymphatic tissue and these substances with antigenic and mitogenic properties [6] may influence the regulation of the local immune response.

Further studies identifying and locating bacteria and bacterial products as well as characterization of the crypt epithelium [7, 8] are needed for the understanding of bacterial uptake and processing in upper respiratory tract lymphatic tissue.

References

1   Holmberg H, Holme T, Krook A, Olsson T, Sjöberg L, Sjöberg AM: Detection of C-polysaccharide in *Streptococcus pneumoniae* in the sputa of pneumonia patients by an enzyme-linked immunosorbent assay. J Clin Microbiol 1985;22:111–115.
2   Sjögren AM, Holme T: A highly specific two-site ELISA for pneumococcal C-polysaccharide using monoclonal and affinity-purified polyclonal antibodies. J Immunol Methods 1987;102:93–100.
3   Van Nieuwkerk EBJ, De Wolf CJM, Kamperdijk EWA, van der Baan S: Lymphoid and nonlymphoid cells in the adenoid of children with otitis media with effusion: a comparative study. Clin Exp Immunol 1990;79:233–239.
4   Ruokonen J, Sandelin K, Mäkinen J: Adenoids and otitis media with effusion. Ann Otol 1979;88:166–171.
5   Brodsky L, Moore L, Stanievich J: The role of *Hemophilus influenzae* in the pathogenesis of tonsillar hypertrophy in children. Laryngoscope 1988;98:1055–1060.
6   Rynnel-Dagöö B: Polyclonal activation to immunoglobulin secretion in human adenoid lymphocytes induced by bacteria from nasopharynx in vitro. Clin Exp Immunol 1978;34:402–410.
7   Bland P: MHC class II expression by the gut epithelium. Immunol Today 1988;9: 174–178.
8   Brandtzaeg P: Immune Functions and Immunopathology of Palatine and Nasopharyngeal Tonsils. New York, Raven Press, 1987, pp 63–106.

Dr. Britta Rynnel-Dagöö, Department of Otorhinolaryngology,
Karolinska Institute, Huddinge University Hospital, S–141 86 Huddinge
(Sweden)

Galioto GB (ed): Tonsils: A Clinically Oriented Update.
Adv Otorhinolaryngol. Basel, Karger, 1992, vol 47, pp 124–128

Intraepithelial γ-δ T Cells in Normal and Hypertrophic Rhinopharyngeal Tonsils

Oreste Gallo[a], *Daniele Bani*[b], *Lucio Rucci*[a], *Omero Fini-Storchi*[a]

[a] Second Otorhinolaryngological Clinic and [b] Department of Human Anatomy
and Histology, Section of Histology, University of Florence, Italy

The epithelium overlying mucosal tissue does not act as a complete mechanical barrier to macromolecules or particulate antigens. On the contrary, there is increasing agreement that the epithelium may play a central role in regulating the penetration of foreign antigens and the interaction between antigens and lymphoid cells in the mucosa, possibly by trapping antigens from the exterior and carrying them to the underlying lymphoid tissue. In this context, recent studies on GALT revealed that the epithelium of the Peyer's patches contains relatively high numbers of lymphocytes expressing CD8 antigen and γ-δ T-cell receptor (TCR) [1–4]. Because these cells have been shown to have cytolytic activity against epithelial cells modified antigenically by viral infection or neoplastic transformation [2], it was proposed that such cells could also be important in controlling penetration of antigens by killing epithelial cells bearing exogenous molecules on their surface [1, 5]. It is tempting to speculate that γ-δ TCR+ lymphocytes may represent a common mechanism of immune surveillance at every immunological frontier. Here we report that numerous CD8+ lymphocytes, together with a minority of γ-δ TCR+ cells, can also be found in the epithelium of rhinopharyngeal tonsils, and that they are likely involved in the regulation of antigen uptake.

Materials and Methods

Tissue from rhinopharyngeal tonsils was taken at surgery from 10 children, aged from 4 to 11 years, with adenoidal enlargement and from 4 age-matched healthy subjects treated surgically for unrelated diseases of the rhinopharynx. Subjects with a history of asthma, bronchitis, or IgE-mediated allergy were excluded from our series. Some tissue

Table 1. Primary antisera used

Antiserum against	Working dilution	Source	Type
CD3	1:20	Coulter	mouse monoclonal
CD8	1:20	Ortho	mouse monoclonal
CD4	1:20	Coulter	mouse monoclonal
γ-δ TCR	1:30	T-cell science	mouse monoclonal
HLA-Dr	1:100	Becton-Dickinson	mouse monoclonal
CD1a	1:20	Ortho	mouse monoclonal
S-100	not diluted	Ortho	rabbit polyclonal

fragments from each specimen were frozen in liquid nitrogen and cut with a cryostat in 6-μm thick sections; these were air-dried, fixed in cold acetone and processed for immunocytochemistry by using either the APAAP technique (for mouse monoclonal primary antibodies) or the ABC/AP technique (for rabbit polyclonal anti-S-100 antiserum). The antisera employed are listed in table 1. Proper positive and negative controls were included in every immunostaining reaction. In each case, 500 different cells comprised in the thickness of the epithelial lamina were counted under a light microscope with a × 40 objective; the number of lymphoid cells positive to CD3, CD8, CD4 and γ-δ TCR was registered and the ratio positive cells/total cells was calculated. Statistical analysis of the differences between the normal subjects and those with adenoidal enlargement was carried out using the Student's t test for unpaired values. $p < 0.05$ was considered significant.

The remaining tissue fragments from each subject were fixed in cold 4% glutaraldehyde in 0.1 M cacodylate buffer, pH 7.4, at room temperature and postfixed in 1% OsO_4 in 0.1 M phosphate buffer, pH 7.4, at 4 °C. They were then dehydrated in a graded acetone series, passed through propylene oxide and embedded in Epon 812. Ultrathin sections were stained with uranyl acetate and alkaline bismuth-subnitrate and examined under a Siemens Elmiskop 102 electron microscope at 80 kV.

Results

Immunophenotypical analysis (table 2) showed that, in both normal and enlarged adenoids, several CD3+ lymphocytes populated the epithelial layer. Moreover, in the same zone CD8+ cells were present in relatively large numbers, whereas CD4+ cells were scarce. Immunocytochemistry also revealed that γ-δ TCR+ lymphocytes were present in the epithelium of rhinopharyngeal tonsils in both healthy subjects and children with enlarged adenoids (fig. 1). It is noteworthy that the ratio γ-δ TCR+ cells/total

Table 2. Semiquantitative analysis of the immunostained intraepithelial cells

Antisera against	Normal adenoids	Enlarged adenoids
CD3	0.22 ± 0.01	0.25 ± 0.02
CD8	0.17 ± 0.02	0.2 ± 0.02
CD4	0.07 ± 0.01	0.06 ± 0.01
γ-δ TCR	0.007 ± 0.003	0.0198 ± 0.002

cells was significantly higher in the enlarged adenoids than in the normal ones ($p < 0.01$). In the subepithelial areas, numerous dendritic cells positive to CD1a or S-100 could be found; these cells constitutively expressed HLA-Dr antigens. By electron microscopy, intraepithelial lymphocytes, often with large cytoplasms and unusually abundant organelles, were frequently found tightly apposed to epithelial cells with features of degenerating cells, i.e. condensation of the cytoplasmic matrix, nuclear pyknosis and ruptures of the plasma membrane (fig. 2). Deep clefts of the epithelial lamina, apparently originating from cell death, could be found in the enlarged adenoids. They were especially frequent in areas of massive lymphoid infiltration of the epithelium. In the subepithelial zone, cells with the features of dendritic accessory cells and apposed closely to the surrounding lymphocytes were usually found in both normal and enlarged adenoids.

Discussion

The present findings indicate that numerous CD8 cytotoxic/suppressor T lymphocytes are present in the epithelium of rhinopharyngeal tonsils, together with a minor population of γ-δ TCR+ cells, which also have cytotoxic activity [6]. This fits well with our ultrastructural findings suggesting a destruction of epithelial cells by intraepithelial lymphocytes. It is conceivable that intraepithelial cytotoxic lymphocytes may specifically destroy epithelial cells which have bound alloantigens at their surface. Taken together, the present data and those of the literature on the GALT [1–5] suggest that intraepithelial cytotoxic lymphocytes may play a role in cell-mediated immune surveillance at the epithelial frontiers by exerting a restriction of antigen uptake. In spite of their relatively low number as

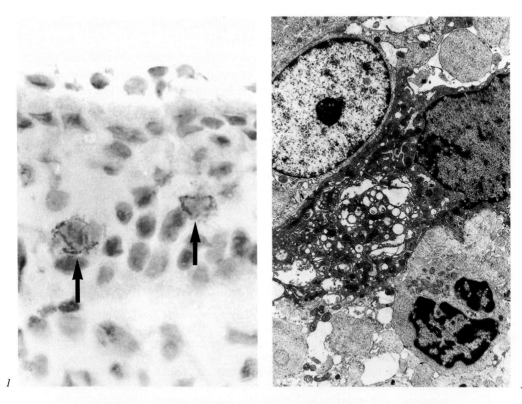

Fig. 1. Enlarged adenoid. γ-δ TCR⁺ T lymphocytes can be seen within the epithelium (arrows). APAAP method. × 1,200.

Fig. 2. Enlarged adenoid. A degenerating epithelial cell with nuclear pyknosis and condensation of the cytoplasmic matrix is seen in close contact with a lymphocyte. EM. × 5,100.

compared with the bulk of the intraepithelial lymphocytes, it is noteworthy that γ-δ TCR⁺ cells are present in higher amounts in the enlarged adenoids than in normal ones, and that clefts of the epithelial lamina, apparently originating from killing of epithelial cells by lymphocytes, can usually be found in the enlarged adenoids, whereas in the normal ones cannot. One could hypothesize that increased numbers of γ-δ TCR⁺ cells may lead to enhanced cytotoxic activity against epithelial cells, which result in a loss of the epithelial integrity, thus allowing an uncontrolled permeation of antigens and infectious agents. This may eventually lead to an imbalance of the immune response and concurrent hyperplasia of the lymphoid tissue, which is typical of adenoidal enlargement [7].

Basing on the present findings, it is unlikely that the epithelial cells of rhinopharyngeal tonsils are actively engaged in antigen presentation, as proposed by previous authors [8–10]. In fact, in our cases, the low number of CD4+ lymphocytes in the epithelium, the expression of few or even no HLA-Dr antigens on epithelial cells and the presence of numerous dendritic accessory cells expressing HLA-Dr antigens constitutively and in close contact with lymphocytes in the subepithelial area suggest that epithelial cells are not substantially involved in antigen processing and presentation to lymphocytes.

References

1 Bonneville M, Janeway CA Jr, Ito K, Haser W, Ishida I, Nakanishi N, Tonegawa S: Intestinal intraepithelial lymphocytes are a distinct set of gamma-delta T cells. Nature 1988;336:479–481.

2 Goodman T, Lefrançois L: Expression of the gamma-delta T cell receptor on intestinal CD8+ intraepithelial lymphocytes. Nature 1988;333:855–858.

3 Haas W, Kaufman S, Martinez CA: The development and function of gamma-delta T cells. Immunol Today 1990;11:340–343.

4 Brandtzaeg P, Halstensen TS, Kettt K, Krajci P, Kvale D, Rognum O, Scott H, Sollid LM: Immunobiology and immunopathology of human gut mucosa: humoral immunity and intraepithelial lymphocytes. Gastroenterology 1989;97:1562–1584.

5 Janeway CA Jr: Frontiers of the immune system. Nature 1988;333:804–806.

6 Moretta L, Pende D, Bottino C: Human CD3+, 4−, 8−, WT31− T lymphocyte population expressing the putative T cell receptor gamma gene product. A limiting dilution and clonal analysis. Eur J Immunol 1987;17:1229–1234.

7 Friedmann I, Michaels J, Gerwat J: The microscopic anatomy of the nasopharyngeal tonsil by light and electron microscopy. ORL 1972;34:195–209.

8 Gallo O, Bani D, Rucci L, Fini-Storchi O: Does the epithelium play a central role in the immune function of rhinopharyngeal tonsils? An immunocytochemical and ultrastructural study. Int J Pediatr Otorhinolaryngol 1991;22:219–229.

9 Karchev T, Kabachev P: M cells in the epithelium of the nasopharyngeal tonsil. Rhinology 1984;22:201–210.

10 Fujiyoshi T, Watanabe T, Ichimiya I, Mogi G: Functional architecture of the nasopharyngeal tonsils. Am J Otolaryngol 1989;10:124–131.

Dr. Oreste Gallo, Clinica Otorinolaringologica II, Policlinico di Careggi,
V.le G.B. Morgagni, 85, I–50134 Firenze (Italy)

Galioto GB (ed): Tonsils: A Clinically Oriented Update.
Adv Otorhinolaryngol. Basel, Karger, 1992, vol 47, pp 129–133

A Role of Tonsillar Lymphocyte for Focal Infection

With Special Reference to Lymphocyte Adhesion to Vessels in Dermis

Yukari Akagi, Takaaki Kimura, Masaru Kunimoto, Kiyonori Kuki, Toshihide Tabata

Department of Otorhinolaryngology, Wakayama Medical College, Wakayama City, Japan

The pathogenesis of palmoplantar pustulosis (PPP), which is one of the secondary diseases of tonsil with focal infection [1], is still unknown, particularly about its early stage. It was previously reported that demonstration of T-lymphocyte infiltration around the pustules on the plantar skin of PPP suggested an important contribution of cell-mediated immunity to the onset of PPP [2].

In the present study, the adhesion of tonsillar lymphocytes to the vessels surrounding the pustule and the expression of ICAM-1 (intercellular adhesion molecule-1), one of the adhesion molecules on endothelial cells [3], were investigated by the adhesion technique and immunohistochemical staining of plantar skin of PPP patients.

Materials and Methods

Palatine tonsils, plantar skins and peripheral blood were obtained from PPP patients during tonsillectomy under general anesthesia.

Lymphocyte Adhesion to Plantar Skin

The adhesion technique is the modification of the method by Jalkanen and Butcher [4] (fig. 1). The extracted tonsillar tissue was sliced into thin pieces in phosphate-buffered saline (PBS), and filtered through stainless mesh. The filtrate was washed with PBS, centrifuged over gradients of Ficoll-Hypaque, and lymphocytes were suspended in RPMI

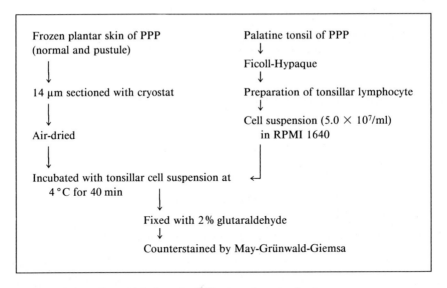

Fig. 1. Experimental design of tonsillar lymphocyte adhesion.

1640 containing 10% FCS (5×10^7 lymphocytes/ml). Peripheral blood lymphocytes were also isolated in the same way, and suspended in RPMI 1640 (5×10^7 lymphocytes/ml). Plantar skin was frozen with *n*-hexane, to $-80\,^{\circ}$C, and sliced into 14-μm sections with a cryostat. The lymphocyte suspension mentioned above was then placed over each section and slides were placed on a rotating table at $4\,^{\circ}$C, for 40 min. After incubation, the sections were fixed for 10 min in 2% glutaraldehyde, washed with PBS, and stained by the May-Grünwald-Giemsa method.

Immunohistochemical Staining of Plantar Skin

The frozen plantar skin was sliced into 4-μm sections. After air-drying and fixation with acetone at $4\,^{\circ}$C, for 10 min, the sections were stained by the avidin-biotin-peroxidase complex (ABC) method, using anti-ICAM-1 monoclonal antibody as the primary antibody, and biotinized anti-mouse IgG antibody as the secondary antibody.

Results

Lymphocyte Adhesion to the Plantar Skin

The infiltrating cells were observed from dermis to the base of pustules by hematoxylin and eosin (HE) staining (fig. 2). In the pustule sites, the tonsillar lymphocytes adhered to the vessels in dermis under the pus-

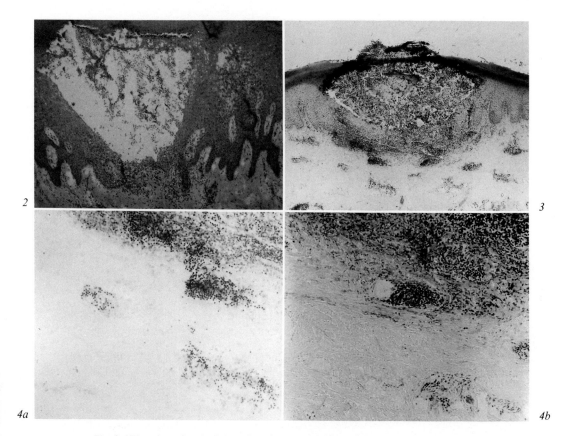

Fig. 2. HE stains of pustules on the plantar skin. 10 × 3.3.

Fig. 3. Microscopic feature of tonsillar lymphocyte adhesion to the pustule. May-Grünwald-Giemsa. 4 × 3.3.

Fig. 4. The comparative demonstration of lymphocyte adhesion to the plantar skin with pustules. May-Grünwald-Giemsa. 10 × 3.3. a Tonsillar lymphocytes. b Peripheral blood lymphocytes.

tule and the epidermis at the base of pustule (fig. 3). In other sites, however, only a few lymphocytes adhered in both dermis and epidermis. Compared with peripheral blood lymphocytes, the adhesion of tonsillar lymphocytes seemed stronger (fig. 4). Moreover, tonsillar lymphocytes adhered to the vessels running through the dermal papilla (fig. 5).

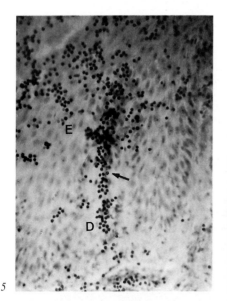

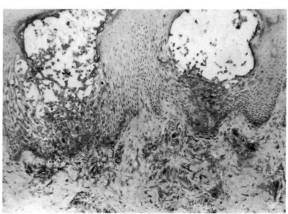

5

6

Fig. 5. The tonsillar lymphocytes adhesion to the vessel running through papilla of dermis. May-Grünwald-Giemsa. 20 × 3.3. E = Epidermis; D = dermis; arrow = adhering tonsillar lymphocyte.

Fig. 6. Immunohistochemical staining of plantar skin with pustule by anti-ICAM-1 monoclonal antibody: ICAM-1 expressed on the vessels in dermis and on the epidermis at the base of pustule.

Immunohistochemical Staining of Plantar Skin

It was revealed by immunohistochemical staining of plantar skin that ICAM-1 expressed strongly on the vessels in dermis involved papilla surrounding the pustule and on the epidermis at the base of pustule (fig. 6).

Discussion

Various studies have been reported regarding the pathogenesis of PPP, but much is yet unknown. Kimura et al. [2] suspected the involvement of T lymphocytes in the tissue injury of PPP, by infiltrating T lymphocytes into the plantar skin of PPP patients using immunohistochemical staining method. The migration of lymphocytes into perivascular tissue begins with their adhesion to high endothelial venule [5]. In 1983, Gallatin et al. [6] found the receptor on lymphocytes that recognizes the endothelial cells.

From our study of tonsillar lymphocyte adhesion to the pustule sites involving dermal papilla, it is suggested that some of the infiltrating lymphocytes in these sites would originate from the palatine tonsil as focus, and that the intercellular edema, an early stage of the pustule formation [7], would result from the injury of keratinocytes by tonsillar lymphocytes through the vessel in dermal papilla. Moreover, the ICAM-1 expression in these sites proposed the possible contribution for adhesion molecules to the tonsillar lymphocyte adhesion to the endothelial cell.

From these findings, it is considered that cell-mediated immunity would play an important role in the onset of PPP as humoral immunity.

References

1   Andrews GC, Machacek GF: Pustular bacterids of the hand and feet. Arch Dermatol 1935;32:837–847.
2   Kimura T, Fujiwara K, Tabata T, et al: Study on the onset of tonsil with focal infection – with special reference of palmoplantar pustulosis. J Jpn Soc Tonsil Problem 1990;29:133–138.
3   Rothlein R, Dustin ML, Marlin SD, et al: A human intercellular adhesion molecule-1 (ICAM-1) distinct from LFA-1. J Immunol 1986;137:1270.
4   Jalkanen ST, Butcher EC: In vitro analysis of the homing properties of human lymphocytes. Blood 1985;66:577–582.
5   Gowans JL, Knight EJ: The route of recirculation of lymphocytes in the rat. Proc R Soc Lond [B] 1964;159:257.
6   Gallatin WM, Weissman IL, Butcher EC: A cell-surface molecule involved in organ-specific homing of lymphocytes. Nature 1983;304:30–34.
7   Uehara M, Ofuji S: The morphogenesis of pustulosis palmaris et plantaris. Arch Dermatol 1974;109:518–520.

Dr. Y. Akagi, Department of Otorhinolaryngology, Wakayama Medical College, 7-Bancho 27, Wakayama City (Japan)

Galioto GB (ed): Tonsils: A Clinically Oriented Update.
Adv Otorhinolaryngol. Basel, Karger, 1992, vol 47, pp 134–141

Evolution of the Bacterial Flora in Recurrent Adenotonsillitis

Therapeutic Implications

E. Mevio[a], *E. Giacobone*[b], *P. Galioto*[a], *D. Perano*[a], *A.G. Bulzomi*[a]

[a] Department of Otorhinolaryngology, and [b] Department of Microbiology, University of Pavia, IRCCS San Matteo, Pavia, Italy

In the last 10 years, there has been an increasingly greater number of reports of an evolution in the pharyngotonsillar microbial flora in which the presence of beta-lactamase-producing microorganisms resistant to antibiotics has been increasing. Beta-lactamase-producing microorganisms in the oropharynx include a large number of pathogenic organisms (*Staphylococcus, Haemophilus, Branhamella, Fusobacterium,* etc.) and of normal saprophytes of the oropharynx itself which would together be responsible for 'indirect pathogenesis' by inactivating antibiotics and therefore allowing growth of pathogens [3, 8, 11, 21, 23]. The increase in beta-lactamase-producing strains is the result of a selection induced by treatment with beta-lactamines which have been the drugs of first choice in the treatment of inflammations of the upper respiratory tracts. In addition, the more or less frequent use of similar substances can induce in the same individual the phenomenon of resistance. Recent works that have studied the bacterial flora in children affected by inflammations of the upper respiratory tracts after treatment with penicillin V, amoxicillin or cefalospor have demonstrated a sharp decline in the presence of streptococci and pneumococci and the appearance of beta-lactamase-producing strains.

Another factor to consider when choosing treatment for oropharyngeal infections is the difficulty involved in distinguishing the causative agent or agents. In fact, many authors have pointed out the existence of important differences between the bacterial flora on isolates from the surface of tonsils and that found deep within the tonsil tissue [2, 5, 7, 14, 19]. As a result, the use of pharyngeal cultures with the aim of identifying the pathogenic agents appears to be an unreliable method. However, other more searching methods like needle aspiration are not commonly recommended.

Only a more thorough understanding of the bacterial flora of the tonsils and its more recent evolutions can best lead to an appropriate antimicrobial therapy and resolve as well those recurrent bouts of inflammation for which there is no other choice than surgery.

Methods

Forty children, aged between 2 and 13 years, were selected to participate in the study. All were admitted to our clinic for adenotonsillectomy following a history of recurrent adenotonsillitis (i.e., having at least 5 episodes in the past year) not responsive to medical treatment. The medical history was gathered and included duration of infection, number of episodes, yearly frequency, allergies if any, therapy already received, and date of last administration of antibiotics.

Routine preoperative examination included a radiography of the thorax, ECG, hematological profile including a differential white blood count, ESR, antistreptolysin titer, C-reactive protein, electrophoresis of serum proteins, indices of coagulation as well as those of hepatic and renal function.

During surgery cultures of exudate were taken (Cultiplast Transport Swab with Stuart's transport medium). Samples were taken from the floor of the nasal cavities, the palate, and the surface of the tonsils. Immediately after the adenoids and the tonsils were removed a part of their surfaces was first electrically cauterized and then incised in order to take samples from within their tissues. Before surgery a blood sample was taken for blood culture. This was also repeated at the end of surgery. Both blood samples were introduced directly into the culture medium 'Liquid blood culture bottle B-S Roche'.

All the samples collected were transported immediately to the Department of Microbiology where they were introduced into the following mediums: (1) CNA blood agar to determine the presence of hemolytic streptococci; (2) mannite salt agar to determine the presence of staphylococci; (3) McConkey agar to determine the presence of enterobacteria and nonglucose fermenting microorganisms; (4) chocolate agar to determine the presence of certain troublesome bacteria; (5) thioglycolate culture medium to determine the presence of anaerobic microorganisms; after incubation at 37 °C for 24–48 h introduction in blood agar under conditions of anaerobiosis.

Results

The following is a list of the more important findings that we obtained:

(1) There is a significant difference between the microbial flora of the adenoids and that of the tonsils. In more specific terms, some bacteria (*Staphylococcus intermedius,* beta-lactamase-producing *Staphylococcus haemolyticus* and *Haemophilus influenzae* and *parainfluenzae*) were found

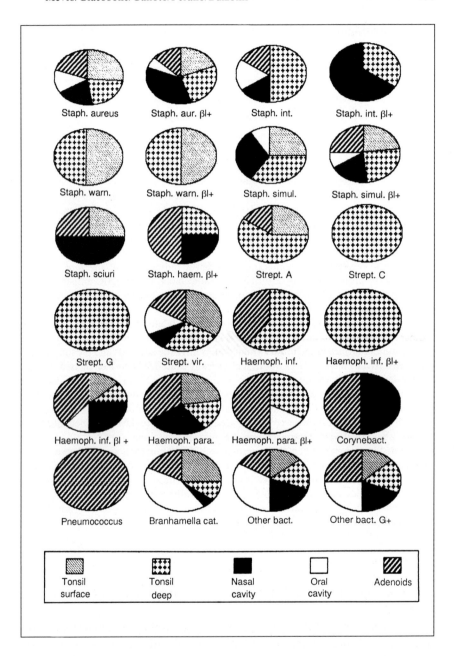

Fig. 1. Difference between the microbial flora the adenoids, tonsils and the oral and nasal cavity.

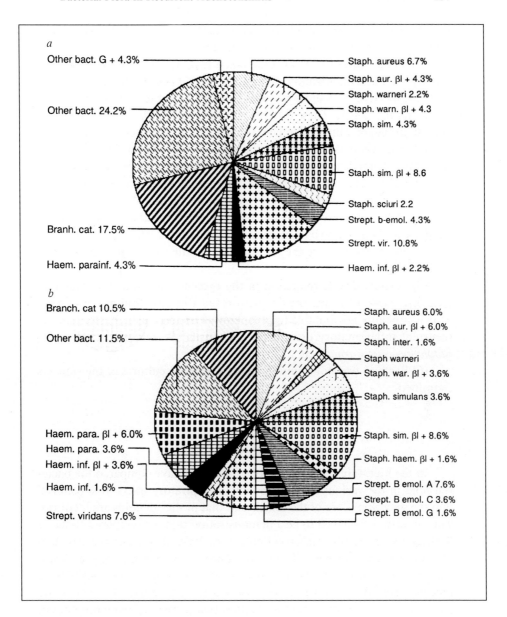

Fig. 2. Comparison between the cultures taken from the surface (*a*) and those taken from deep within the tonsil tissue (*b*).

in greater percentage and others (*Corynebacterium* and *Diplococcus pneumoniae*) exclusively in the adenoids (fig. 1).

(2) The cultures of the exudate taken from the nasal cavities and the oral cavity were significantly different in their bacterial flora when compared, respectively, to those cultures isolated from the surface of the adenoids and the tonsils. These differences could perhaps be due to the different conditions in which the mucosal barriers find themselves in each site.

(3) The comparison between the cultures taken from the surface and those taken from deep within the tonsil tissue shows a significant difference in bacterial populations. In particular, some species (*Streptococcus* C and G, *H. influenzae,* etc.) are found only deep within the tonsils (fig. 2a, b).

(4) Beta-lactamase-producing bacteria were isolated in 40% of the children studied. These bacteria were isolated deep within the tonsil tissue in all these subjects, while they were found on the surface in only one half of them (fig. 2a, b).

(5) A considerable reduction in the presence of group A beta-hemolytic *Streptococcus* in the tonsils, with respect to past findings, was seen. This is probably attributable to preoperative opportunistic bacteria in the recurrent inflammatory diseases of the tonsils (*Branhamella catarrhalis, Staphylococcus warneri,* etc.).

(6) Bacteria was not found in any of the blood cultures of the subjects examined.

Conclusions

In the literature there are many studies that have compared the bacterial flora in the various areas of the upper respiratory tracts. It is believed that the microbial flora of the tonsils and that of the adenoids are identical. This, in turn, is believed to be a demonstration that the lymphoid tissue of Waldeyer's ring is of common colonization. While this seems perfectly logical, doubts are legitimate if one only thinks, for example, of the classic situation in which children immune to inflammation of the tonsils have repeated episodes of otitis media associated with adenoid hypertrophy and/or recurrent rhinitis. Our results show that there is a greater presence in the adenoids with respect to the tonsils of some of the bacteria species noted for being responsible for tubotympanic pathologies (beta-lactamase-producing and non-beta-lactamase-producing *H. influenzae* and parainfluenzae, *Diplococcus pneumoniae*). These data concord with those of other studies which have evaluated the bacterial flora of the adenoids and that of the endotympanic secretion during an episode of secretory otitis media [12].

It should be noted that other types of bacteria are found either exclusively or preferentially in the adenoids (*Corynebacterium,* beta-lactamase-producing *S. haemolyticus).* As far as the bacterial flora of the tonsils is concerned, two important findings should be pointed out: (1) the exclusive or preponderant presence of certain bacterial species and (2) the difference in the flora between the surface and deep tissue of the tonsils. For example, all streptococci are localized preferentially in the tonsils. It is interesting to note that Lancefield's group A *Streptococcus* [2–4, 13, 15] is found less frequently while the group C and A *Streptococcus* and *Streptococcus viridans,* once considered not to be pathogenic [6, 9], are found in increasing number with respect to past findings. According to several authors, these 'emerging pathogens' and in particular their localization within the tonsil tissue are responsible for the recurrent episodes of inflammation despite treatment with penicillin or one of its derivatives [3, 15, 19, 20]. Therefore, the presence of beta-lactamase-producing aerobic and anaerobic bacteria within the tonsil tissue seems to be a very important phenomenon to be taken into consideration. Their existence impedes treatment with penicillin and allows not only their own anomalous development but also that of strains usually sensitive to penicillin therapy. Indicative of this are the reports concerning *B. catarrhalis* and *H. influenzae.*

In 1970, when *Neisseria catarrhalis* was renamed *B. catarrhalis,* in honor of the American microbiologist Branham, this bacteria was considered a commensal microorganism of little importance. It was, in fact, commonly found in healthy individuals and when it appeared in pathologies of the upper respiratory tracts it was always associated with other pathogenic microorganisms. Later, it was considered an emerging pathogen in otitis, sinusitis and pulmonary infections [16, 22]. In 1977, the first strains of beta-lactamase-producing *Branhamella* were reported. Currently, 70% of cultures have this quality [8].

Type B and type non-B *H. influenzae* have lately been mentioned more frequently as a pathogenic agent of the tonsils. The isolation of this microorganism deep within the tissue of tonsils is a more frequent finding in 10-year-old children (44%) than in older subjects (19%) [17]. Consequently they represent one of the principal pathogenic agents of tonsillitis in the first years of life. Other authors have highlighted its role in the pathogenesis of adenoid hypertrophy and the sleep apnea that follows. The presence of these microorganisms brings about an unusual variation in the

T helper/T suppressor ratio which results in hypertrophy of the Waldeyer's ring [1].

All these considerations have both diagnostic and therapeutic implications. As far as diagnosis is concerned, it is easily understandable from what has been said that a pharyngeal culture, even if done correctly, is of relatively little significance as it gives only a picture of the superficial flora.

The indications from our study concerning the choice of therapy for recurrent and nonrecurrent inflammation of Waldeyer's ring are particularly interesting. It is evident that an ideal antibiotic should present the following characteristics:

(1) A high capacity to diffuse into tissue substance so that at more than sufficient doses it penetrates within the tissue of the tonsils (often its structure and vascularization are altered as a result of previous inflammation and subsequent reparative processes) and eliminates the pathogens situated here.

(2) A resistance to beta-lactamase which is produced by some types of bacteria that are continually becoming more common.

(3) Combined action against emerging pathogens such as *Haemophilus* and *Branhamella* otherwise free to carry out their action on the very same sites or to provoke complications in other areas (otitis, tracheitis, etc.).

Some of these considerations bring up questions concerning the validity of the classic therapeutic protocol of recurrent tonsillitis, in other words the use of benzathine penicillin. The action of this drug has been found to be ineffective for the vast majority of pathogens in subjects undergoing such treatment. The possible alternatives are either repeated cycles of an antibiotic having more specific characteristics [12, 18] or prolonged administration of such a drug at low doses as has been suggested by some authors.

References

1   Brodsky L, Moore L, Stanievich J: The role of *Haemophilus influenzae* in the pathogenesis of tonsillar hypertrophy in children. Laryngoscope 1988;98:1055–1060.
2   Brook I, Yocum P, Friedman EM: Aerobic and anaerobic bacteria in tonsils of children with recurrent tonsillitis. Ann Otol Rhinol Laryngol 1981;90:261–263.
3   Brook I: The presence of beta-lactamase-producing bacteria as a guideline in the management of children with recurrent tonsillitis. Am J Otolaryngol 1984;5:382–386.
4   Cantarella G, Mascheroni E, Tocalli L, Guastella C, Pasargiklian I: Studio microbiologico del parenchima tonsillare in bambini affetti da tonsilliti recidivanti. Otorinolaringol Ital 1987;37:487–490.

5 Chiaradia V, Pascoli L, Cavarzerani A, Sacilotto C, Beduz R, Santini GF: Flora batterica nelle tonsilliti croniche. Otorinolaringol Ital 1986;36:157–160.
6 Cimolai N, Edford RW, Bryan L, Anand C, Breger P: Do the beta-haemolytic non-group A streptococci cause pharyngitis? Rev Infect Dis 1988;10:587–601.
7 De Dio RM, Tom LWC, McGowon KL, Wetmare RF, Handler SD, Potsic WP: Microbiology of the tonsils and adenoids in a pediatric population. Arch Otolaryngol Head Neck Surg 1988;114:763–765.
8 Eliasson I, Holst E, Molstad S, Kamme C: Emergence and persistence of beta-lactamase-producing bacteria in the upper respiratory tract in children treated with beta-lactam antibiotics. Am J Med 1990;88(suppl 5A):519–559.
9 Hayden GF, Murphy TF, Handley JO: Non-group A streptococci in the pharynx. Am J Dis Child 1989;143:794–797.
10 Marchant CD: Spectrum of disease due to *Branhamella catarrhalis* in children with particular reference to acute otitis media. Am J Med 1988(suppl 5a):15–17.
11 Molstad S, Eliasson I, Hovelins B, Komme C, Schalen C: Beta-lactamase production in the upper respiratory tract flora in relation to antibiotic consumption: a study in children attending day nurseries. Scand J Infect Dis 1988;20:329–334.
12 Palva T, Malmberg H, Lehtinen T: Effect of erythromycin on adenoid bacteria. Acta Otolaryngol (Stockh) 1986;101:348–352.
13 Peter G, Smith AL: Group A streptococcal infections of the skin and pharynx. N Engl J Med 1977;271:365–370.
14 Rosen G, Samuel J, Vered I: Surface tonsillar microflora versus deep tonsillar microflora in recurrent acute tonsillitis. J Laryngol Otol 1977;91:911.
15 Ross PW: Bacteriological monitoring in penicillin treatment of streptococcal sore throat. J Hyg (Camb) 1971;69:355–360.
16 Shuring PA, Marchant CD, Kim CH, et al: Emergence of beta-lactamase-producing strains of *Branhamella catarrhalis* as important agents of acute otitis media. Pediatr Infect Dis 1983;2:34–38.
17 Styernquist-Desatnik A, Prellner K, Schalen C: Colonization by *Haemophilus influenzae* and group A streptococci in recurrent acute tonsillitis and tonsillar hypertrophy. Acta Otolaryngol (Stockh) 1990;109:314–319.
18 Sundberg L, Eden T, Ernstson S: Penetration of erythromycin in Waldeyer's ring-adenoid tissue. Acta Otolaryngol (Stockh) 1981;384(suppl):3–9.
19 Toner JG, Stewart TJ, Campbell JB, Hunter J: Tonsil flora in the very young tonsillectomy patients. Clin Otolaryngol 1986;11:171–174.
20 Tuner K, Nord CE: Beta-lactamase-producing anaerobic bacteria in recurrent tonsillitis. J Antimicrob Chemother 1982;10(suppl):153–156.
21 Tuner K, Nord CE: Beta-lactamase-producing microorganisms in recurrent tonsillitis. Scand J Infect Dis 1983;39(suppl):83–85.
22 Wald ED, Milmoe GJ, Bowen AD, Ledesma-Medina J, Salamon N, Bluestone CD: Acute maxillary sinusitis in children. N Engl J Med 1981;304:749–754.
23 Weber M, Conroy MC, Mory F, Burdin YC, Wayoff M: Sensibilité à l'association amoxicilline-acide clavulanique de la flore amygdalienne profonde isolée au cours d'amygdalites chroniques. Ann Otollaryngol Chir Cervicofac 1988;105:143–146.

Emilio Mevio, Via Gravellone 37, I–27100 Pavia (Italy)

Galioto GB (ed): Tonsils: A Clinically Oriented Update.
Adv Otorhinolaryngol. Basel, Karger, 1992, vol 47, pp 142–145

Interfering α-Streptococci as a Protection against Recurrent Streptococcal Pharyngotonsillitis

Kristian Roos[a], Stig E. Holm[b], Eva Grahn[b], Lena Lind[c]

[a] ENT Department, Lundby Hospital, Göteborg; [b] Bacteriological Department, Umeå, and [c] Bacteriological Department, Göteborg, Sweden

Recurrences after antibiotic treated streptococcal pharyngotonsillitis are a common finding, although the number of these recurrences can vary depending on which antibiotic was used [1–3]. These recurrences are a great problem, especially in certain epidemiological situations as in schools, day-care centers, military camps and within the family.

Different reasons for these high recurrence rates has been given. Thus, patient compliance and the importance of a full 10 days' course of antibiotics in streptococcal pharyngotonsillitis has been stressed by Schwartz et al. [1] and Strömberg et al. [2]. The significance of the absorption of antibiotics and its ability to penetrate to the infected tonsillar tissue in relation to treatment failure of streptococcal tonsillitis have been discussed before [4–6]. The presence in the throat of bacteria, aerobes as well as anaerobes, producing antibiotic inactivating enzymes [7–9], as well as resistance to erythromycin [10, 11] has also been connected with recurrences. Bacterial tolerance has also been suggested as a cause of treatment failure of streptococcal tonsillitis [12]. Recurrent, streptococcal pharyngotonsillitis can also be due to a new infection, as a reinfection with the same streptococcal type cannot be differentiated from a true treatment failure.

We would like to add one further reason to recurrent streptococcal pharyngotonsillitis, namely a disturbed normal throat flora and especially the lack of the interfering α-streptococcal flora. Microorganisms in the flora have an influence upon each other in different ways, like changing the pH, competing for essential nutritient factors or by producing antibacterial substances, e.g. bacteriocins. The competition for receptor sites on epithelial cells is probably also of significance for the establishment of an invading bacteria. Interference between microorganisms in the throat may thus play an important role for the protection against invading bacteria. This was shown earlier by Sanders et al. [13], who found interference between viridans streptococci and group A streptococci in the respiratory tract. Sprunt et al. [14] implanted an α-streptococcal strain in the throats of neonates in order to diminish an overgrowth of gram-negative bacteria. An increased resistance versus repeated streptococcal infections in the throat was also noted by Grahn and Holm [15] in family members with a throat flora containing high numbers of α-streptococci with interfering activity against the group A streptococcus causing an epidemic outbreak. Roos et al. [9] noticed significantly less interfering α-streptococci in patients with recurrent streptococcal group A tonsillitis compared to healthy individuals, carrying the same β-streptococcal type.

In an earlier open study [16] we selected four α-streptococcal strains (3 *Streptococcus sanguis* and 1 mitis strain) with good growth-inhibiting activity against 84–98% of clinical isolates of β-streptococci. A pool of these four α-strains was given as a spray into the mouth of 31 patients suffering from recurrent streptococcal group A tonsillitis. None of these patients recurred within 3 months.

The aim of the present study was to document the beneficial effect of colonization with a selection of α-streptococci on recurrences in patients with streptococcal tonsillitis in a double-blind randomized clinical study.

Materials and Methods

The present study included 36 patients, 5–40 years of age, who suffered from recurrent streptococcal group A tonsillitis. They all had a history of at least one streptococcal tonsillitis within the last 2 months. The present acute tonsillitis was diagnosed by a clinical picture of streptococcal tonsillitis, a positive rapid test and a positive group A streptococcal culture. 34 patients were treated with penicillin V, 1 with erythromycin and 1 with dicloxacillin for 10 days. All drugs were given in standard doses orally for 10 days. The patients were randomized to supplementary treatment with a pool of the above mentioned α-streptococci given as a spray in the throat twice a day for 10 days. This treatment started immediately after the course of antibiotics was ended. 19 patients received placebo and 17 α-streptococci. The patients were followed clinically and bacteriologically for 3 months.

Results

Within 2 months, 7 out of the 19 patients in the placebo group recurred, but none of the patients treated with α-streptococci. After 3 months a total of 11 out of the 19 in the placebo group recurred, but only 1 out of the 17 in the α-treated group had a recurrence. These differences are significant. All 11 patients in the placebo group recurred with the same streptococcal type, while the patient who recurred in the α-treated group had changed to a new type. Furthermore, the originally given α-streptococcal strains could not be reisolated from this patient at the time of recurrence.

Discussion

Recurrent streptococcal pharyngotonsillitis is a multifacetted phenomenon. Our study indicates a role for interfering α-streptococci in recurrent streptococcal pharyngotonsillitis. We would like to focus the attention on the important normal throat flora and the interfering activity of certain α-streptococci against certain β-streptococci. It seems likely that implantation of these α-streptococci offered a protective effect against renewed streptococcal throat infections. We would thus like to point out that recolonization at the end of antibiotic treatment in patients with recurrent streptococcal pharyngotonsillitis seems to offer a new way to lower the rate of recurrences.

References

1   Schwartz RH, Wientzen RL, Pedreira F, Ferioli EJ, Mella GW, Guandolo VL: Penicillin V for group A pharyngotonsillitis. A randomized trial of seven vs. ten days' therapy. JAMA 1981;246:1790–1795.
2   Strömberg A, Schwan A, Cars O: Five versus ten days' treatment of group A streptococcal pharyngotonsillitis: a randomized controlled clinical trial with phenoxymethylpenicillin and cefadroxil. Scand J Infect Dis 1988;20:37–46.
3   Holm SE, Roos K, Strömberg A: Rate of recurrence in streptococcal pharyngotonsillitis after treatment with cefadroxil and phenoxymethylpenicillin. Pediatr Infect Dis J 1991;10(suppl):68–71.
4   Roos K, Grahn E, Ekedahl C, Holm SE: Pharmacokinetics of phenoxymethylpenicillin in tonsils. Scand J Infect Dis 1986;18:125–130.
5   Roos K, Brorson J-E: Concentration of phenoxymethylpenicillin in tonsillar tissue. Eur J Clin Pharmacol 1990;39:417–418.

6   Roos K, Holm SE, Ekedahl C: Treatment failure in acute streptococcal tonsillitis in children over the age of ten and in adults. Scand J Infect Dis 1985;17:357–365.

7   Kundsin RB, Miller JM: Significance of the *Staphylococcus aureus* carrier state in the treatment of disease due to group A streptococci. N Engl J Med 1964;271;1395–1397.

8   Brook I, Yocum P, Calhoun L: Beta-lactamase-producing Bacteroides species recovered from children. Possible clue to failure of penicillin treatment. Lancet 1981;i:332.

9   Roos K, Grahn E, Holm SE: Evaluation of beta-lactamase activity and microbial interference in treatment failures of acute streptococcal tonsillitis. Scand J Infect Dis 1986;18:313–319.

10 Maruyama S, Yoshioka H, Fujita K, Takimoto M, Satake Y: Sensitivity of group A streptococci to antibiotics. Prevalence of resistance to erythromycin in Japan. Am J Dis Child 1979;133:1143–1145.

11 Zackrisson G, Lind L, Roos K, Larsson P: Erythromycin-resistant beta-hemolytic streptococci group A in Göteborg. Scand J Infect Dis 1988;20:419–420.

12 Grahn E, Holm SE, Roos K: Penicillin tolerance in beta-streptococci isolated from patients with tonsillitis. Scand J Infect Dis 1987;19:421–426.

13 Sanders C, Nelsen G, Sanders E: Bacterial interference. II. Epidemiological determinants of the antagonistic activity of the normal throat flora against group A streptococci. Infect Immun 1977;16:599–603.

14 Sprunt K, Leidy G, Redman W: Abnormal colonization of neonates in an ICV: Conversion to normal colonization by pharyngeal implantation of alpha-streptococcus strain. Pediatr Res 1980;14:308–313.

15 Grahn E, Holm SE: Bacterial interference in the throat flora during a streptococcal outbreak in an apartment house area. Zentralbl Bact Hyg [A] 1983;256:72–79.

16 Roos K, Grahn E, Holm SE, Johansson H, Lind L: Interfering alpha-streptococci as a protection against recurrent streptococcal tonsillitis in children. Int J Pediatr Otorhinolaryngol 1992, in press.

Kristian Roos, MD, PhD, ENT Department, Lundby Hospital,
Wieselgrensplatsen 2A, S–417 17 Göteborg (Sweden)

Galioto GB (ed): Tonsils: A Clinically Oriented Update.
Adv Otorhinolaryngol. Basel, Karger, 1992, vol 47, pp 146–150

Bacteriology of Tonsils in Children: Comparison between Recurrent Acute Tonsillitis and Tonsillar Hypertrophy

M. François[a], E. Bingen[b], Th. Soussi[a], Ph. Narcy[a]

[a] ORL Department, Hôpital Robert-Debré, and
[b] Department of Microbiology, Faculty Bichat, University Paris VII, Paris, France

Many children exhibit temporary hypertrophy of tonsils during acute tonsillitis, then the size of the tonsils usually returns to normal. The size of tonsils is not significantly different in children having tonsillectomy for recurrent acute tonsillitis (RT) and children having adenoidectomy alone [1]. Nevertheless, some children develop tonsillar hypertrophy (TH). This may lead to obstructive sleep apnea. TH is due to an increase of the lymphoid elements and not to an increase of the supportive connective tissue stroma. Brodsky et al. [2] showed that the number of T-helper, T-suppressor and B-cells per gram of tonsil is markedly greater in diseased tonsils than in controls. They found a positive correlation of the number of *Haemophilus influenzae* (HI) per gram of tonsil to tonsil weight. In contrast, Brook [3] found more HI, *Staphylococcus aureus* and *Bacteroides fragilis* in adenoids from children with chronic adenotonsillitis than with adenoid hypertrophy. However, bacteriology of upper respiratory tract infections is different in France and in the USA.

The aim of our study was to compare the bacteriology of tonsils in children under 5 years of age undergoing tonsillectomy for TH or RT.

Materials and Methods

Between March 1989 and April 1991, we studied the bacteriology of tonsils in children under 5 years of age undergoing tonsillectomy in the ENT Department at Robert Debré's Hospital, Paris, France. Children who had received any antibiotic during the 2 weeks preceding surgery were excluded from this study. Patients were divided into three groups. A first group, with TH (70 children); a second group with RT (39 children)

Table 1. Culture isolates from tonsillar surface specimens as related to indications for tonsillectomy in 120 children under 5 years of age (* p < 0.01)

	TH	RT	TH + RT
Number of tonsils	70	39	11
Number of isolates (%) in:			
Haemophilus influenzae	33 (47)*	30 (77)*	7 (64)
Haemophilus parainfluenzae	11 (16)	2 (5)	0
Streptococcus pyogenes	13 (19)*	1 (3)*	0
Streptococcus pneumoniae	5 (7)	6 (15)	0
Staphylococcus aureus	4	0	0
Branhamella catarrhalis	0	0	0

defined as more than 3 tonsillitis during the previous 6 months or more than 5 during the past year; a third group (11 children) with both RT and TH. The mean ages of the children in the 3 groups were respectively 42, 49 and 44 months.

Bacteriology

A tonsillar surface specimen was collected on a swab immediately before surgery, with the patient under general anesthesia. On removal the tonsil was dipped into a povidone-iodine solution for 5 min, then rinsed with sterile saline solution and transported in a sterile tube to the laboratory. There the tonsil was aseptically homogenized. For a quantitative colony count a 0.01-ml loop was used to inoculate the following media: sheep blood agar (5%) supplemented with colistin and nalidixic acid, Mueller-Hinton agar (Diagnostic Pasteur), mannitol salt agar, chocolate agar with polivitex (Biomérieux, France) and MacConkey's agar (Diagnostic Pasteur). The plates were incubated for 48 h at 37 °C aerobically (MacCarkey, mannitol salt agar and Mueller-Hinton agar plates), anaerobically (blood agar plates) or under 5% CO_2 (chocolate agar plates). Bacteria were identified by conventional methods.

The bacteriological findings in the three groups were compared using χ^2 test, p values < 0.01 being considered significant.

Results

Tables 1 and 2 list the number of each isolate in surface and core cultures in the three groups. In some tonsils there were two different strains of HI, so the number of isolates may be more important than the number of tonsils, such as in culture isolates from tonsillar core in the group with TH + RT. In the core tissue of tonsils, there was no significant difference in culture isolates between the 3 groups. There was more HI and less *Strepto-*

Table 2. Culture isolates from tonsillar core tissue as related to indications for tonsillectomy in 120 children under 5 years of age

	TH	RT	TH + RT
Number of tonsils	70	39	11
Number of isolates (%) in:			
Haemophilus influenzae	54 (77)	33 (85)	12 (100)
Haemophilus parainfluenzae	5 (7)	6 (15)	0
Streptococcus pyogenes	17 (24)	6 (15)	1
Streptococcus pneumoniae	10 (14)	8 (21)	0
Staphylococcus aureus	8 (11)	5 (13)	2 (18)
Branhamella catarrhalis	0	1	0

Table 3. Number of isolates related to tonsillar bacterial load in 120 children under 5 years of age (number of organisms in 1 g: $\log_{10}$ CFU)

		Number of isolates, CFU/g							
		$< 10^2$	10^3	10^4	10^5	10^6	10^7	10^8	mean
Haemophilus influenzae									
TH	70	21	7	10	24	10	0	3	3.8
RT	39	10	4	5	13	6	5	0	4.1
TH + RT	11	1	1	6	4	0	1	0	4.9
Streptococcus pyogenes									
TH	70	53	3	1	5	5	3		
RT	39	33	1	2	2	1	0		
TH + RT	11	10	0	0	0	1	0		
Streptococcus pneumoniae									
TH	70	60	2	6	0	2			
RT	39	31	1	2	4	1			
TH + RT	11	11	0	0	0	0			

coccus pyogenes on the tonsillar surface in the group with RT than in the group with HT. Table 3 summarizes the results of the bacteriological load of tonsils in colony forming units per gram of tonsil (CFU/g). Sensitivity to antibiotics of microorganisms isolated in core cultures of enlarged tonsils is indicated in table 4.

Table 4. Percentage of efficacy of oral antimicrobial agents on microorganisms isolated from core cultures of enlarged tonsils from 70 children under 5 years of age (E = effective, N = noneffective)

	E	N
Ampicillin	74	26
Amoxicillin + clavulanate potassium	97	3
Cefalotin	80	20
Cefuroxime	97	3
Cefotaxime	97	3
Erythromycin	46	54
Trimethoprim + sulfamethoxazole	50	50

Discussion

General indications for tonsillectomy in children are TH or RT. The pathogenesis of persistent TH is still unknown. It is possible that the underlying pathologic condition is infection of the tonsil. The results of Brodsky et al. [2] support an etiological role of HI in the pathogenesis of TH in children, especially β-lactamase producers. In fact, HI is isolated from the core of tonsils in 27–62% of tonsillectomies in children [4–6]. Our study confirms the high incidence of HI in tonsil core microflora in children. HI was isolated in 58% of the cases in surface cultures and in 83% of the cases in core cultures. Surow et al. [7] reported a total absence of HI in the core cultures of children in whom RT was an indication for surgery, whereas HI was cultured from 35% of the enlarged tonsils, but only in 2% of the surface specimens. Other authors such as DeDio et al. [8] and Kielmovitch et al. [9] reported no difference between TH and RT in regard to HI colonization of the core tissue. In our study we found that more tonsils have HI on their surface in the RT group (77%) than in the HT group (47%). In the core tissue, we found a mean load of HI of $8 \cdot 10^3$ CFU/g in enlarged tonsils and 10^4 CFU/g in tonsils removed for RT, which is not statistically different.

Moreover, we found more tonsils with *S. pyogenes* on their surface in group 1 with TH (19%) than in group 2 with RT (3%, p < 0.01). In the core tissue, there was also more *S. pyogenes* in group 1 with TH (24%) than in group 2 with RT (15%), but the statistical analysis shows no significant difference.

Oral antibiotics are frequently ineffective in vitro on microorganisms isolated from the core of enlarged tonsils. Only 46% of isolates were sensitive to erythromycin and 50% to trimethoprim-sulfamethoxazole. If a prophylactic antibiotic coverage is intended for a tonsillectomy, e.g. in a child with cardiac disease, these results will have to be considered. An oral cephalosporin such as cefuroxime-axetil or the combination amoxicillin-clavulanate potassium seems more appropriate than phenoxy-methyl penicillin or amoxicillin alone in case of tonsillectomy for enlarged tonsils.

References

1   Barr GS, Crombie IK: Comparison of size of tonsils in children with recurrent tonsillitis and in controls. BMJ 1989;298:804.
2   Brodsky L, Moore L, Stanievich J: The role of *Haemophilus influenzae* in the pathogenesis of tonsillar hypertrophy in children. Laryngoscope 1988;98:1055–1060.
3   Brook I: Aerobic and anaerobic bacteriology of adenoids in children: a comparison between patients with chronic adenotonsillitis and adenoid hypertrophy. Laryngoscope 1981;91:377–382.
4   Brook I, Yocum P, Friedman EM: Aerobic and anaerobic bacteria in tonsils of children with recurrent tonsillitis. Ann Otol Rhinol Laryngol 1981;90:261–263.
5   Weber M, Conroy MC, Mory F, Burdin JC, Wayoff M: Sensibilité à l'association amoxicilline-acide clavulanique de la flore amygdalienne profonde isolée au cours d'amygdalites chroniques. Ann Oto-Laryng (Paris) 1988;105:143–146.
6   Timon CI, McAllister VA, Walsh M, Cafferkey MT: Changes in tonsillar bacteriology of recurrent acute tonsillitis: 1980 vs. 1989. Resp Med 1990;84:395–400.
7   Surow JB, Handler SD, Telian SA, Fleisher GR, Baranak CC: Bacteriology of tonsil surface and core in children. Laryngoscope 1989;99:261–266.
8   DeDio RM, Tom L, McGowan KL, Wetmore RF, Handler SD, Potsic WP: Microbiology of the tonsils and adenoids in a pediatric population. Arch Otolaryngol Head Neck Surg 1988;114:763–765.
9   Kielmovitch IH, Keleti G, Bluestone CD, Wald ER, Gonzalez C: Microbiology of obstructive tonsillar hypertrophy and recurrent tonsillitis. Arch Otolaryngol Head Neck Surg 1989;115:721–724.

Dr. M. François, Service ORL, Hôpital Robert-Debré, 48, Bld Sérurier,
F–75019 Paris (France)

Galioto GB (ed): Tonsils: A Clinically Oriented Update.
Adv Otorhinolaryngol. Basel, Karger, 1992, vol 47, pp 151–160

Epstein-Barr Virus in Waldeyer's Lymphatic Tissue

Masaru Kunimoto[a, b]*, Shinji Tamura*[a, b]*, Osamu Yoshie*[b]*,
Toshihide Tabata*[a]

[a] Department of Otorhinolaryngology, Wakayama Medical College,
Wakayama City, and [b] Shionogi Institute for Medical Science, Mishima,
Settsu-shi, Osaka, Japan

Epstein-Barr virus (EBV) is a ubiquitous B lymphocyte-tropic human herpes virus. Most people apparently have primary infection during early childhood without noticeable symptoms and the virus persists in the hematopoietic system throughout life with intermittent excretion in saliva. Primary infection in young adults, however, often causes the self-limiting lymphoproliferative disease, infectious mononucleosis. EBV is also closely associated with human malignancies, such as endemic Burkitt's lymphoma, undifferentiated nasopharyngeal carcinoma and EBV-associated lymphomas in immunocompromised patients [1]. Furthermore, the list of EBV-associated diseases is still growing [2–5].

Recent studies have revealed the existence of two type A and B EBV [6, 7] through divergence of the BamHI WHY region of EBV genome, which encodes the EBV nuclear antigen 2 (EBNA-2) and is essential for EBV-induced B-cell transformation [8]. Compared to transformation induced by the prototypic A variant, those induced by B variant grow and expand inefficiently [9]. Therefore, it may be inaccurate to determine the distribution and incidence of the type B variant in an ordinary hematopoietic system and saliva through immortalization of lymphoblastoid cell lines.

Polymerase chain reaction (PCR) is a powerful procedure for detection of a specific DNA sequence in a small amount of sample [10]. By using

PCR, we have developed a simple method for sensitive detection and typing of EBV. The universal primers are consensus to both EBNA-2A and -2B sequences [11], but the amplified sequences from these two types are different in size, and therefore, easily distinguished by gel electrophoresis and ethidium bromide staining.

The PCR was employed for detection and typing of EBV in Waldeyer's lymphatic tissues and lymphocytes deviced from patients with various types of tonsillitis.

Materials and Methods

Cells and Samples

B95-8 and Raji (both EBV type A-positive), Jijoye and AG876 (both type B-positive), AKATA (EBV-positive, type unknown) [12] and BJAB and K562 (both EBV-negative) were maintained in RPMI-1640 supplemented with 10% fetal bovine serum. Tonsillar tissues were obtained from tonsillectomy of chronic tonsillitis and focal infection of the tonsil with PPP or biopsy of infectious mononucleosis. Lymphocytes from the tonsils were collected by Ficoll-Paque (Pharmacia) separation after mincing tonsillar tissues from 5 cases of chronic tonsillitis, 5 cases of focal infection of the tonsil with PPP, 2 cases of hypertrophic tonsil and 2 cases of adenoid vegetation. Isolation of DNA from cultured cells and tissue specimens was carried out as described.

Preparation of DNA

Cellular DNA samples used as standards were prepared by digestion with proteinase K and RNase extraction with phenol and chloroform/isoamyl alcohol, and precipitation with ethanol as described previously [13]. For determination of detection sensitivity of PCR, each cell mixture was washed 3 times, suspended with 30 µl of a buffer (10 mM Tris-HCl, pH 7.4, 1 mM EDTA) containing 0.05% Triton X-100 and lysed by boiling for 10 min. After centrifugation at 7,000 g for 10 min, supernatants were used for PCR.

Polymerase Chain Reaction

Oligonucleotides used for primers and probes were synthesized in a DNA synthesizer (Cyclone, MilliGen/Biosearch, USA) and purified by Nemseorb Prep cartridges (E.I. du Pont de Nemours & Co., USA) and HPLC. Primer sequences were 5'-TTTCACCAA-TACATGAACC-3' and 5'-TGGCAAAGTGCTGAGAGCAA-3' and the probe sequence was 5'-CAATGTATCCCAAATAAATG-3'. DNA samples were denatured at 94 °C for 10 min, and placed in 100 µl of the reaction mixture containing 50 mM KCl, 10 mM Tris-HCl, pH 8.3, 1.5 mM MgCl$_2$, 0.01% gelatin, 0.5 µg of each primer, 0.3 mM of each dNTP and 2.5 units of Taq-polymerase. Amplification was carried out by 40 cycles of denaturation at 94 °C for 1 min, annealing at 51 °C for 2 min and extension at 72 °C for 3 min in a DNA Thermal Cycler (Perkin-Elmer Cetus). After amplification, each reaction mixture was extracted once with phenol and once with chloroform-isoamyl alcohol. One-tenth of each reaction mixture was then analyzed by electrophoresis on a 6% polyacrylamide gel and stained with ethidium bromide.

Table 1. Sequence of oligonucleotide primers and probes for universal PCR synthesized from the U2 region of EBV

Oligonucleotide	Sequence	Base positions[1]
Primers		2771–2789
(Sense)	+ 5'-TTTCACCAATACATGAACC	3149–3130
(Antisense)	– 5'-TGGCAAAGTGCTGAGAGCAA	
Probes		
(Sense)	+ 5'-CAATGTATCCCAAATAAATG	2994–3013

[1] The base positions are those from Dambaugh et al. [11].

Southern Blot Hybridization

For hybridization with probes, DNA fragments separated by gel electrophoresis were denatured with 1.5 M NaCl and 0.5 M NaOH and transferred onto a Hybond-N nylon membrane (Amersham, UK) with 1.5 M NaCl and 0.25 M NaOH. Prehybridization was carried out at 37 °C with 5 × SSPE, 0.01% SDS, 1× Denhardt's solution and 200 µg/ml of salmon sperm DNA. Hybridization was carried out at 37 °C in the same solution containing a probe labeled with ^{32}P-ddATP by using a 3'-end-labeling kit (Amersham). Membranes were washed for 1 h with three changes of 5× SSPE and 0.01% SDS. Autoradiography was carried out with Fuji X-ray films at –80 °C.

Results

Specificity and Detection Sensitivity of Universal PCR

A single set of universal primers suitable for detection and typing of EBV and probe were synthesized from a conserved sequence in the BamHI WYH of both EBV strains. The amplified sequences were different in size because of a large deletion of the type A EBV (table 1, fig. 1). As shown in figure 2, the type of EBV was easily determined by gel electrophoresis and ethidium bromide staining. The detection sensitivity of the universal PCR was assessed using serially diluted Raji cells (type A-positive) or AG876 cells (B type-positive) with a constant number of BJAB cells (EBV-negative). As shown in figure 3, universal PCR was capable of producing a band detectable by ethidium bromide staining when the reaction mixture contained DNA from at least 10 Raji or AG876 cells. Subsequent Southern blot hybridizations using the oligonucleotides probe might increase the detection sensitivity 10-fold.

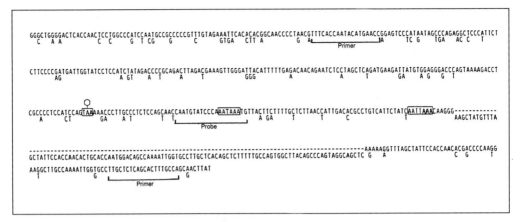

Fig. 1. Amplified region of PCR with a single pair of the universal primers. The amplified sequence of the B95-8 is shown on the upper A lines. Difference in the sequence of AG876 is shown comparatively on the B line. A hyphen indicates a deleted base.

Fig. 2. Gel separations and Southern blot analysis of EBV sequences amplified with a single pair of universal primers. After separation by electrophoresis, PCR products were analyzed by ethidium bromide stains (*a*) and Southern blot hybridization using a 3′-end-labeled oligonucleotide probe (*b*). The lanes were as follows: M = PhiX174 DNA digested with HaeIII; 1 = B95-8 (type A-positive); 2 = Raji (type A-positive); 3 = AKATA (EBV type unknown); 4 = K562 (EBV-negative); 5 = BJAB (EBV-negative); 6 = Jijoye (type B-positive); 7 = AG876 (type B-positive).

Fig. 3. Detection sensitivity of universal PCR determined by ethidium bromide staining and Southern blot analysis. DNAs from serial 10-fold dilutions of type A-positive Raji cells ranging from 1×10^5 cells to 1 cell with a constant number of EBV-negative BJAB cells (2.5×10^5 cells) were amplified by universal (*a*). DNAs from serial 10-fold dilutions of type B-positive AG876 cells ranging from 1×10^5 cells to 1 cell with BJAB (2.5×10^5 cells) were amplified by universal PCR (*b*). The lanes were as follows: M = PhiX174 DNA digested with HaeIII; 1 = 1×10^5 Raji or AG876 cells + 2.5×10^5 BJAB cells; 2 = 1×10^4 Raji or AG876 cells + 2.5×10^5 BJAB cells; 3 = 1×10^3 Raji or AG876 cells + 2.5×10^5 BJAB cells; 4 = 1×10^2 Raji or AG876 cells + 2.5×10^5 BJAB cells; 5 = 1×10 Raji or AG876 cells + 2.5×10^5 BJAB cells; 6 = $1 \times$ Raji or AG876 cells + 2.5×10^5 BJAB cells; 7 = 2.5×10^5 BJAB cells.

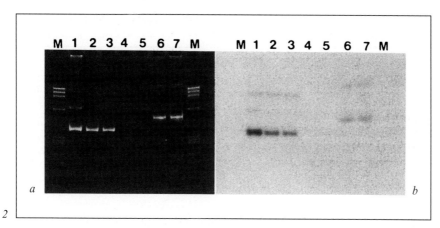

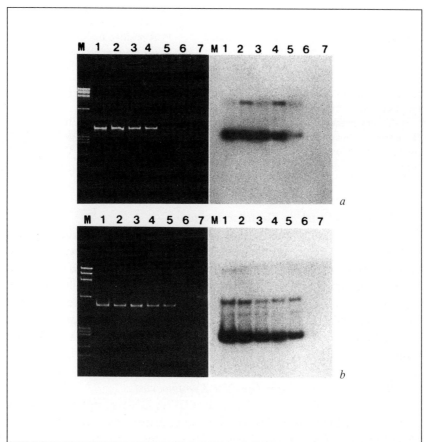

Table 2. Detection and typing of EBV in tonsillar tissues of patients with various types of tonsillar diseases

Disease	Cases	PCR positive for			
		type A	type B	both	none
Chronic tonsillitis	9	0	0	0	9
Focal infection of tonsil					
with palmoplantar pustulosis	16	2	0	0	14
Infectious mononucleosis	2	2	0	0	0

Table 3. Detection and typing of EBV in tonsillar lymphocytes of patients with various types of tonsillar diseases

Disease	Cases	PCR positive for			
		type A	type B	both	none
Chronic tonsillitis	5	1	0	0	4
Focal infection of tonsil					
with palmoplantar pustulosis	5	2	0	0	3
Hypertrophic tonsil	2	2	0	0	0
Adenoid vegetation	2	0	0	0	2

Detection of EBV in Tonsillar Tissues

DNA samples obtained from tonsillar tissue specimens from patients with various tonsillitis were subjected to PCR amplification with the universal primers. All the tested patients were confirmed to be EBV seropositive. Representative results are shown in figure 4, and the results for all 25 cases are summarized in table 2. Weak bands of type A EBV were detected in 2 cases of PPP. In 2 cases of infectious mononucleosis, strong bands of type A EBV were found that showed a high EBV content in the tonsillar tissues.

Detection of EBV from Tonsillar Lymphocytes

Universal PCR was used to detect EBV in DNA samples of lymphocytes separated from tonsillar tissues from patients with hypertrophic tonsil, chronic tonsillitis, adenoid vegetation and focal infection of the tonsil

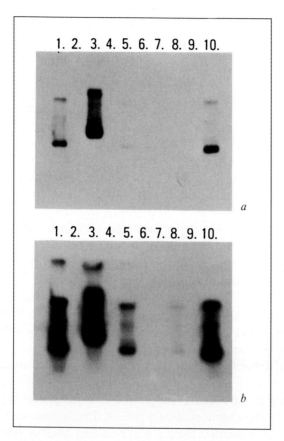

Fig. 4. PCR detection and typing of EBV tonsillar tissues from patients with chronic tonsillitis, focal infection of palmoplantar pustulosis and infectious mononucleosis. Samples were subjected to PCR amplifications using universal primers. Products were analyzed by Southern blot hybridization. Autoradiography of 1-day exposure (*a*) and 5-day exposure (*b*) at −80 °C. The lanes were as follows: 1 = B95-8 (type A-positive); 2 = BJAB (EBV-negative); 3 = AG876 (type B-positive); 4 = chronic tonsillitis; 5–9 = focal infection with palmoplantar pustulosis; 10 = infectious mononucleosis.

with PPP. All the tested patients were confirmed to be EBV seropositive. The results from 14 cases are summarized in table 3. A type EBV bands were detected in 1 case of chronic tonsillitis, 2 cases of focal infection with PPP, both of 2 cases of hypertrophic tonsil but none from adenoid vegetation, even though the positive bands were weak.

Discussion

Classically, the presence of EBV genotype in a small number of specimens was determined by Southern blot analysis or Western blotting after a spontaneous outgrowth of B lymphoblastoid cells or of immortalization of human umbilical cord B lymphocytes. These methods, however, take a long period of time for getting a result, and may be false-negative in the case of type B EBV which is inefficient for immortalization of human B lymphocytes compared with type A [9]. PCR, which is often capable of detecting even a single copy of target sequence, have come to be applied more and more for detection of EBV sequences [14–19].

In the present study, we could detect and type EBV in the tonsillar tissues and lymphocytes without establishing lymphoblastoid cells using PCR. Our universal PCR was proved to be useful for one-step detection of type A and type B EBV and high sensitivities. Sixbey et al. [14] also developed a universal PCR for detection and typing of EBV using primers synthesized from EBNA-2. Their primers were chosen from sequences consensus to both types but encompassing sequences highly divergent between the two types. After PCR amplification, the determination of EBV types was accomplished by hybridization analysis using type-specific probe.

It is well known that EBV DNA was detected in peripheral blood lymphocytes of an infectious mononucleosis patient. Employing our universal PCR for DNA from tonsillar tissues, a very strong band of type A EBV was shown in 2 cases of infectious mononucleosis. This result shows the enormous increment of EBV in the tonsil tissues. On the other hand, there is no data about direct analysis of EBV types and detection in the Waldeyer's lymphatic tissue; however, the tonsil was rich in B lymphocyte. Analyzing the DNA directly prepared from the tonsillar tissues of 25 seropositive cases, the existence of type A EBV was detected in 2 cases. Analyzing the DNA prepared from 14 seropositive cases, the existence of type A was detected in 5 cases. These results might indicate that the proportion of EBV-infected cells was mostly very low in the patient without severe immunological dysfunction; however, tonsil is one of the B lymphocyte-enriched organs. In the present study, EBV was detected in 9 cases, which are all type A strains and no type B EBV was detected in tonsil. These results might indicate that the proportion of type B EBV was very low in tonsil of the Kansai area in Japan.

Note Added in Proof

Additional data about tonsil and EB virus reactivation was described satisfactorily in Kunimoto M, Tamura S, Tabata T, Yoshie O: One-step typing of Epstein-Barr virus by polymerase chain reaction: Predominance of type 1 virus in Japan. J Gen Virol 1992;73: 455–461.

Acknowledgements

We are grateful to Dr. K. Takada and Dr. A.B. Rickinson for providing AKATA and AG876, respectively. We also thank Dr. Y. Hinuma, the Director of Shionogi Institute for Medical Science, for his constant advice and encouragement.

References

1 Dillner J, Kallin B: The Epstein-Barr virus proteins. Adv Cancer Res 1988;50:95–158.

2 Greenspan JS, Greenspan D, Lennette ET, Abrams DI, Conant MA, Petersen V, Freese UK: Epstein-Barr virus replicates within the epithelial cells of oral 'hairy' leukoplakia, an AIDS-associated lesion. N Engl J Med 1985;313:1564–1571.

3 Fox RI, Pearson G, Vaughan JH: Detection of Epstein-Barr virus-associated antigens and DNA in salivary gland biopsies from patients with Sjögren's syndrome. J Immunol 1986;137:3162–3168.

4 Weis LM, Strickler JG, Warnke RA, Puritilo DT, Sklar J: Epstein-Barr viral DNA in tissues of Hodgkin's disease. Am J Pathol 1987;129:86–91.

5 Harabuchi Y, Yamanaka N, Kataura A, Imai S, Kinoshita T, Mizuno F, Osato T: Epstein-Barr virus in nasal T-cell lymphomas in patients with lethal midline granuloma. Lancet 1990;335:128–130.

6 Aldinger HK, Delius H, Freese UK, Clarke J, Borkamm GW: A putative transforming gene of Jijoye virus differs from that of Epstein-Barr virus prototypes. Virology 1985;141:221–234.

7 Zimber U, Aldinger HK, Lenoir GM, Vuillaume M, Knebel-Doeberitz MV, Laux G, Desgranges C, Wittmann P, Freese UK, Schneider U, Bornkamm GW: Geographical prevalence of two types of Epstein-Barr virus. Virology 1986;154:56–66.

8 Skare J, Farley J, Strominger JL, Fresen KO, Cho MS, zur Hausen H: Transformation by Epstein-Barr virus requires DNA sequences in the region of BamHI fragments Y and H. J Virol 1985;55:286–297.

9 Rickinson AB, Young LS, Rowe M: Influence of the Epstein-Barr virus nuclear antigen EBNA-2 on the growth phenotype of virus-transformed B cells. J Virol 1987;61:1310–1317.

10 Saiki RK, Gelfand DH, Stoffel S, Scharf SJ, Higuchi R, Horn GI, Mullis KB, Erlich HA: Primer-directed enzymatic amplification of DNA with a thermostable DNA polymerase. Science 1988;239:487–491.

11 Dambaugh T, Hennessy K, Chamnankit L, Kieff E: U2 region of Epstein-Barr virus DNA may encode Epstein-Barr nuclear antigen 2. Proc Natl Acad Sci USA 1984;81:7632–7636.

12 Takada K, Horinouchi K, Ono Y, Aya T, Osato T, Takahashi M, Hayasaka S: An Epstein-Barr virus-producer line Akata: Establishment of the cell line and analysis of viral DNA. Virus Genes 1991;5:147–156.

13 Sambrook J, Fritsch EF, Maniatis T: Molecular Cloning: A Laboratory Manual, ed 2. New York, Cold Spring Harbor Laboratory Press, 1989.

14 Sixbey JW, Shirley P, Chesney PJ, Buntin DM, Resnick L: Detection of a second widespread strain of Epstein-Barr virus. Lancet 1989;ii:761–765.

15 Saito I, Servenius B, Compton T, Fox R: Detection of Epstein-Barr virus DNA by polymerase chain reaction in blood and tissue biopsies from patients with Sjögren's syndrome. J Exp Med 1989;169:2191–2198.

16 Telenti A, Marshall WF, Smith TF: Detection of Epstein-Barr virus by polymerase chain reaction. J Clin Microbiol 1990;28:2187–2190.

17 Gopal MR, Thomson BJ, Fox J, Tedder RS, Honess RW: Detection by PCR of HHV-6 and EBV DNA in blood and oropharynx of healthy adults and HIV-seropositives. Lancet 1990;i:1598–1599.

18 Chang YS, Tyan YS, Liu ST, Liu ST, Tsai MS, Pao CC: Detection of Epstein-Barr virus DNA sequences in nasopharyngeal carcinoma cells by enzymatic DNA amplification. J Clin Microbiol 1990;28:2398–2402.

19 Crouse CA, Pflugfelder SC, Cleary T, Demick SM, Atherton SS: Detection of Epstein-Barr virus genomes in normal lacrimal glands. J Clin Microbiol 1990;28:1026–1032.

Dr. M. Kunimoto, Department of Otorhinolaryngology, Wakayama Medical College, 7 Bancho 27, Wakayama City, Wakayama 640 (Japan)

Galioto GB (ed): Tonsils: A Clinically Oriented Update.
Adv Otorhinolaryngol. Basel, Karger, 1992, vol 47, pp 161–167

Experimental Study of the Pathological Changes of Rabbit Tonsils Exposed to Anthracite Coal Briquette Gas

Jin Young Kim, Chul Hee Lee, Myung Whun Sung, Yang-Gi Min, Pil Sang Chung

Department of Otolaryngology, Seoul National University, College of Medicine, Seoul, Korea

As air pollution is becoming a great danger to the human being, many researchers have studied the effect of air pollutants on human health. These studies have focused on several air pollutants, such as carbon monoxide (CO), sulfur dioxide (SO_2), nitrogen dioxide (NO_2), and hydrogen dioxide (H_2S). Anthracite coal briquette is a unique traditional fuel commonly used in Korea. This is sometimes very dangerous because it produces a large amount of CO, SO_2, NO_2, and H_2S during combustion, especially in hypoxic condition.

Although the pharynx is the area of the first contact not only with many biological agents but noxious air pollutants as well, the toxic effect of air pollutants on the tonsil has been neglected in general. The authors tried an experiment using concentrated anthracite coal briquette gas in order to examine the morphological change of the tonsils.

Materials and Methods

Fifty healthy rabbits were used as subjects. The animals were exposed to the anthracite coal briquette gas using a gas exposure chamber, in which the concentration of the toxic gases was as follows: CO 700–1,500 ppm, SO_2 2–5 ppm, NO_2 0–2.5 ppm, and H_2S 0–2 ppm.

The animals were divided into three groups: control, acute exposure, and chronic exposure. In the acute exposure group, the animals were exposed to this gas for 1 or 3 h and the animals were sacrificed immediately, 3 days, and 7 days after exposure. In the chronic exposure group, the animals were exposed to the gas for 20 min/day during 1, 2 or 3 weeks.

The tonsils and adjacent mucosa were examined under a light microscope with HE staining and parts of specimens were fixed in 2.5% glutaraldehyde and 1% osmium tetroxide for electron microscopic examination.

We picked up and scored the four most predominant histological changes in tonsillar crypts, tonsillar surface epithelium, crypt luminal exudates, and follicular hyperplasia. For the former three items, the changes were graded into four scales and statistically analyzed by ridit (relative to an identified distribution) method. For the follicular hyperplasia, the relative size of the germinal center to the lymphoid follicle was calculated and analyzed by the Kruskal-Wallis method. Electron microscopic examination was also carried out for representative specimens after the light microscopic examination.

Results

Light Microscopic Findings

Control Group. Most specimens showed a mild lymphocytic infiltration and edema and a small amount of exudates in the tonsillar crypt. On average, the germinal center occupied 34.7% of the lymphoid follicle.

Acute Exposure Group. Immediately after the exposure, almost all specimens revealed a moderate to severe inflammatory reaction in the tonsillar parenchyma and a large amount of exudates in the crypt and many neutrophils were seen (fig. 1). Inflammatory reaction in the epithelium was less conspicuous. Activation of the germinal center was so marked that the area ratios were 68.2% for 1-h exposed animals and 70.2% for 3-h exposed animals, revealing highly significant differences between the control and exposed groups (p < 0.01).

Although the change immediately after the exposure was very intense, the amount of the exudates in the crypt was reduced and the inflammatory reactions were also significantly recovered in both subgroups along the time elapse. The size of the germinal center also significantly decreased to 51.3% after 3 days and 50.7% after 7 days in the 1-h exposure subgroup; the 3-h exposure subgroup showed the same changes, 50.1% after 3 days and 48.5% in 7 days.

Chronic Exposure Group. All specimens disclosed severe inflammatory reactions in the crypt epithelium with more plasma cells than the acute exposure group. The amount of the exudates in the crypt was also increased. The change of the surface epithelium was evident only in the 3-week subgroup. The average sizes of the germinal centers were 41.7% in the 1-week subgroup, 50.8% in the 2-week subgroup, and 57.1% in the 3-week subgroup. These figures were significantly different from the control group.

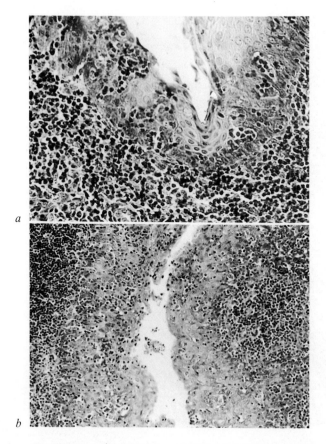

Fig. 1. Crypt epithelium in control (*a*) and 3-h exposure group (*b*), showing severe infiltration of inflammatory cells and edema in the latter. $a \times 375$; $b \times 190$.

Pharyngeal Mucosa. There were no remarkable inflammatory changes in the pharyngeal mucosae included in the specimens that were significant.

Electron Microscopic Findings

Control Group. The surface squamous epithelium showed its characteristic regular arrangement and the individual cell was covered with microridges (fig. 2). The desmosomes were clearly seen between cell membranes.

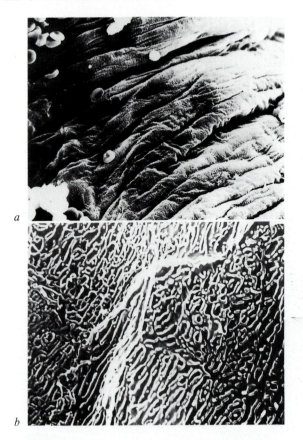

Fig. 2. Scanning electron microscopic findings of tonsils from control animals, showing flat and regular pattern of surface epithelium (*a*) and microridges (*b*). *a* × 940; *b* × 6,600.

Fig. 3. Scanning electron microscopic findings of 3-h exposure group, revealing severe desquamation (*a*), and blunting and obliteration of microridges (*b*). *a* × 940; *b* × 6,600.

Fig. 4. Transmission electron microscopic findings of control (*a*) and 3-h exposure group (*b*). *a* Flat cellular pattern and uniform development of microridges are seen. × 5,600. *b* Desquamation and loss of microridges of the surface epithelium are seen and new microridges are developing in the replacement cells. × 9,400.

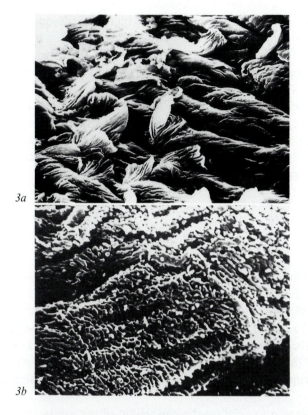

3a

3b

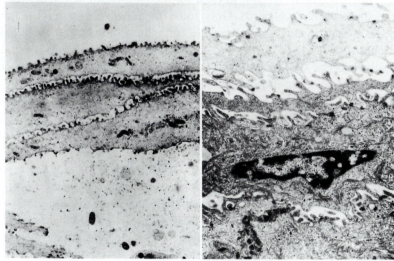

4a

4b

Acute Exposure Group. As the exposure time is increased, desquamation of the epithelium became evident and the roughening and loss of the microridges were seen (fig. 3). In the basal replacement cells, there was new development of the microridges (fig. 4). These changes slowly recovered to nearly normal state at 7 days after the exposure.

Chronic Exposure Group. This group also showed loss of regularity of the microridges in size and direction, and desquamation and separation of the surface epithelium, which became severer as the exposure durations were lengthened. The desmosomes became less distinct and the distance between the cells was increased in several layers.

Discussion

In this study we found that the tonsils react not only to many biological agents but also to the physical and chemical stimuli, such as air pollutants. Whereas the pathological changes of the respiratory epithelium by a single gas consisted of a loss of cilia, desquamation and edema, the tonsil demonstrated the infiltration of the inflammatory cells in the surface and crypt epithelium and in the exudates. These findings may be due to the histological and functional difference between the tonsil and the respiratory tissue.

Microridges are known to exist on the epithelium of the uterine cervix, cornea, and vocal cords. Gray and Titze [2] suggested that the microridges make the mucus overlying the epithelium thinner and more tightly adherent to it. They also found that an excessive mechanical irritation resulted in the loss of microridges on the vocal cords. The desmosomes became less distinct in the basal layer and eventually the epithelium was separated. A loss of regularity of the microridges was noted by electron microscopic examination before any changes were identified by light microscope. This may be one of the earliest changes of the tonsil exposed to noxious gas.

Many epidemiological studies revealed that various irreversible pathologic states can be caused by acute and chronic exposure to air pollutants. This experiment confirmed that anthracite coal briquette gas can cause inflammatory reaction in the tonsil. Furthermore, chronic daily exposure to this gas might be a cause of chronic tonsillopharyn gitis in Korea. We need a further epidemiological study to clarify this point.

References

1 Gardner DE, Coffin DL, Pinigin MA, et al: Role of time as a factor in the toxicity of chemical compounds in intermittent and continuous exposures. I. Effects of continuous exposure. J Toxicol Environ Health 1977;3:811–820.
2 Gray S, Titze I: Histologic investigation of hyperphonated canine vocal cords. Ann Otol Rhinol Laryngol 1988;97:381–388.
3 Kodama A, Hashino T: Scanning electron microscopic study of human tonsillar crypt. Pract Otolaryngol 1977;70:479–486.
4 Saito H, Ikematsu T: Tonsils and environmental pollution – Influence of ozone upon rabbit tonsil and its histological study. Jpn J Tonsil 1975;14:91–95.
5 Summer W, Sher LD, Randle MW: Inhalation of irritant gas. Clin Chest Med 1981; 2:273–281.

Jin Young Kim, MD, Department of Otolaryngology, Seoul National University, College of Medicine, 28 Yongon-Dong, Chongno-Gu, Seoul 110-744 (Korea)

Galioto GB (ed): Tonsils: A Clinically Oriented Update.
Adv Otorhinolaryngol. Basel, Karger, 1992, vol 47, pp 168–171

Alpha-Streptococci-Inhibiting Beta-Streptococci Group A in Treatment of Recurrent Streptococcal Tonsillitis

Helena Lilja[a], *Eva Grahn*[a], *Stig E. Holm*[a], *Kristian Roos*[b]

[a] Department of Clinical Microbiology, University of Umeå, and
[b] ENT Department, Lundby Hospital, Göteborg, Sweden

The recurrence rate after penicillin treatment of streptococcal tonsillitis has been reported to be 10–25% [1] and several factors have been proposed to contribute to this [2]. One important factor is ecological disturbances following antibiotic treatment. The normal bacterial flora is an important barrier towards invading beta-hemolytic streptococci group A (GAS). We demonstrated earlier in vitro that alpha-streptococci can inhibit GAS in vitro [3] and that the absence of interfering alpha-streptococci correlated to treatment failure in streptococcal tonsillitis [4]. Therefore we have isolated from throat samples obtained from healthy individuals four alpha-streptococci with a strong growth-inhibiting capacity against clinical isolates of GAS. The aim of this study was to see if the isolated alpha-streptococci inhibit GAS independent of their serotype and geographic area of recovery.

Material and Methods

Bacterial Strains
Four alpha-streptococci with broad growth-inhibiting capacity versus GAS [3] were used in the present study. These represented three *Streptococcus sanguis* II and one *Streptococcus mitis* according to the API Strep Test (France). 392 GAS strains were isolated from patients with tonsillitis from four different cities in Sweden: A-D (A = Uppsala, B = Umeå, C = Göteborg, D = Boden). The GAS strains were T-typed using T-typing sera (Institute of Sera and Vaccines, Prague, Czechoslovakia) and SOR-tested, all according to Maxted and Widdowson [5].

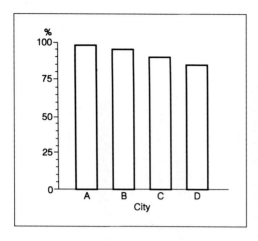

Fig. 1. Total inhibition of 392 GAS strains by four alpha-streptococci. A = Uppsala, B = Umeå, C = Göteborg, D = Boden.

Interference

GAS and alpha-streptococci were grown in a trypticase-yeast medium at 37 °C. Minidrops of the alpha-streptococcal strains (containing 10^5 CFU/ml) were transferred to blood agar plates (25 strains on each plate) by a Steers' steel pin replicator and allowed to dry. A sample of a GAS strain was applied adjacent to each of the alpha-streptococci and the plates were incubated in 5% CO_2 at 37 °C. After one night's incubation the plates were examined for interference between the microorganisms. Inhibition of GAS growth was recorded as positive (+) and noninhibition of GAS or inhibition of the alpha-streptococci were recorded as negative (–). The combined GAS inhibiting capacity of all four alpha-streptococci was designated 'total inhibition.'

Results

Twenty-one different serotypes of GAS were found among the 392 isolates. Among those types, T1M1, T12M12 and T28 were the most frequent ones. The growth inhibition afforded by the four alpha-streptococci together (total inhibition) varied between 84 and 98% of the GAS isolates from the four geographic areas (fig. 1). The inhibitory capacity of alpha 2 and 3 was high against all GAS isolates but varied for alpha 4 significantly with the geographic area from which the GAS were recovered (fig. 2). All four alpha-streptococci had the capacity to inhibit the growth of GAS independent of serotype but the inhibition was less pronounced against the T1M1 isolates (fig. 3).

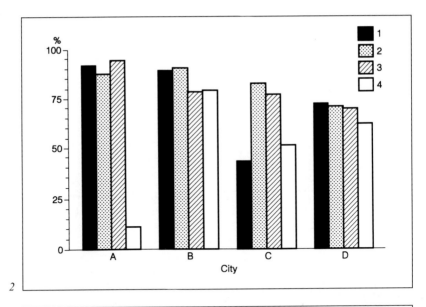

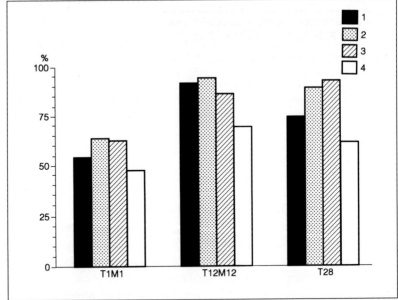

Fig. 2. Inhibiting capacity on GAS afforded by the four individual alpha-strepto-cocci (1–4). A = Uppsala, B = Umeå, C = Göteborg, D = Boden.

Fig. 3. Inhibiting capacity of the four alpha-streptococci on various GAS sero-types.

Conclusions

Although the four alpha-streptococci individually inhibited the growth of GAS to a various extent (11–98%) they together had the capacity to inhibit 84–98% of the 392 clinical isolates recovered from various geographic areas in Sweden. In a preliminary study these four alpha-streptococci have been successfully used for colonization to hinder further recurrences of streptococcal tonsillitis [6]. The present study underlines the importance of using more than one inhibiting alpha-streptococcal strain in such recolonization studies in order to account for differences in growth-inhibiting capacity afforded by individual alpha strains.

References

1   Kaplan EL, Gastanaduy AS, Huwe BB: The role of the carrier in treatment failures after antibiotic therapy of group A streptococci in the upper respiratory tract. J Lab Clin Med 1981;98:326–335.
2   Holm SE, Grahn E: Recurrence of streptococcal tonsillitis after penicillin treatment – a multifacetted problem. Res Clin Forums 1991;12:37–48.
3   Grahn E, Holm SE, Ekedahl C, Roos K: Interference of α-hemolytic streptococci isolated from tonsillar surface on β-hemolytic streptococci. A methodological study. Zentralbl Bakteriol Hyg I [A] 1983;254:459–468.
4   Roos K, Grahn E, Holm SE: Evaluation of beta-lactamase activity and microbial interference in treatment failures of acute streptococcal tonsillitis. Scand J Infect Dis 1986;18:313–319.
5   Maxted WR, Widdowson JP: The protein antigens of group A streptococci; in Wannamaker LW, Matsen JM (eds): Streptococci and Streptococcal Diseases. New York, Academic Press, 1972, pp 252–264.
6   Roos K, Grahn E, Holm SE, Johansson H, Lind L: Interfering alpha-streptococci as a protection against recurrent streptococcal tonsillitis in children. Int J Pediatr Otorhinolaryngol 1992, in press.

Prof. Stig E. Holm, Department of Clinical Bacteriology, University of Umeå, S–901 87 Umeå (Sweden)

Galioto GB (ed): Tonsils: A Clinically Oriented Update.
Adv Otorhinolaryngol. Basel, Karger, 1992, vol 47, pp 172–175

Clinical Differentiation of Peritonsillar Cellulitis from Abscess

Kalpesh S. Patel, Vasilis Delis, Manuel Oyarzabal

Department of Otorhinolaryngology, Royal Sussex County Hospital,
Brighton, UK

Peritonsillar abscess (PTA) is one of the commonest deep abscesses in the head and neck region. Management of this potentially lethal condition remains controversial and includes incision and drainage or permucosal needle aspiration. Failure to yield pus occurs in up to 50% of cases [1] either because the correct diagnosis is peritonsillar cellulitis (PTC) or because there has been failure to localize the abscess within the peritonsillar space.

Distinguishing PTA from PTC has important clinical implications since cellulitis is managed with antibiotics alone whereas the optimal management of an abscess is drainage of pus. We carried out a detailed prospective study on patients presenting with peritonsillar infections to see if clinical features will differentiate PTA from PTC thereby obviating unnecessary surgical intervention in the PTC patients.

Methods

Fifty-six patients (ages 14–33, mean 22.3; 31 male, 25 female) presenting with peritonsillar infections over a 12-month period were studied. The parameters shown in table 1 were recorded. In addition to clinical features, the white cell count was measured. After application of topical 10% Xylocaine local anaesthetic, drainage was attempted with an 19-gauge needle and 10-ml syringe. Aspiration was attempted at 3 locations to include posterior or inferiorly positioned abscesses. These were (1) supratonsillar, (2) midtonsillar, and (3) infratonsillar, just above the retromolar trigone. Failure to yield pus was considered to suggest PTC.

Table 1. Clinical features recorded for each patient

History	Examination
Age	Temperature
Duration of sore throat	Voice
Dysphagia	Side involved
Odynophagia	Trismus (interincisor distance, mm)
Drooling of saliva	Pharyngotonsillar bulge (graded I–III)[1]
Voice change	
Otalgia	
Fever	
Antibiotic treatment	
Previous tonsillitis	
Previous peritonsillar infection	

[1] Grades: I = minimal deviation of the uvula; II = deviation of the uvula and tonsil but not occluding oropharynx; III = complete occlusion of the oropharynx.

Results

In 36 patients (64%) pus was aspirated whereas in 20 patients (36%) pus was not found. All patients improved clinically with intravenous antibiotics. No patients required repeated aspiration. Comparison of symptoms and signs is shown in tables 2 and 3. No statistical differences were seen between the two conditions except in respect to the degree of pharyngotonsillar swelling.

Discussion

The optimal management of PTA has remained controversial for many decades. Ideally pus should be drained since antibiotics will not penetrate the abscess cavity in sufficient concentrations and will fail to resolve the infection in the majority of cases. However, antibiotics alone would be appropriate in the presuppurative or cellulitis stage thereby obviating the need for surgical intervention. This is particularly important in children or uncooperative adults.

Table 2. Comparison of clinical features

Symptom/sign		PTA, %	PTC, %	χ^2
Dysphagia		92	90	p > 0.05
Odynophagia		100	100	p > 0.05
Drooling of saliva		67	65	p > 0.05
Voice change		83	80	p > 0.05
Otalgia		92	85	p > 0.05
Fever		61	70	p > 0.05
Antibiotic treatment		58	70	p > 0.05
Previous tonsillitis		42	35	p > 0.05
Previous peritonsillar infection		6	10	p > 0.05
Pharyngotonsillar bulge[1]	I	19	30	p > 0.05
	II	53	65	p > 0.05
	III	28	5	*p < 0.05*

[1] Grades I–III as explained in table 1.

Table 3. Comparison of clinical parameters with t test

Clinical parameter	PTA		PTC		Student's t test
	mean	SD	mean	SD	
Age, years	23.7	6.4	20.9	6.9	p > 0.05
Duration of sore throat, days	4.6	2.9	4.2	3.4	p > 0.05
Temperature, °C	37.9	1.5	38.2	1.6	p > 0.05
White cell count, $\times 10^9$/litre	15.6	5.5	16.1	6.4	p > 0.05
Trismus, mm	26.8	6.9	24.7	7.2	p > 0.05

In addition to minimizing patient discomfort, avoiding drainage procedures also negates the risk of trauma to aberrant vessels or dissemination of infection.

Attempts have been made to differentiate PTA from PTC on clinical grounds with variable results. Shoemaker et al. [2] concluded that increased age, presence of dysphagia, and drooling of saliva were more likely to be associated with abscess whereas trismus was a greater predictor of cellulitis. Conversely, Fried and Forrest [3] found trismus and salivary drooling to be prevalent in PTA, and that bilaterality of symptoms were more often seen in PTC. Snow et al. [1] found that trismus, uvular oedema, and palatal swelling were highly associated with PTA whereas otalgia and odynophagia were not discerning factors. Brodsky et al. [4] studied a paediatric population and found no one single factor which distinguished PTC from PTA at the time of presentation.

Conclusions

This study suggests that (1) PTA cannot be differentiated from PTC on clinical parameters alone; (2) the presence of severe pharyngotonsillar swelling is more likely to be associated with PTA, and (3) that drainage should be attempted at presentation to avoid complications of PTA.

References

1   Snow DG, Campbell JB, Morgan DW: The management of peritonsillar sepsis by needle aspiration. Clin Otol 1991;16:245–247.
2   Shoemaker M, Lampe RM, Weir MR: Peritonsillitis: Abscess or cellulitis. Paediatr Infect Dis 1986;5:435–439.
3   Fried MP, Forrest JL: Peritonsillitis. An evaluation of current therapy. Arch Otolaryngol Head Neck Surg 1981;107:283–286.
4   Brodsky L, Sobie SR, Korwin D, Stanievich JF: A clinical prospective study of peritonsillar abscess in children. Laryngoscope 1988;98:780–783.

Dr. Kalpesh S. Patel, FRCS, Department of Otolaryngology,
Royal Sussex County Hospital, Eastern Road, Brighton BN2 5BE (UK)

Table 3. Isolation rates (in %) for groups A and B

Organism	Day 1		Day 2		Day 5	
	A	B	A	B	A	B
Streptococcus milleri	68	62	68	67	38	44
Streptococcus mutans	58	53	48	51	40	47
Staphylococcus albus	62	67	66	60	45	55
Staphylococcus aureus	38	28	30	34	28	30
Neisseria sp.	36	43	30	38	18	23
Streptococcus pneumoniae	24	35	22	20	18	17
Haemophilus influenzae	28	36	27	29	15	15
Haem Streptococcus (B, C, D, F)	14	18	13	15	13	9
Diphtheroids sp.	10	14	8	12	8	6
Bacteroides fragilis	87	78	84	80	80	71
Bacteroides melaninogenicus	73	75	70	67	58	53
Bacteroides oralis	48	54	40	42	37	33
Fusobacterium sp.	29	26	38	32	26	29

Table 4. Isolation rates (in %) from group C (D = diathermy; L = ligation)

Organism	Day 1		Day 2		Day 5	
	D	L	D	L	D	L
Streptococcus milleri	58	65	62	57	51	64
Streptococcus mutans	52	57	48	62	56	59
Staphylococcus albus	57	61	62	71	61	54
Staphylococcus aureus	36	45	40	30	30	27
Neisseria sp.	35	48	42	44	36	28
Streptococcus pneumoniae	23	28	20	25	18	21
Haemophilus influenzae	33	29	27	26	17	23
Haem Streptococcus (B, C, D, F)	16	19	12	11	9	11
Diphteroids sp.	12	10	8	10	6	6
Bacteroides fragilis	90	83	78	81	72	75
Bacteroides melaninogenicus	78	67	74	71	58	60
Bacteroides oralis	46	57	40	38	36	32
Fusobacterium sp.	28	22	20	20	24	20

Table 5. Factors which influence the composition of oral microflora [4]

Anatomical site	Antimicrobial drugs
Surface	Oral or systemic disease
Salivary composition	Dental treatment
Salivary flow rate	Dental appliances
Diet	Hormonal factors
pH, pO_2	Genetic factors
Microbial nutrition	Smoking
Microbial adherence	Oral hygiene

diathermy and 1 following ligation. There were no clinical features of infection. Swabs taken from these patients grew no pathogenic organisms and had a similar microbial profile to non-haemorrhage patients.

Discussion

The microbiology of the oral cavity is complex with commensal anaerobes outnumbering the aerobes by a factor of 10–1,000:1. The significance of anaerobic bacteria as part of the normal flora and their role in a variety of infections has become more widely appreciated in recent years. A number of factors affect the microbial flora which are shown in table 5. Saliva probably plays an important role in influencing the oral flora. Thus the commonly given advice following tonsillectomy to encourage early oral intake not only promotes the physical removal of potentially infected eschar from the tonsillar fossae, but also increases salivary flow and therefore takes advantage of its antimicrobial properties. In view of the numerous factors affecting the flora of the oral cavity, it seems unlikely that haemostatic technique has a major influence.

Conclusions

To conclude: (1) the flora of the tonsillar fossa is complex and compares with other parts of the oral cavity; (2) the method of haemostasis does not appear to influence the microbial flora, and (3) the role of infection in secondary haemorrhage requires further study.

References

1   Handler SD, Miller L, Richmond KH, Baranak CC: Post-tonsillectomy haemorrhage: Incidence, prevention and management. Laryngoscope 1986;96:1243–1247.
2   Phillips JJ, Thornton RD: Tonsillectomy haemostasis: Diathermy or ligation. Clin Otol 1989;14:419–424.
3   Telian SA, Handler SD, Fleisher GR, Baranak CC, Whetmore RF, Potsic WP: The effect of antibiotic therapy on recovery after tonsillectomy in children. Arch Otolaryngol Head Neck Surg 1986;112:610–615.
4   Hardie JM, Shah HN: Factors controlling the microbial flora of the mouth. Eur J Chem Antibiot 1982;2:3–11.

Dr. Kalpesh S. Patel, FRCS, Department of Otolaryngology,
Royal Sussex County Hospital, Eastern Road, Brighton BN2 5BE (UK)

Galioto GB (ed): Tonsils: A Clinically Oriented Update.
Adv Otorhinolaryngol. Basel, Karger, 1992, vol 47, pp 181–185

Recurrent Pharingotonsillitis: Epidemiological Observations at the Center of Preventive Medicine ORL USL BA/2

Clinical and Anatomopathological Situations

G. De Cillis, F. Inchingolo, M. D'Urso

Hospital of Canosa di Puglia, ORL Ward (Head: Dr. *G. De Cillis*),
Social Center of Pediatric Audiology, Canosa, Italy

The Social Center of Pediatric Audiology was added to our ORL Ward 15 years ago. It carries on not only activities of preventive audiological medicine, but also activities of prevention of the chronic inflammatory pathology of the superior respiratory tracts in school-age children. Throughout the school year, about 1,000 children come with their teachers who have previously received a first list of questions. After the clinical ORL test the audiometric test follows. Those children who show symptoms of acute, inflammatory chronic pathology, auditory deficit or linguistic troubles are asked to come again for a second test. This test takes place in the presence of a child's parents. They also answer questions of other lists. After studying the topographic distribution of the schools we noted that the majority of IRR and hypoacusis occur in those children who live in the most suburban and poorest areas of the town. This remark is very important for the primary prevention of transmissive hypoacusis of the school age. There are social, economic and cultural differences between suburban and urban areas. In Canosa there are not any residential quarters in the suburban areas, only public housing. This is meaningful to explain the fact that the phlogistic pathology of the middle ear has been pounded out above all in these areas. The children who attend suburban schools show (more than the others) acute, subacute or chronic affections of the superior respiratory tracts, relapsing tonsillitis, acute relapsing or chronic otitis. They are also disregarded by their family and treated in an irrational way. Because of their agrarian activity, the parents usually give little importance to these processes; they also have more children, so they do not consider in the right way the inflammations of the rhinopharynx, relapsing otalgies, and tonsillitis of the pharynx. They think that the hearing defects are simply effects of inattention. Clinical observations, conversations with the parents, and information from primary school teachers, family doctors, pediatric specialists and school doctors, have pointed out very important statistics about familiar conditions, diffusion of pathology, and about the way of applying therapy at home. In the three centers of Canosa, Minervino and Spinazzola, the diffusion of IRR shows meaningful differences among the children who come from areas characterized by different social levels. In a sample survey of 1,355 children we found IRR in 18.5%. For many years we have been studying the etiopathogenetic factors which determine the relapse of the pharyngotonsillar inflammations. Anatomic, environmental, and hereditary factors are the main causes, but we have also realized that the inappropriate application of the antibiotic therapy (in its use and abuse) and the avoidance of the surgical operation may have a peculiar importance for the relapses. We are persuaded that the bad use and abuse of antibiotics (as it happens in nonbactericidal manifestations) may hamper the synthesis of the antibodies and delay the acquisition of immunity, then if an antibiotic therapy is scanty in quantity and is applied for a short time, it can turn acute inflammations into latent inflammations which can easily provoke a relapse. The antibiotic failures are caused by human factors or by factors linked to the medicine, germs, or host [1].

The daily activity of the department and the continuous observations of the Social Center show how often the pharyngotonsil and upper respiratory tract's infectious pathology, with its effects on the hearing apparatus and the risk of rheumatic disease drastically lowered during an antibiotic era but always feared in case of failure in therapy, is underestimated by parents and sometimes by misinformed physicians.

Materials and Methods

Our studies have confirmed the danger of a wrong therapy and the advantages of appropriate surgical treatment. As in many relapsing pharyngotonsillitis children (with no immunologic deficit), the therapy, repeated a short time after the last inflammation, did not stop relapsing (4–6 in 2 years). We studied the lymphatic organs to observe their

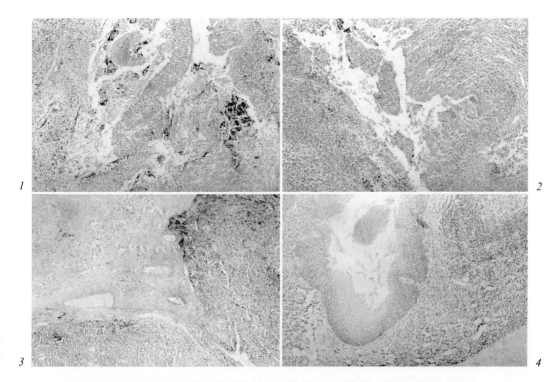

Fig. 1. Crypt's abscesses with necrotic material in the crypt and inflammatory surrounding.

Fig. 2. Crypt's abscesses: inflammatory diffused perifollicular infiltration.

Fig. 3. Chronic atrophic tonsillitis: atrophy of lymphatic tissue with signs of necrosis.

Fig. 4. Crypt of tonsil covered by floored composed epithelium with amorphous material in the crypt without inflammation.

histological changes [2] due to the numerous inflammations which, we suppose, might have explained the failure of antibiotic therapy. We chose 155 subjects aged 18 months to 14 years (during the last 7 years of hospital activity) each of them with 4–6 pharyngotonsil inflammations in the last 2 years. We cut their tonsils 3 or 4 weeks after the last inflammation. Among those children there were some with relapsing throat and ear inflammation (they had had their adenoids cut elsewhere), and some with respiratory troubles during sleep [3], who had not been treated surgically because they were too young. I suppose some with relapsing pharyngotonsil inflammation had been treated with a repeated antibiotic therapy, in fact their parents had been told that 'we do not cut tonsils anymore ...' [4].

Results and Conclusions

The histological diagnoses of the lymphatic organs examined have been: chronic atrophic tonsillitis, chronic nonspecific tonsillitis, subacute chronic nonspecific tonsillitis, subacute chronic hyperplastic tonsillitis; the alterations of greater importance: atrophic follicular ulceration, necrosis (microabscesses), diffused inflammation, hyperplasias, fibrosis.

Anatomopathological observations demonstrated the impossibility of the antibiotic to seep through the tonsillar tissue sufficiently, at this point impaired and distraught in its structure by numerous previous inflammations and the easy recurrences. Some very significant findings are shown in figures 1–4. Besides, we analyzed a group of 66 control children for 6–8 months treated rationally and with recent antibiotics (amox-clav) [5] in the precocious phase of relapse (more advantageous than treatment of the frank symptoms): we had 19 successes and 47 failures. After a correct antibiotic therapy, sometimes with immunostimulation, a recurrence suggested operation was necessary. Our study demonstrates how antibiotic therapy does not reduce the incidence of the recurrent pharyngotonsillitis; with tonsillectomy we have a reduction of the episodes until the disappearance within 6–18 months. It is obvious that the sclerosis of the germinative centers that happens in the tonsils with recurrent inflammations, determines insufficient defensive capacity. In our opinion the surgical decision in recurrent pharyngotonsillitis is based on: number of recurrences (especially if increased in time) was 4–6 in the last 2 years, serious infection, inflammation of the lymph nodes of the neck, clear symptoms of general resentment (pallor, asthenia, slight fever, etc.) that sometimes anticipate metafocal manifestations, always dangerous in the case of therapeutic failure [4, 6, 7–9].

References

1   Gardner P, Provine HT: Failure of Antibiotic Therapy. Manual of Acute Bacterial Infections; Early Diagnosis and Treatment. Boston, Little Brown, 1975.

2   Cellesi C, Mattei C, Piccini A, Sossolini A, Sensini I: Bacteriological, histopathological and clinical remarks on 100 chronic tonsillitis in children. Valsanva 1978;54: 90–99.

3   De Cillis G, Inchingolo F, D'Urso M: Night obstructive apnea and ORL surgery. Our questionnaire on the screenings of risk patients. Atti del LXXVII Congresso Nazionale SIO 1990, pp 386–389.

4 Fini Storchi O, Giannelli A, et al: Decrease of annual influence and reasons of tonsillectomy and adenoidectomy: Report on 39–526 children. Acta Otorhinolaryngol Ital 1982;2:607–626.

5 Brook I, Yocum P, Shah K: Beta-lactamase producing bacteroides species recovered from children: possible clue to failure of penicillin treatment. JAMA 1980;244: 1696–1699.

6 Aliprandi G: Tonsillectomy: an everlasting problem. Polso 1982;7:48–53.

7 Bernabei L, Carmi G: The chronic tonsillitis. Topical aspects of an ancient problem. Attual Otorinolaringol 1980;17:26.

8 Paradise JL, Bluestone CD, Bachman RZ: History of recurrent sore throat as an indication for tonsillectomy. N Engl J Med 1978;288:409–413.

9 Sala O, Marchiori C, Martini A, Soranzo G: Directions for tonsillectomy. Fed Med 1984;37:10.

Dr. G. De Cillis, via F. D'Aragona, 4, I–70051 Barletta (Italy)

Galioto GB (ed): Tonsils: A Clinically Oriented Update.
Adv Otorhinolaryngol. Basel, Karger, 1992, vol 47, pp 186–188

Role of *Haemophilus influenzae* and Group A Streptococci in Recurrent Tonsillar Infection or Hypertrophy

A. Stjernquist-Desatnik[a], *C. Schalén*[b]

Department of [a] Oto-Rhino-Laryngology and [b] Medical Microbiology,
University of Lund, Sweden

High tonsillar core isolation rates of *Haemophilus influenzae* and group A streptococci (GAS) both among cases of recurrent acute tonsillitis and of tonsillar hypertrophy have been reported from several studies [1, 2]. These findings might suggest that, in addition to GAS, *H. influenzae* may be actively involved in recurrent acute tonsillitis, and that both species may also be involved in tonsillar hypertrophy. Since core culture is only possible in cases of tonsillectomy, no information is available as to recovery rates in healthy individuals.

Material and Methods

One hundred and twenty-six patients who underwent tonsillectomy because of recurrent acute tonsillitis (more than 5 episodes annually for over 2 years, 59 patients), tonsillar hypertrophy (with no history of recurrent tonsillitis, 30 patients) or sleep apnea (judged by neurophysiological findings, 37 patients) were evaluated by tonsillar core culturing. The sleep apnea patients served as controls, since none of them had tonsillar hypertrophy at ENT examination or any history of recurrent acute tonsillitis, and thus their tonsillar core flora could be regarded as normal. For tonsillar core tissue culture, the tonsils were first flame-scorched, cut aseptically and a piece of tissue stroked across the agar surface as previously described [3].

Group bacteriological data were compared using the χ^2 test with continuity correction, p values below 0.05 being considered significant.

Table 1. Bacterial isolation rates from tonsillar core tissue as related to indication for tonsillectomy

	Recurrent acute tonsillitis		Tonsillar hypertrophy		Sleep apnea
	all patients (59)[1]	patients >20 years (28)	all patients (30)	patients >20 years (2)	patients >20 years (37)
H. influenzae	12*	7**	11***	0	1
Group A streptococci	10	5	6	0	2
Group C streptococci	0	0	3	1	0
Group G streptococci	2	0	0	0	1
B. catarrhalis	1	0	2	0	1
Pneumococci	1	0	2	0	1

χ^2 test, as related to isolation rate in patients with sleep apnea.
* $p < 0.05$; ** $p < 0.02$; *** $p < 0.01$
[1] Total number of patients with this indication for tonsillectomy is shown in parentheses.

Results

The isolation rate of *H. influenzae* was much lower among sleep apnea controls (2.7%) than among either the patients with recurrent acute tonsillitis (20.3%) ($p < 0.05$) or those with tonsillar hypertrophy (36.7%) ($p < 0.01$), as was that of GAS, 5.4% versus 16.9 and 20% respectively (though the latter differences were not statistically significant). The isolation frequencies of *Branhamella catarrhalis,* pneumococci, group C and G streptococci did not differ between the three groups (table 1).

Culture Findings in Patients over 20 Years of Age

Of the 59 patients with recurrent acute tonsillitis, 28 were over 20 years of age. Of these patients, 25% exhibited growth of *H. influenzae,* as compared with 2.7% of the sleep apnea controls ($p < 0.02$). GAS was recovered in 5/28 of the patients with recurrent acute tonsillitis, as compared with 2/37 of the sleep apney controls.

Conclusion

The high tonsillar core recovery rates of *H. influenzae* and GAS both
in patients with recurrent acute tonsillitis and in those with tonsillar hypertrophy, as compared with normal controls, suggests the possible involvement of these bacteria in both conditions.

References

1   Brodsky L, Moore L, Stanievich J: The role of *Haemophilus influenzae* in the patho-
    genesis of tonsillar hypertrophy in children. Laryngoscope 1988;98:1055–1060.
2   Kielmovitch IH, Keleti G, Bluestone CD, Wald ER, Gonzales C: Microbiology of
    obstructive tonsillar hypertrophy and recurrent tonsillitis. Arch Otolaryngol Head
    Neck Surg 1989;115:721–724.
3   Stjernquist-Desatnik A, Prellner K, Schalén C: Colonization by *Haemophilus
    influenzae* and group A streptococci in recurrent acute tonsillitis and in tonsillar
    hypertrophy. Acta Otolaryngol (Stockh) 1990;109:314–319.

Dr. A. Stjernquist-Desatnik, Department of Oto-Rhino-Laryngology,
University Hospital, S–221 85 Lund (Sweden)

Galioto GB (ed): Tonsils: A Clinically Oriented Update.
Adv Otorhinolaryngol. Basel, Karger, 1992, vol 47, pp 189–192

Microbial Flora and Lymphocytes in Nasopharyngeal Lymphatic Tissue in Children

Amos Piccini [a], *Cesare Biagini* [a], *Isaia Sensini* [a], *Alessandra Zanchi* [b], *Manuela Uberti* [b], *Gloria Regoli* [b], *Angela Barberi* [b], *Carla Cellesi* [b], *Alessandro Fantoni* [b]

[a] Istituto di Clinica ORL e
[b] Istituto di Malattie Infettive, Università degli Studi di Siena, Italia

Airway obstruction secondary to adenoid tissue hypertrophy and recurrent or chronic adenoiditis with otitis and rhinitis are common problems in the pediatric population. Several studies have investigated the microbial flora of adenoids in both groups of patients [1, 2], that had no significant differences between the type of pathogens. The pathogens most frequently isolated were *Staphylococcus aureus* and *Haemophilus* species [3–5].

The aim of the present study was to investigate the role of the microbial flora and local cellular immunity in the hypertrophy and phlogosis of the adenoid tissue.

Materials and Methods

From January to June 1991, 24 children (aged between 4 and 12) who had undergone adenoidectomy at the ORL Institute of Siena were studied. One group (13) showed upper airway obstruction only and the other (11) showed chronic or recurrent adenoiditis with hypertrophy. The anatomic specimens were immediately transported to the laboratory to be processed.

Bacteriological Study. One gram of adenoid tissue from each patient was homogenized in 10 ml of saline solution and centrifuged. The sediment, diluted 1/10 in saline solution, was inoculated onto blood agar, blood agar-CNA, chocolate agar and chocolate agar-bacitracin. After 24 h of incubation at 37 °C the bacterial strains developed were counted and identified.

Immunological Study. The adenoid tissue, homogenized in 10 ml of saline solution, was centrifuged on Lymphoprep and the mononucleated cells were tested in order to

determine the percentage of the lymphocyte population. The percentage of the B lymphocytes was evaluated by means of fluoresceinated antibodies (IgD-IgM) (direct immunofluorescence method).

The percentage of T3, T4, and T8 lymphocytes was evaluated by means of the
indirect immunofluorescence method (addition of two different series of antibodies to the
cellular suspension: the first, monoclonal against lymphocyte antigens; the second, fluoresceinated against antibody proteins).

Results

The bacteriological findings are given in tables 1 and 2. Table 1 shows
a higher frequency of saprophytes or pathogens in the obstruction than in
the infection group. *H. influenzae* prevails in the obstruction group,
whereas *S. pneumoniae* prevails in the infection group.

As shown in table 2, we found at least one or more pathogens in all
(100%) of the cases of the infection group and in 69% of the cases of the
obstruction group. The difference is not statistically significant because of
the small number of cases.

The immunological findings are given in table 3, which shows the percentage of lymphocyte cells in the two groups studied. No differences are
noted between cells in either group.

Conclusions

The present study in accordance with other works has shown a higher
frequency of saprophyte flora from adenoid tissue in both groups of children. *H. influenzae* was isolated in our specimens more frequently than in
others. On the contrary, *S. aureus* was rarely isolated. These discrepancies
may be partially due to the brief period of study. The high frequency of
pathogens in the two groups could in theory justify an antibiotic treatment
for both. However, the antimicrobial therapy appears ineffective against
the pathogens (poor concentration of drug?) and against the saprophytes
(drug resistance?). Indeed we do not know the real role of the saprophyte
and pathogenic flora in recurrent adenoid phlogosis and secondary hypertrophy.

The immunological findings confirm that the adenoid tissue is a B-
lymphoid organ. Indeed the percentage of B lymphocytes is higher in adenoid tissue than in the blood. The percentage of T3 lymphocytes is in

Table 1. Bacteriologic findings in adenoid tissue after adenoidectomy

Isolates	Obstruction group (n = 13)	Infection group (n = 11)
No pathogenic *Neisseria* species	12	9
α-Hemolytic streptococci	10	7
γ-Hemolytic streptococci	8	5
Haemophilus spp., not *H. influenzae*	8	5
Staphylococcus, not *S. aureus*	2	4
Staphylococcus aureus	1	1
Corynebacterium spp.	1	–
Propionibacterium spp.	1	–
Haemophilus influenzae	10	6
Streptococcus pneumoniae	5	7
β-Hemolytic streptococci		
Group A	3	3
Group B	1	–
Group F	1	–
Total isolates	64	47

Table 2. Pathogens in adenoid tissue after adenoidectomy

Isolates	Obstruction group (n = 13)	Infection group (n = 11)
Pathogens (one or more strains)	9 (69%)	11 (100%)

Table 3. Percentage of lymphocyte cells in adenoid tissue after adenoidectomy

Lymphocytes	Obstruction group	Infection group
B	26%	28%
T3 (CD3)	34%	38%
T4 (CD4)	24%	23%
T8 (CD8)	7%	7%

agreement with other authors [6] and the T subsets are lower but proportional to those in the blood. The low percentage of T8 cells (suppressor) confirms the activity in antibody production by this organ.

References

1 De Dio RM, Tom LWC, McGowan KL, Wetmore RF, Handler SD, Potsic WP: Microbiology of the tonsils and adenoids in a pediatric population. Arch Otolaryngol Head Neck Surg 1988;114:763–765.
2 Brook I: Aerobic and anaerobic bacteriology of adenoids in children: a comparison between patients with chronic adenotonsillitis and adenoid hypertrophy. Laryngoscope 1981;91:378–382.
3 Kielmovitch IH, Keleti G, Bluestone GD, Wald ER, Gonzales C: Microbiology of obstructive tonsillar hypertrophy and recurrent tonsillitis. Arch Otolaryngol Head neck Surg 1989;115:721–724.
4 Bieluch VM, Chasin WD, Martin ET, Tally FP: Recurrent tonsillitis: histologic and bacteriologic evaluation. Ann Otol Rhinol Laryngol 1989;98:332–335.
5 Surow JB, Handler SD, Telian SA, Fleisher GR, Baranak CC: Bacteriology of tonsil surface and core in children. Laryngoscope 1989;99:261–266.
6 Lafont S, Haguenauer JP, Leval J, Revillard JP: Physiologie du tissu lymphoïde pharyngé; in Encycl Méd Chir (Paris) Otorhinolaryngol 1987;7:20498/A10, pp 1–8.

Dr. A. Piccini, Istituto di Clinica ORL, Università degli Studi di Siena,
I-53100 Siena (Italy)

Galioto GB (ed): Tonsils: A Clinically Oriented Update.
Adv Otorhinolaryngol. Basel, Karger, 1992, vol 47, pp 193–195

The Concept of Focal Infection of Tonsil

Toshihide Tabata

Department of Otorhinolaryngology, Wakayama Medical College,
Wakayama, Japan

The concept of focal infection was initially proposed by Pässler [1] at the beginning of this century. In 1939, Gutzeit and Parade [2] documented clinically that chronic inflammation in localized areas of the body could produce organic or functional injuries at distant sites where there were no clinical symptoms. However, there has been no clear evidence to support the concept of focal infection of tonsil.

The upper respiratory tract and oral cavity including the tonsil and teeth are commonly exposed to germs. There is no doubt that the tonsil, which consists of lymphoid tissue with crypt structure characteristics that present lymphoepithelial symbiosis, is exposed to infection at all times.

Recent advances in immunology have revealed the immunological function of tonsil, which contributes greatly to self-defense, because the tonsil contains all the lymphocyte sets necessary for immunosurveillance. In addition, it has become obvious that tonsil with chronic inflammation plays an important role in the occurrence of secondary diseases in the form of focal infection.

Japan has been active in this type of study, and many reports on basic and clinical research have been published. Referring to previous reports on the immunopathogenesis of focal infection of tonsil, a hypothesis is set forth in figure 1.

The tonsillar epithelium exposed to germs may change its surface antigenicity, stimulating the immunosurveillance system to respond by producing autoantibodies. The autoantibodies from the tonsil circulate through the vessels and finally precipitate onto surface tissue antigens in distant regions, causing a cross-reaction. Therefore, Arthus-type tissue

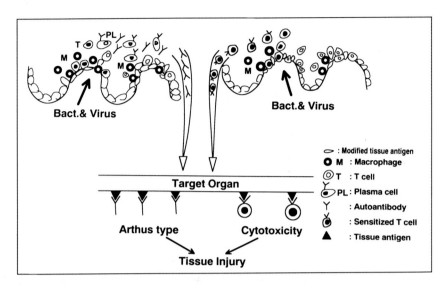

Fig. 1. Schematic drawing of tissue injury due to focal infection of tonsil.

injuries will, through the autoimmune system, be able to induce related diseases. On the other hand, if cell-mediated immunity is involved, the effector lymphocytes sensitized with modified epithelial antigen of tonsil due to germ infection will contribute to tissue injury at distant organs by cytotoxicity.

In Japan, experimental studies on the mechanism of focal infection, with special reference to immunology, have long been carried out. It is commonly accepted that the palmoplantar pustulosis of chronic, recurring disorders of the palm and sole is due to focal infection of tonsil, because tonsillectomy has been shown to be effective since the first report by Andrews et al. [3] in 1935. Therefore, numerous fundamental studies concerning the pathogenesis of this disease have been performed. It is clear that the immunopathogenesis, not only immune complexes of the Arthus-type, but also cytotoxicity of effector lymphocytes is closely related to the onset of disease.

Furthermore, it has been recognized that IgA nephropathy, which was reported by Berger [4] in 1969 and is assumed to be an immune complex-mediated glomerulonephritis, and chronic arthritis involving sternocosto-clavicular hyperostosis, as reported by Köhler in 1975 [5], are also closely related to chronic inflammation of the upper respiratory tract, including tonsil, because tonsillectomy is commonly effective. The pathogenesis, however, is not clear.

References

1   Pässler H: Über die Beziehungen einiger septischer Krankheitszustände zu chroni-
    scher Infektion der Mundhöhle. Verh Kongr Inn Med 1909;26:321.
2   Gutzeit K, Parade GW: Fokalinfektion. Ergeb Inn Med Kinderheilk 1939;57:613.
3   Andrews GC, Machalk GH: Pustular bacterid of the hand and feet. Arch Dermatol
    Syphilol 1953;32:837.
4   Berger J: IgA glomerular deposits in renal disease. Transplant Proc 1969;I:939.
5   Köhler H: Sterno-Kosto-Klavikularhyperosteose – ein bisher nicht beschriebenes
    Krankheitsbild. Dtsch Med Wochenschr 1975;100:1519.

T. Tabata, MD, Department of Otorhinolaryngology, Wakayama Medical College,
Nanaban-cho 27-banchi, Wakayama 640 (Japan)

Galioto GB (ed): Tonsils: A Clinically Oriented Update.
Adv Otorhinolaryngol. Basel, Karger, 1992, vol 47, pp 196–202

Focus Tonsils and Skin Diseases with Special Reference to Palmoplantar Pustulosis

Kiyonori Kuki, Takaaki Kimura, Yasuhiro Hayashi, Toshihide Tabata

Department of Otolaryngology, Wakayama Medical College,
Wakayama City, Japan

Pustulosis palmaris et plantaris (PPP) is a chronic recurrent pustular dermatosis localized to the palms and soles, and is characterized by the appearance of sterile, intraepidermal pustules [1]. The etiology of PPP is still not known, and the relation to psoriasis vulgaris is controversial. The dermatological synonyms of PPP include pustulosis palmoplantaris, persistent palmoplantar pustulosis, and pustular psoriasis of the extremities.

Treatment of PPP is associated with difficulty. The two conventional methods of treatment are corticosteroids and the removal of foci based on a focal infection theory. In 1935, Andrews and Machacek [2] described a close relationship of PPP to the presence of foci of bacterial infection, mainly on the teeth and tonsils. They stressed the importance of the tonsils as the focus of infection. Since then, tonsillectomy has played an important role in the treatment of this refractory dermatosis [3]. There are however opposing views on the validity of focal infection theory of PPP [4].

We studied 231 patients with PPP for therapeutic effectiveness of tonsillectomy on this disease. We also examined keratin and antikeratin antibodies both in the tonsils and on the skin of patients with PPP to clarify the relationship between the tonsils and this skin disorder.

Materials and Methods

Part I: We sent questionnaires to 231 patients, 118 men and 113 women (men:women = 1.04:1), who had been examined for the relationship between tonsils and the development of PPP in the Department of Otolaryngology, Wakayama Medical College Hospital, between 1980 and 1990. We received valid replies from 181 patients, who were divided into 119 tonsillectomized patients and 62 nontonsillectomized patients.

The effect of tonsillectomy was judged on a 4-grade scale: 'completely healed', 'markedly improved', 'partially improved' and 'unchanged'. These grades depended on Noda and Ura's [5] report. 'Completely healed' means the disappearance of eruptions; 'markedly improved', disappearance of pustules and vesicles without oral or topical treatment; 'partially improved', partial disappearance of pustules and vesicles, allowing their persistence to a level of 50% or more before tonsillectomy, and 'unchanged', the condition remained unchanged or worsened. Of these, 'completely healed' and 'markedly improved' were regarded as 'effective tonsillectomy', and 'partially improved' and 'unchanged' as 'ineffective tonsillectomy'.

Part II: To clarify the relationship between the tonsils and PPP, we performed an immunological study, placing a focus on keratin and keratin antibodies. We performed an enzyme-linked immunosorbent assay (ELISA) to examine antikeratin antibody in the sera by Hayashi and Tabata's [6] method.

Results

Part I: The ages of men ranged from 14 to 73 (average 43.21), and the ages of women ranged from 18 to 78 (average 45.56) (fig. 1).

Bacteriological examination of the tonsillar crypts: The tonsillar crypts were examined for microbiological inhabitants in 189 patients whose cultures revealed the following pathogenic and nonpathogenic microorganisms: *Streptococcus viridans* in 126 patients; *Staphylococcus aureus* in 21; *Streptococcus hemolyticus* in 15; *Streptococcus pyogenes* in 6; *Neisseria* in 6, and *Klebsiella pneumoniae* in 4 patients.

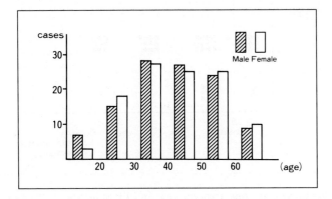

Fig. 1. Age and sex distribution of 231 PPP patients.

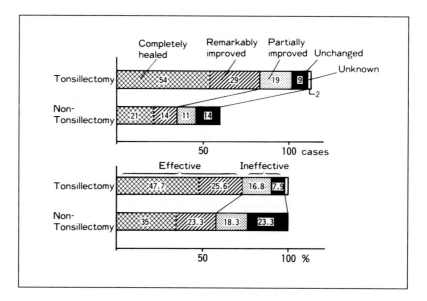

Fig. 2. Therapeutic effect of tonsillectomy for PPP patients.

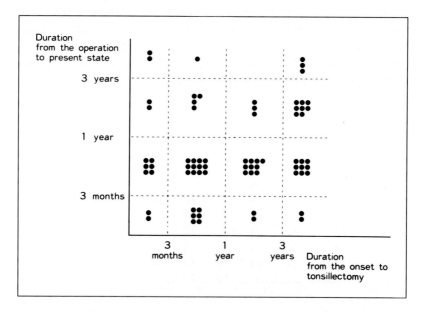

Fig. 3. Relation between the time from the onset of PPP to tonsillectomy and the course of healing.

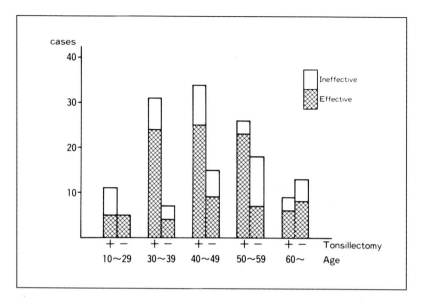

Fig. 4. Relation between patients' ages and the effect of tonsillectomy.

Therapeutic effect of tonsillectomy (fig. 2): Of the 117 tonsillectom-ized patients, 'completely healed' and 'markedly improved' were noted in 87 patients (76%). Of the 62 nontonsillectomized patients, 'completely healed' and 'markedly improved' were noted in 36 (58%). The rate of effectiveness in the tonsillectomized patient group was therefore higher than the rate in the nontonsillectomized patient group. The rate of 'un-changed' was 7% in the tonsillectomized patient group and 21% in the nontonsillectomized patient group.

Relation between the time from the onset of PPP to tonsillectomy and the course of healing (fig. 3): Of 83 of the 87 'completely healed' and 'markedly improved' put together, 50 (60%) got rid of pustules within 1 year, and 72 (82%) within 3 years, after tonsillectomy.

Relation between patients' ages and the effect of tonsillectomy (fig. 4): The effect of tonsillectomy on the treatment of PPP was relatively high in the patients who were elderly at the onset of the disease.

Relation between the history of tonsillitis and the effect of tonsillecto-my: The experience of tonsillectomy was confirmed in 16 patients, in whom the rate of effectiveness of tonsillectomy was 88%. Meanwhile, the

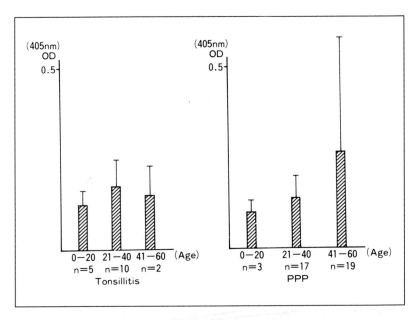

Fig. 5. Antikeratin antibody titers of IgG in the sera of patients with recurrent tonsillitis and patients with PPP.

rate of effectiveness of tonsillectomy in those who had not experienced tonsillitis was 68%.

Part II: The levels of antikeratin antibody in the serum (fig. 5): Aged patients with PPP had significantly higher IgG antibody titers than the control patients who consisted of adult patients with recurrent tonsillitis.

Changes in serum antikeratin antibody titers in patients with PPP (fig. 6): Titers of both IgG and IgM antibodies began to decrease after tonsillectomy.

Discussion

Andrews and Machacek's [2] report in 1935 has heretofore prompted many Japanese researchers to investigate into the etiology of PPP. Many of them have agreed to the effect of tonsillectomy on this refractory skin disorder taking account of the focal infection theory. There are however

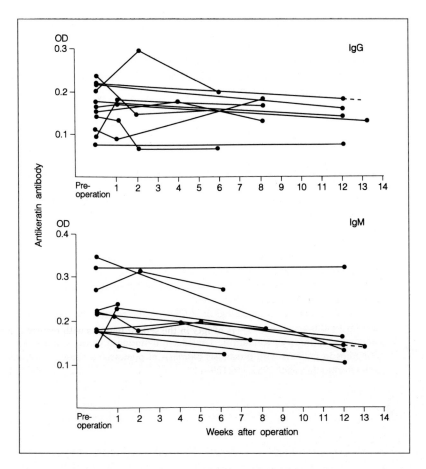

Fig. 6. Changes in serum antikeratin antibody titers (IgG and IgM) in patients with PPP after tonsillectomy.

opposing views to the reported effect of tonsillectomy, which classify the effect of tonsillectomy as a nonspecific surgical intervention. We examined 138 patients with PPP for the effect of tonsillectomy on the course of PPP by questionnaires. Analyses of the 118 replies showed that three fourths of the tonsillectomized patients had either completely healed or markedly improved.

We however have had no rigid criteria for the indication for tonsillectomy in the treatment of PPP. The serum titers of keratin antibody in patients with PPP were higher than those in the control patients and tended to decrease after tonsillectomy. This finding suggests an important role of the antikeratin antibody in the development of PPP [6, 7]. Further investigation is necessary for tonsillectomy to be classified as a reliable means of the treatment of PPP.

References

1   Uehara M, Ofuji S: The morphogenesis of pustulosis palmaris et plantaris. Arch Dermatol 1974;109:518–520.
2   Andrews GC, Machacek GF: Pustular bacterids of the hands and feet. Arch Dermatol Syphilis 1935;32:837–847.
3   Ono T: Evaluation of tonsillectomy as a treatment for pustulosis palmaris et plantaris. J Dermatol 1977;4:163–172.
4   Hellgren L, Mobacken H: Pustulosis palmaris et plantaris. Prevalence, clinical observation and prognosis. Acta Dermatovenereol 1971;51:284–288.
5   Noda Y, Ura M: Pustulosis palmaris et plantaris due to tonsillar focal infection. Acta Otolaryngol 1983(suppl 401):22–30.
6   Hayashi Y, Tabata T: Immunological studies on the relation between tonsil and pustulosis palmaris et plantaris. Acta Otolaryngol 1988(suppl 454):227–236.
7   Yamanaka N, Shido F, Kataura A: Tonsillectomy-induced changes in anti-keratin antibodies in patients with pustulosis palmaris et plantaris: a clinical correlation. Arch Otorhinolaryngol 1989;246:109–112.

Dr. K. Kuki, Department of Otolaryngology, Wakayama Medical College, 27-7 Bancho, Wakayama 640 (Japan)

Galioto GB (ed): Tonsils: A Clinically Oriented Update.
Adv Otorhinolaryngol. Basel, Karger, 1992, vol 47, pp 203–207

The Effect of Tonsillectomy and Its Postoperative Clinical Course in IgA Nephropathy with Chronic Tonsillitis

Yu Masuda, Shinichiro Tamura, Nobuyoshi Sugiyama

Department of Otolaryngology, Okayama University Medical School, Okayama, Japan

IgA nephropathy has a high incidence in chronic glomerulonephritis and 20% of the patients suffering from this disease in Japan are thought to develop into renal failure. The pathogenesis of this disease is considered to be associated with the tonsils, especially in cases with chronic tonsillitis.

We present new data mainly concerning long-term results of tonsillectomy for IgA nephropathy cases with chronic tonsillitis.

Materials and Method

Twenty-six cases of IgA nephropathy, associated with chronic tonsillitis and all considered on the clinical effect of tonsillectomy using the postoperative effect on the proteinuria as a standard, took part in the study. Postoperative changes of several clinical symptoms and immunological factors were also investigated to obtain further recognition of the postoperative effect on this disease.

Results

We used postoperative changes of urinary findings for the judgement of the clinical effect of tonsillectomy. Table 1 shows the postoperative clinical effect in all cases, according to our judgement. The improved case results in 46.2% at the time of 2 years after operation, but 50% at the time of 1 year after operation. In other words, the clinical effect deteriorates from year to year after the operation.

Table 1. General view of clinical effect (2 years after the operation) in 26 IgA nephropathy cases with chronic tonsillitis

Grade of effect		Cases
Improved cases	excellent	5 ⎫ 46.2%
	good	7 ⎭
Not improved cases	unchanged	13
	worse	1

One year after the operation, 10 of 20 cases improved.

Table 2. Clinical effect in hematuria (n = 26)

Grade	Preoperative cases	Postoperative cases	
		after 1 year	after 2 years
0	0 ⎫ 7.7%	4 ⎫ 46.2%	2 ⎫ 69.2%
1	2 ⎭	8 ⎭	16 ⎭
2	8	6	3
3	16	8	5
Total	26	improved cases 16 61.5%	improved cases 19 73.1%

On the other hand, postoperative changes of hematuria were observed (table 2). The slight grade cases including grade 0 and 1 are 7.7% of all cases. However, the slight grade cases increased to 46.2% at the time of 1 year after operation and it increased to 69.2% at the time of 2 years after operation.

The postoperative changes of renal function in 13 cases are shown in table 3. We had 10 cases with preoperative renal hypofunction and 6 of them were improved to normal renal function at the time of 1 year after operation. Furthermore, several immunological factors were measured to investigate changes of levels after the operation.

A preoperative high level of serum IgA was observed in 13 cases (table 4). The mean level in preoperative high level cases decreases at the time of 2 years after operation and there is a significant difference between

Table 3. Changes in renal (Ccr) function (n = 13)

Case No.	Sex	Age	Grade of histo- pathol.	Ccr, l/day		Effect
				preop.	postop. (1 year)	
5	F	59	P1	85	108	FD/improved
7	F	23	1	74	62	FD
10	M	15	2	65	112	FD/improved
11	M	14	1	90	71	FD
14	F	39	3	95	115	FD/improved
15	F	15	1	82	86	FD
16	F	19	3	147	121	
17	F	30	2	97	115	FD/improved
18	F	61	1	88	117	FD/improved
19	M	18	2	186	132	
20	F	29	1	125	103	
24	F	28	3	73	72	FD
25	F	54	2	62	98	FD/improved
Mean				97.6 ± 35.4	100.9 ± 21.7 (NS)	6/10 improved

Normal limit of Ccr: > 100 l/day. FD = Functional disturbance.

Table 4. Changes in serum IgA level of 13 cases with high level of sIgA (mean ± SD)

	Preoperatively	2 years postoperatively	
Mean of sIgA level, mg/dl	450.7 ± 71.6	356.8 ± 92	$p < 0.01$
Cases with high level of sIgA	13	6	

Normal sIgA level < 350 mg/dl.

them. Besides, the number of the high level cases decreases postoperatively, such as from 10 to 6 cases. It means that the other 7 cases begin to have a normal level of serum IgA postoperatively. We have few cases with a preoperative high level of polymeric IgA. However, the number of high level cases clearly decreases at the time of 2 years after operation. We have also very few cases to evaluate the postoperative clinical effect on CIC level.

Table 5. Findings of renal biopsies

	Histological findings						Immunofluorescent patterns					
	MC	MM	GS	adhe-sion	cres-cent	int. scarring	IgA	IgG	IgM	C3	Clq	fibrin-ogen
Case 1												
Preop.	+	+f	–	–	–	–	+	–	–	–	–	+
Postop.[1]	–	±f	–	–	–	–	+	–	+	+	+	+
Case 2												
Preop.	2+	+	–	+	–	–	+	–	–	+	–	+
Postop.	–	+	–	+	–	–	+	–	–	–	–	–
Case 3												
Preop.	2+	2+d	+	+	+	+	+	–	–	+	–	–
Postop.	–	+f	+	+	+
fibrous	+	+	–	–	–	–	–

Grades: + = mild; 2+ = moderate; d = diffuse global; f = focal segmental.
MC = Proliferation of mesangial cell; MM = increase of mesangial matrix; GS = global sclerosis; int. scarring = interstitial scarring.
[1] Postoperative biopsies were performed 2 years after operation.

At the end of this report, 3 cases who underwent follow-up renal biopsies 2 years after operation are presented. The postoperative clinical effect by tonsillectomy was excellent in these 3 cases.

The histopathological and immunofluorescent findings before and 2 years after operation are shown in table 5. The rebiopsy findings reveal the tendency of histological improvement in mesangial cell and matrix. Also in immunofluorescent patterns, depositions of C3 and fibrinogen postoperatively disappear or decrease. However, the IgA deposition clearly continues in all cases, in spite of a general decrease of activity in this disease.

Discussion

From our experience of postoperative observations in the tonsillectomized cases of IgA nephropathy with chronic tonsillitis, 60% or more of operated cases were improved in urinary findings and serum IgA level and levels of several other immunological factors [1, 3]. Furthermore, in some cases the CH_{50} level decreased to the normal range after operation [4]. This improvement of clinical findings led us to think tonsillectomy is useful for removing the source of pathogenetic IgA production. However, the clinical effect deteriorates from year to year after the operation, as shown in table 1. Besides, our study of follow-up renal biopsy showed that IgA deposition continues in spite of the improvement of clinical signs. It may mean that removed tonsils give place to other tonsils in production of pathogenetic IgA.

Conclusions

To conclude: (1) tonsillectomy may be clinically and pathogenetically effective in IgA nephropathy with chronic tonsillitis; (2) some of the improved cases show recurrence of clinical symptoms 1 year or more after the operation, and (3) IgA deposition in the mesangial areas in the kidney continues even after tonsillectomy.

References

1   Sugiyama N, Masuda Y: Effect of tonsillectomy in 8 cases with IgA nephropathy accompanied with chronic tonsillitis. Jpn J Tonsil 1983;22:132–137.
2   Sugiyama N, Masuda Y: Relationship between IgA nephropathy and tonsillectomy. Clinical and immunological study. Jpn J Tonsil 1985;24:237–243.
3   Masuda Y, Terasawa K, Kawakami S, Ogura Y, Sugiyama N: Clinical and immunological study of IgA nephropathy before and after tonsillectomy. Acta Otolaryngol (Stockh) 1988(suppl 454):248–255.
4   Masuda Y, Uno K, Ogura Y, Komoda K: The effect of tonsillectomy on IgA nephropathy – A case report. Jpn J Tonsil 1984;23:118–122.

Dr. Yu Masuda, Department of Otolaryngology, Okayama University Medical School, 2-5-1, Shikata-cho, Okayama 700 (Japan)

Galioto GB (ed): Tonsils: A Clinically Oriented Update.
Adv Otorhinolaryngol. Basel, Karger, 1992, vol 47, pp 208–212

On Arthropathy with Special Reference to Sternocostoclavicular Hyperostosis

Fumiaki Shido, Makoto Hamamoto, Yasushi Kukuminato,
Akikatsu Kataura

Department of Otolaryngology, Sapporo Medical College, Sapporo, Japan

It is well known that the palatine tonsils may play an important role as a focus in the pathogenesis of secondary diseases in the skin, bone, joint, and kidney. A number of clinical reports suggest that the various independent diseases such as pustulosis palmaris et plantaris (PPP), psoriasis vulgaris (PV), sternocostoclavicular hyperostosis (SCCH), rheumatoid arthritis (RA), and IgA nephropathy, may have a tonsillar origin and be improved by tonsillectomy.

In the present paper, we report on the effect of tonsillectomy in the treatment of osteoarthropathy with special reference to SCCH, a newly proposed clinical entity by Köhler et al. [1].

Patients and Methods

We performed tonsillectomy for the treatment of 64 patients with SCCH, which were combined with PPP in 76.6%, 14 patients with RA, which were combined with PPP in 21.4% and SCCH in 28.6%, and 22 patients with seronegative arthritis, which were combined with PPP in 31.8%, SCCH in 36.4%, and erythema in 27.3%. On the basis of clinical data from the patients followed up over 6 months after tonsillectomy, we evaluated the clinical effects against the secondary diseases by the operation.

Fig. 1. Typical appearance of the swelling in bilateral sternoclavicular joints of a 54-year-old female patient with SCCH.

Fig. 2. Abnormal uptake of technetium-99m in the right clavicular bone and bilateral sternoclavicular joints of a 58-year-old female patient with SCCH.

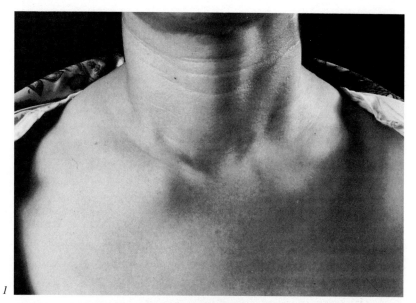

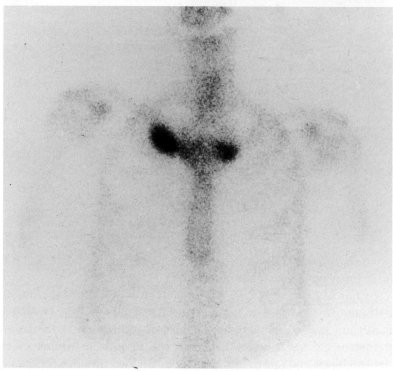

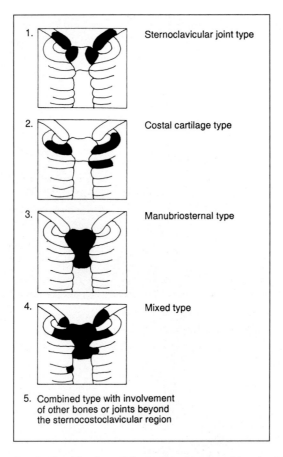

1. Sternoclavicular joint type

2. Costal cartilage type

3. Manubriosternal type

4. Mixed type

5. Combined type with involvement
   of other bones or joints beyond
   the sternocostoclavicular region

Fig. 3. Classification of five regional types of involved lesions in a patient with SCCH.

Results

Sex Differences. Sex differences in osteoarthropathy are found to be three times more dominant in females.

Clinical Types of SCCH. The patients with SCCH had the swelling of sternum, clavicles and/or sternocostoclavicular joints (fig. 1). The bone scintigram showed the abnormal uptake of technetium in the lesions of sternocostoclavicular bones and joints (fig. 2) with or without other peripheral bones and joints. SCCH could be divided into five regional types based on mainly the involved lesion such as sternoclavicular joint type, costal cartilage type, manubriosternal type, mixed type, and combined type with involvement of other bones or joints beyond the sternocostoclavicular region (fig. 3).

Effect of Tonsillectomy in the Treatment of SCCH. The results of the clinical observations of 52 cases with SCCH showed 50% or more improvement of the sternocostoclavicular pain in 84.6% of the patients after tonsillectomy.

Effect of Tonsillectomy in the Treatment of RA. The results of the clinical observations of 12 cases with RA showed 50% or more improvement of the joint pain in 83.3% of the patients after tonsillectomy.

Effect of Tonsillectomy in the Treatment of Seronegative Arthritis. The results of the clinical observations of 18 cases with seronegative arthritis showed 50% or more improvement of the joint pain in 88.9% of the patients after tonsillectomy.

Effect of Tonsillectomy in the Treatment of PPP Combined with SCCH. Considering the clinical observations in 43 SCCH cases with PPP, 50% or more improvement in the skin lesion was recognized in 83.7% of patients after tonsillectomy. The long-term result of improvement rate in patients with PPP was found to progress well according to time course, until 80% of disappearance and 100% of improvement by 51 months after tonsillectomy.

Discussion

Clinical Entity

PPP, which is characterized by the sterile pustules on the palms and/or soles, appears to be the most common secondary disease in the tonsillar focal infections [2].

SCCH, which is characterized by the hyperostosis of the sternum and middle part of the clavicle, synostosis of the sternoclavicular joint with involvement of the two first ribs as well as a thickening and increase in breadth of the sternum, is a new clinical entity reported first by Köhler et al. [1] in 1975. SCCH tends to be complicated with PPP, both of which may be improved by tonsillectomy. Although Sonozaki et al. [3] reported the complex of PPP and SCCH as pustulotic arthro-osteitis (PAO), we consider the PAO as a disease complex in tonsillogenic dermatoosteoarthropathy caused by a common pathogenetic origin in the tonsils.

Diagnostic Criteria

The diagnostic criteria in SCCH as a secondary disease of tonsillar focal infections were established under the basis of comparative evaluations between the preoperative examination and the postoperative clinical course as follows: (a) clinical episodes of anamnestic tonsillitis which caused or exacerbated the sternocostoclavicular pain; (b) a positive result of body temperature or significant increase of sternocostoclavicular pain in the provocation test of tonsils by using a direct ultra-short wave method; (c) significant relief of sternocostoclavicular pain in negation test of tonsils by local injections with Impletol solution.

Effect of Tonsillectomy in the Treatment of Osteoarthropathy

Although Köhler et al. [1] suggested that infectious diseases generally worsened the symptoms, the pathogenesis of SCCH has yet been unclear. Umetani et al. [4] first described that the symptoms of 2 patients with SCCH were improved after tonsillectomy.

Our results revealed that SCCH, RA, seronegative arthritis, and PPP tended to be combined with each other and had a close relationship with tonsil focus. These findings suggest that RA, seronegative arthritis as well as SCCH may have a tonsillar origin and be improved by tonsillectomy.

References

1 Köhler H, Uehlinger E, Kutzner J, Weihrauch TR, Wilbert L, Schuster R: Sterno-kosto-klavikuläre Hyperostose – ein bisher nicht beschriebenes Krankheitsbild. Dtsch Med Wschr 1975;100:1519–1523.
2 Yamanaka N, Shido F, Kataura A: Tonsillectomy-induced changes in anti-keratin antibodies in patients with pustulosis palmaris et plantaris: a clinical correlation. Arch Otorhinolaryngol 1989;246:109–112.
3 Sonozaki H, Mitsui H, Miyanaga Y, Okitsu K, Igarashi M, Hayashi Y, Matsuura M, Azuma A, Okai K, Wakashima M: Clinical features of 53 cases with pustulotic arthro-osteitis. Ann Rheum Dis 1981;40:547–553.
4 Umetani Y, Ono T, Igarashi F, Endo T, Yamagishi M, Suzuki M, Ino H, Takahashi H, Tojo T, Murasawa A: Two cases of sterno-, costo-clavicular hyperostosis supposed of the tonsillar focal infection. Jpn J Tonsil 1980;19:82–87.

Dr. F. Shido, Department of Otolaryngology, Sapporo Medical College, S-1, W-16, Chuo-ku, Sapporo 060 (Japan)

Galioto GB (ed): Tonsils: A Clinically Oriented Update.
Adv Otorhinolaryngol. Basel, Karger, 1992, vol 47, pp 213–221

Immunohistochemical Comparison between Multinucleated Giant Cells Which Appear Frequently in the Tonsils of Patients with Pustulosis palmaris et plantaris and in Other Granulomatous Inflammatory Lesions

Makoto Kawaguchi[a], *Takeshi Sakai*[a], *Shin Ishizawa*[a],
Fuyumi Shimoda[b], *Kazuhisa Kitagawa*[c], *Tomoaki Kaji*[d],
Fumitomo Koizumi[a]

[a] Second Department of Pathology, Faculty of Medicine, Toyama Medical and
Pharmaceutical University; [b] Section of Japanese Oriental Medicine,
Toyama Medical and Pharmaceutical University Hospital, and Departments of
[c] Otolaryngology and [d] Dermatology, Toyama Prefectural Central Hospital,
Toyama, Japan

Pustulosis palmaris et plantaris (PPP) is a well-known skin disease closely related to tonsillar focal infections. Tonsillectomy is a frequently applied remedy which is very effective in curing this disease [1]. Multinucleated giant cells appear in patients with PPP more frequently than in patients with persistent angina. Multinucleated giant cells appear in the lymphepithelial symbiosis and subepithelial areas [2, 3].

Multinucleated giant cells appear in different tissues in various inflammatory states and pathological conditions [4, 5]. The cause and the mechanism of the giant cell's formation in the tonsils of patients with PPP, however, is not known. The origin of the giant cells might be important in solving the tonsil's immunological role in the development of this skin lesion.

In this study, to obtain a precise analysis of the cellular origin of the giant cells, paraffin-embedded sections of the tonsils were immunohistochemically stained with macrophage immunologic markers. CD68 is known as the best macrophage marker [6]. Lysozyme is also a well-known cytoplasmic and lysosomal bacteriolytic enzyme of monocyte/macrophage series [7, 8]. MAC387 detects squamous epithelium and many cells in the monocyte/macrophage series [9]. S-100 protein (S-100) is a marker for a subset of cells known as the dendritic cells of the lymph nodes, which are: Langerhans' cells, interdigitating cells and follicular dendritic cells [10, 11]. Moreover, S-100 is known to have immunoreactivity not only with dendritic cells but also monocyte/macrophage series [12, 13].

We investigated the immunoreactivity of these antibodies to the multinucleated giant cells in the tonsils obtained from patients with PPP. Then, we compared these results of PPP to the immunoreactivity of multinucleated giant cells of other granulomatous lesions, which are tuberculous lymphadenitis, sarcoidosis and foreign body granulomas. The origin and the heterogeneity of these giant cells are discussed in this report.

Materials and Methods

Materials

Four cases of palatine tonsils were obtained from patients with PPP undergoing tonsillectomies. Tuberculous lymphadenitis, sarcoidosis of myocardium and lymph nodes, and foreign body granulomas of the skin were obtained from the files of our routine pathology laboratory. Each 4 cases of these diseases were used in this study. These materials had been fixed in formalin and embedded in paraffin.

Methods

Avidin-biotin complex method was used to stain 3-μm sections using Vectastain Elite ABC Kit (Vector Laboratories, Burlingame, Calif., USA). CD68 (monoclonal mouse anti-human macrophage, KP1), rabbit anti-human lysozyme, MAC387 (monoclonal mouse anti-human myeloid/histiocyte antigen), and rabbit anti-cow S-100 were purchased from Dakopatts, Denmark. Tissue sections were dewaxed, trypsinized (0.1%) at 37°C for 30 min and incubated with 5% goat serum. Tissues were then incubated 30 min with antibodies, CD68 (1:20), lysozyme (1:400), MAC387 (1:400) and S-100 (1:300). Incubation with biotinylated anti-rabbit and anti-mouse IgG was followed by treatment with avidin-biotin peroxidase. Endogenous peroxidase was inhibited by preincubation in 1% H_2O_2 in PBS for 15 min. The sections were finally incubated with 0.03% H_2O_2 and 0.06% 3,3'-diaminobenzidine for 4 min. Two sections of each tissue served as negative controls. In these sections, the primary antibody was replaced by equivalently diluted nonimmune rabbit serum (Dakopatts) and nonimmune mouse IgG (Tago, Calif., USA). No positive reaction was observed in the control sections.

Results

The immunostaining results by CD68, lysozyme, MAC387 and S-100 are summarized in table 1 for each giant cell lesion.

Table 1. Immunoreactivity of multinucleated giant cells

	CD68			Lysozyme			MAC387			S-100		
	−	+	++	−	+	++	−	+	++	−	+	++
PPP (4 cases)	0	1	75[1]	0	5	45	28	5	0	1	31	12
Tuberculous lymphadenitis (4 cases)	0	31	192[1]	3	14	116	87	4	0	74	0	0
Sarcoidosis (4 cases)	0	93	108[1]	0	89	163	104	6	0	77	107	0
Foreign body granuloma (4 cases)	0	6	328[1]	49	21	168	116	56	5	88	22	0

Grades of staining: − = no immunoreactivity; + = slight immunoreactivity; ++ = intense immunoreactivity.
[1] Total number of giant cells which were stained intensely with CD68 from 4 cases in each disease.
One slide of the tissue specimen was observed in each case. The size of each specimen varied, so the counted number of giant cells varied in each case. The other numbers in this table are also calculated and totaled in the same way from 4 cases in each disease.

CD68

CD68 immunoreactivity was found in all of the multinucleated giant cells in the tonsils of PPP, tuberculous lymphadenitis, sarcoidosis and foreign body granulomas (fig. 1).

Lysozyme

Lysozyme was detected in the majority of the giant cells in the lesions of PPP, tuberculous lymphadenitis and sarcoidosis (fig. 2A–C). A few cells did not show lysozyme immunoreactivity in the tuberculous lymphadenitis. In the foreign body granulomas, most of the giant cells showed lysozyme immunoreactivity; however, no reactivity was found in some cells (fig. 2D).

MAC387

The majority of the giant cells of PPP, tuberculous lymphadenitis and sarcoidosis, showed no MAC387 immunoreactivity; however, some giant cells were weakly stained by MAC387 (fig. 3A–C). In the foreign body granulomas, some cells showed intense MAC387 reactivity (fig. 3D).

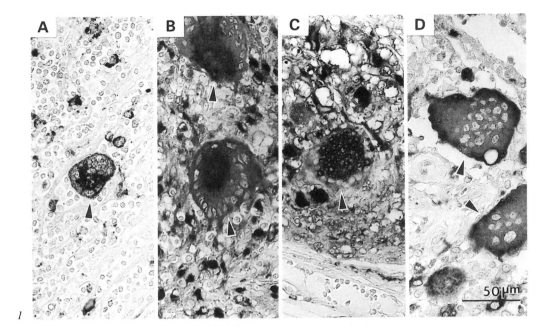

Fig. 1. CD68 immunoreactivity in the giant cells of (*A*) PPP, (*B*) tuberculous lymphadenitis, (*C*) sarcoidosis and (*D*) foreign body granuloma. The giant cells (arrows) of these lesions are all intensely stained. In *A* and *D*, positive macrophages are scattered around the giant cells. In *B* and *C*, epithelioid cells are stained.

Fig. 2. Lysozyme immunoreactivity in the giant cells of (*A*) PPP, (*B*) tuberculous lymphadenitis, (*C*) sarcoidosis and (*D1, 2*) foreign body granuloma. In *A*, the giant cell (arrow) shows intense immunoreactivity. Intensely positive cells and weakly positive dendritic shaped cells are scattered around the giant cell. In *B* and *C*, the giant cells (arrows) and epithelioid cells are stained. The giant cells in *D1* (arrows) showed immunoreactivity; however, the giant cell in *D2* (arrow) does not show any reactivity. In *D2*, note neutrophils around the giant cell are intensely stained.

Fig. 3. MAC387 immunoreactivity in the giant cells of (*A1, 2*) PPP, (*B1, 2*) tuberculous lymphadenitis, (*C*) sarcoidosis and (*D1, 2*) foreign body granuloma. The giant cell in *A1* (arrow) shows weak immunoreactivity; however, the giant cell in *A2* (arrow) does not show any reactivity. The MAC387 immunoreactivity to the tonsillar squamous epithelium indicates that giant cells are typically located near the scattered squamous epithelium. In *B1*, the giant cell (arrow) and epithelioid cells are stained weakly positive. In *B2, C* and *D2*, the giant cells (arrows) do not show any reactivity. The giant cell in *D1* (arrow), however, shows intense immunoreactivity. In *D1* and *D2*, some positive cells are scattered around the giant cells.

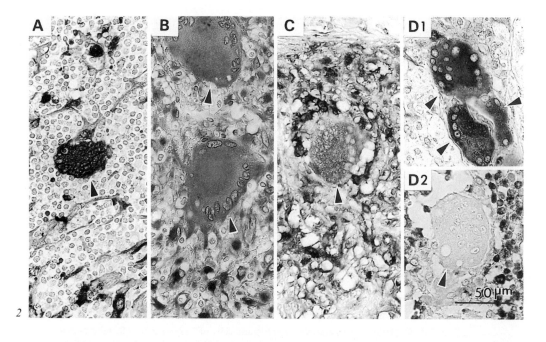

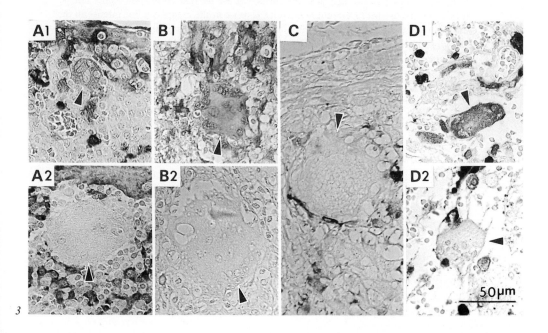

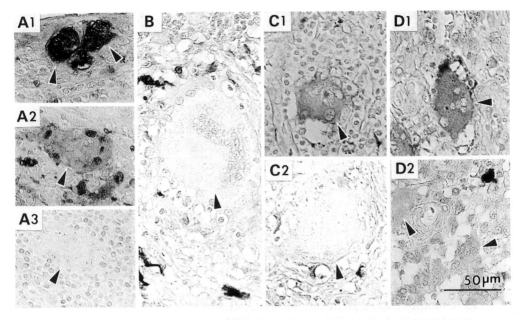

Fig. 4. S-100 immunoreactivity in the giant cells of (*A1–3*) PPP, (*B*) tuberculous lymphadenitis, (*C1, 2*) sarcoidosis and (*D1, 2*) foreign body granuloma. The giant cells in *A1* (arrows) which are located near the surface of the lacunar epithelium, show intense immunoreactivity. In *A2,* immunoreactivity is weak in the cytoplasm but intense in the nuclei. In *A3,* the giant cell (arrow) does not show immunoreactivity. In *B,* the giant cell (arrow) and epithelioid cells do not show immunoreactivity. S-100-positive dendritic cells are scattered around the giant cell. The giant cells in *C1* (arrow) and *D1* (arrow) show a slight immunoreactivity; however, the giant cells in *C2* and *D2* (arrows) do not show any reactivity.

S-100

The majority of giant cells of PPP showed weak to moderately positive S-100 stains in the cytoplasm. Some cells showed intense S-100 immuno-reactivity; however, a very small population of cells did not show any reactivity (fig. 4A). The stains by S-100 were distributed in the cytoplasm and in some nuclei. S-100 immunoreactivity of nuclei varied in degree from cell to cell. In some of the giant cells, none of the nuclei showed S-100 reactivity. In the other types of cells, however, a few to many of the nuclei showed intense reactivity. The giant cells of tuberculous lymphadenitis showed no S-100 immunoreactivity (fig. 4B). Some giant cells of sarcoidosis and foreign body granulomas showed weak S-100 immunoreactivity. Reactivity in the nuclei, however, could not be found in the giant cells of these lesions (fig. 4C, D).

Discussion

The existence of multinucleated giant cells found in the tissues is always considered to be abnormal [4, 5]. We easily observe the inflammatory giant cells, which responded regularly to a wide variety of stimuli. These types of giant cells are thought to be derived from fusion of resident macrophages or their precursors [14, 15].

Approximately 90% of palatine tonsils which were obtained from patients with PPP, contain multinucleated giant cells [3]. The presence of CD68 reactivity and lysozyme in all of the giant cells of PPP provided us considerable support that cells of monocyte/macrophage series fused to form multinucleated giant cells in the tonsils. This is the same as in other granulomatous lesions. The presence of CD68 in the PPP and other granulomatous lesions indicates that CD68 may be the best marker for detecting all multinucleated giant cells in any lesion.

Lysozyme was not present in some of the giant cells in the tuberculous lymphadenitis and foreign body granulomas. Multinucleated giant cells observed in the PPP and other granulomatous lesions were also characterized by the variable immunoreactivity of MAC387 and S-100. These results suggest that the fusion and formation may be induced by some heterogenetic cells.

MAC387 is said to be a more reliable marker for reactive histiocytes (infiltrating macrophages) than lysozyme [9]. MAC387 showed more reactivity in the giant cells of foreign body granulomas than in other granulomatous lesions. It leads us to believe that in the foreign body granulomas, the monocytes and MAC387-positive infiltrating macrophages are likely to fuse together to form giant cells.

Regezi et al. [8] indicate that multinucleated giant cells from various pathologic lesions do not show any S-100 reactivity. Koizumi et al. [3] also state that the giant cells in the tonsils do not show any S-100 reactivity. Our results were different from those of Regezi et al. [8] and Koizumi et al. [3]. It showed that S-100 was detected in the giant cells of PPP and also in other granulomatous lesions. These differences may be related to several factors, such as effects of fixation on antigen preservation or staining procedures.

Takahashi et al. [12] suggest that S-100 alpha subunit immunoreactivity is detected not only in blood monocytes and macrophages, but also in epithelioid cells, Langerhans' giant cells and foreign body giant cells. This supports our immunostaining results using S-100. Takahashi et al. [12] also state that alpha subunit is detected in the cytoplasm, but not in the nuclei of macrophages. In contrast, S-100 beta subunit, which reacts with Langerhans' cells and interdigitating cells, is located throughout the cytoplasm and nuclei. S-100 immunoreactivities of some nuclei in the giant cells of tonsils resembled beta subunits' reactivity. Whether or not interdigitating cells or Langerhans' cells are participants like macrophages in the formation of giant cells, could not be determined from our study alone.

It is concluded that (1) multinucleated giant cells in the tonsils of PPP are probably derived from CD68-positive macrophages; (2) high frequency of S-100 immunoreactivity and the presence of reactivity in the nuclei are characteristic features of multinucleated giant cells in the tonsils from PPP patients, and (3) in the PPP and other granulomatous inflammatory lesions, the formation of multinucleated giant cells may be induced by some heterogenetic cells.

References

1   Ono T, Jono M, Kito M, Tomoa T, Kageshita T, Egawa K, Kuriya N: Evaluation of tonsillectomy as a treatment for pustulosis palmaris et plantaris. Acta Otolaryngol 1983(suppl 401):12–16.
2   Koizumi F, Kurashige Y: Multinucleated giant cells in the palatine tonsil of three patients with pustulosis palmaris et plantaris. Acta Otolaryngol 1983(suppl 401): 75–78.
3   Koizumi F, Kurashige Y, Nakagawa H, Watanabe Y, Kaji T, Kitagawa K: Multinucleated giant cells in the palatine tonsil. (In Japanese.) Jpn J Tonsil 1986;25:163–168.
4   Black MM, Epstein WL: Formation of multinucleate giant cells in organized epithelioid cell granulomas. Am J Pathol 1974;74:263–274.
5   Chambers TJ: Multinucleate giant cells. J Pathol 1978;126:125–148.
6   Pulford KAF, Rigney EM, Micklem KJ, Jones M, Stross WP, Gatter KC, Mason DY: KP1: a new monoclonal antibody that detects a monocyte/macrophage associated antigen in routinely processed tissue sections. J Clin Pathol 1989;42:414–421.
7   Van Furth R, Raeburn JA, van Zwet TL: Characteristics of human mononuclear phagocytes. Blood 1979;54:485–500.

8   Regezi JA, Zarbo RJ, Lloyd RV: Muramidase, α_1-antitrypsin, α_1-antichymotrypsin, and S-100 protein immunoreactivity in giant cell lesions. Cancer 1987;59:64–68.

9   Brandtzaeg P, Dale I, Fagerhol MK: Distribution of a formalin-resistant myelomo-nocytic antigen (L1) in human tissues. Am J Clin Pathol 1987;87:681–699.

10   Takahashi K, Yamaguchi H, Ishizeki J, Nakajima T, Nakazato Y: Immunohisto-chemical and immunoelectron microscopic localization of S-100 protein in the interdigitating reticulum cells of the human lymph node. Virchows Arch [Cell Pathol] 1981;37:125–135.

11   Carbone A, Poletti A, Manconi R, Volpe R, Santi L: Demonstration of S-100 protein distribution in human lymphoid tissues by the avidin-biotin complex immunostain-ing method. Hum Pathol 1985;16:1157–1164.

12   Takahashi K, Isobe T, Ohtsuki Y, Sonobe H, Takeda I, Akagi T: Immunohistochem-ical localization and distribution of S-100 proteins in the human lymphoreticular system. Am J Pathol 1984;116:497–503.

13   Haimoto H, Hosoda S, Kato K: Differential distribution of immunoreactive S-100-α and S-100-β proteins in normal nonnervous human tissues. Lab Invest 1987;57: 489–498.

14   Hassan NF, Kamani N, Meszaros MM, Douglas SD: Induction of multinucleated giant cell formation from human blood-derived monocytes by phorbol myristate acetate in in vitro culture. J Immunol 1989;143:2179–2184.

15   McInnes A, Rennick DM: Interleukin-4 induces cultured monocytes/macrophages to form giant multinucleated cells. J Exp Med 1988;167:598–611.

Dr. M. Kawaguchi, Department of Pathology, Faculty of Medicine, Toyama Medical and Pharmaceutical University, Sugitani 2630, Toyama 930-01 (Japan)

Galioto GB (ed): Tonsils: A Clinically Oriented Update.
Adv Otorhinolaryngol. Basel, Karger, 1992, vol 47, pp 222–226

IgA1 Localization in Tonsillar Follicular Dendritic Cells Is Characteristic of IgA Nephropathy

Chikashi Kusakari[a,b], *Tomonori Takasaka*[a], *Masato Nose*[b],
Masahisa Kyogoku[b]

Departments of [a]Otolaryngology and [b]Pathology,
Tohoku University School of Medicine, Sendai, Japan

IgA nephropathy (IgAN) is thought to represent glomerular deposition of circulating immune complexes containing IgA as the major antibody component [1]. Upper respiratory infection and tonsillitis often precede IgAN and, in some cases, tonsillectomy is an efficient treatment for preventing the progression of IgAN [2].

Thus, tonsils may be a unique organ causing initial and/or progressive events to generate IgA immune complexes in IgAN. To define characteristic pathological features of palatine tonsils in IgAN, the distribution of IgA1 and IgA2 in the tonsils of IgAN was compared with that of non-IgAN patients using immunohistochemical techniques.

Materials and Methods

Tonsil Specimens. Tonsils obtained from the following patients were studied: 12 patients (17–52 years old) with primary IgAN proven by renal biopsy, and 9 patients with chronic tonsillitis without IgAN (5–39 years old).

Immunohistochemistry. Surgical specimens were divided into small pieces and immediately fixed in PLP solution [3]. After being snap-frozen in OCT compound (Miles), serial cryostat sections (6 μm thick) were incubated with monoclonal antibodies for IgA1, IgA2 (anti-human IgA1 and anti-human IgA2; Becton-Dickinson) or follicular dendritic cells (FDC) (Dako DRC-1, Dakopatts). Binding of primary antibodies were then detected by the avidin-biotin complex (ABC) method [4], using the ABC kit PK400 (Vector Labs).

Table 1. Distribution and the relative amount of IgA1- and IgA2-positive cells in IgAN patients and non-IgAN controls

Case	Sex	Age	IgA1		IgA2	
			EF	GC	EF	GC
IgA nephropathy						
1	M	52	++[1]	++	+	–
2	F	30	++	++	+	–
3	F	30	+++	++	+	–
4	M	33	+++	++	+	–
5	M	21	++	+	+	–
6	M	47	+++	++	+	–
7	F	38	++	+	+	–
8	F	17	+++	++	+	–
9	F	30	++	++	+	–
10	M	32	++	+	+	–
11	M	25	++	+	+	–
12	F	20	+	+	+	–
Chronic tonsillitis without IgA nephropathy						
1	M	13	++	–	+	–
2	F	7	++	–	+	–
3	M	18	++	–	+	–
4	M	39	++	–	+	–
5	F	38	++	–	+	–
6	F	5	+	–	+	–
7	F	32	+++	–	+	–
8	M	7	++	–	+	–
9	F	8	+++	–	+	–

EF = Extrafollicular area; GC = germinal center.
[1] A relative amount of positive cells was scored on a – to +++ scale, with – indicating few.

Results

IgA1 was the predominant subclass among IgA-producing cells in palatine tonsils from both IgAN patients and controls (table 1). However, only IgA1, but not IgA2, was stained in the germinal center of tonsils from all patients with IgAN, which was stained in a reticular structure (fig. 1a). This staining was consistent with that of DRC-1-positive cells (fig. 1c). On

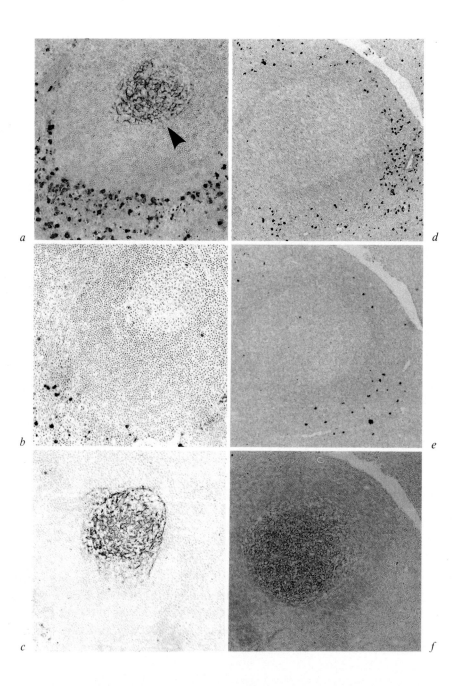

the other hand, both IgA1 and IgA2 staining was negative in the germinal center of tonsils from all the controls tested, while DRC-1-positive cells were distributed in an identical manner to those in tonsils of IgAN patients (fig. 1d–f).

Discussion

Role of IgA subclasses, IgA1 and IgA2, in the pathogenesis of IgAN has been controversial. In the present study we showed that only IgA1 was stained in a reticular pattern in the germinal center of tonsils from IgAN patients, and both IgA1 and IgA2 were negative in the same area of tonsils from non-IgAN controls. These findings indicate that the IgA1 subclass may play an important role in the pathogenesis of IgAN.

IgA1-positive cells in the germinal center of tonsils from IgAN patients showed a distribution identical to that of DRC-1-positive cells, indicating that the cells stained with IgA1 are FDC as far as studied in serial tissue sections. FDC are thought to be located within lymph follicles of secondary lymphoid tissues including tonsils, and to trap immune complexes on their cell surfaces and dendrites. Furthermore, these immune complexes are retained in FDC for a long period [5]. This indicates that the capture of immune complexes by FDC plays an important role in inducing persistent humoral immune responses and B-cell memory. Thus, IgA1 detected on FDC in the tonsils of IgAN patients must be in an immune complex form. These immune complexes may induce persistent immune responses to produce much larger amounts of IgA immune complexes responsible for the onset and progression of IgAN.

Fig. 1. Immunohistochemical staining of tonsils in (*a–c*) a representative IgAN patient and (*d–f*) a representative control. *a, d* Staining for IgA1: a large number of IgA1-positive cells are shown in the tonsil of IgAN patients (*a*). In the germinal center, IgA1 is positive in a reticular structure only in IgAN patients (arrowhead), but not in controls. *b, e* Staining for IgA2: both in IgAN patients and controls, a few IgA2-positive cells are demonstrated. IgA2 is negative in the germinal center both in IgAN patients and controls. *c, f* Staining for FDC: FDC are positive in the germinal center showing a reticular structure both in IgAN patients and controls.

References

1 Berger J: IgA glomerular deposit in renal disease. Transplant Proc 1969;1:934–944.
2 Masuda Y, Terazawa K, Kawakami S, Ogura Y, Sugiyama N: Clinical and immunological study of IgA nephropathy before and after tonsillectomy. Acta Otolaryngol 1988(suppl 454):248–255.
3 McLean IW, Nakane PK: Periodate-lysine-paraformaldehyde fixative: a new fixative for immunoelectron microscopy. J Histochem Cytochem 1974;22:1077–1083.
4 Hsu SM, Raine L, Fanger H: Use of avidin-biotin-peroxidase complex (ABC) in immunoperoxidase techniques: A comparison between ABC and unlabeled antibody (PAP) procedures. J Histochem Cytochem 1981;29:577–580.
5 Szakal AK, Kosco MH, Tew JG: A novel in vivo follicular dendritic cell-dependent iccosome-mediated mechanism for delivery of antigen to antigen-processing cells. J Immunol 1988;140:341–353.

Dr. Chikashi Kusakari, Department of Otolaryngology, Tohoku University,
1-1 Seiryo-machi Aoba-ku, Sendai-shi 980 (Japan)

Adenoids and Tonsil Hypertrophy and Its Complications

Galioto GB (ed): Tonsils: A Clinically Oriented Update.
Adv Otorhinolaryngol. Basel, Karger, 1992, vol 47, pp 227–231

Effect of Adenoidectomy on Eustachian Tube Function

Preliminary Results of a Randomized Clinical Trial[1]

Ellen M. Mandel[a], *Charles D. Bluestone*[b], *Haruo Takahashi*[b],
Margaretha L. Casselbrant[b]

[a] Department of Pediatrics; [b] Division of Pediatric Otolaryngology,
Department of Otolaryngology, University of Pittsburgh School of Medicine,
Department of Pediatric Otolaryngology, Children's Hospital of Pittsburgh,
Pittsburgh, Pa., USA

The effects of adenoidectomy on otitis media with effusion (OME) have been described by several investigators [1–6]. However, even in studies that have shown that adenoidectomy is beneficial, it has not been successful in reducing OME in all the children with OME. If children with OME who might benefit from adenoidectomy can be identified preoperatively by eustachian tube (ET) function testing, it will allow us to spare the child who is unlikely to benefit from adenoidectomy the risks and costs of the procedure. To our knowledge, however, the correlation between the preoperative ET function and the subsequent course of OME has never been analyzed systematically.

To determine if preoperative assessment of ET function could aid in selection of patients who might benefit from adenoidectomy, a randomized controlled study was conducted at the Children's Hospital of Pittsburgh. As part of the analysis of this study, the effect of adenoidectomy on ET function was examined. Furthermore, ET function in a modified condition of patients (during upper respiratory infection (URI)), which might exaggerate ET dysfunction [7], was also analyzed.

[1] This study was supported by Research Grant MCJ-420512, Maternal and Child Health Bureau.

Materials and Methods

Subjects and Enrollment

Subjects were enrolled at the Otitis Media Research Center of the Children's Hospital of Pittsburgh between March 1985 and May 1989. Children between 3 and 12 years of age without any major congenital anomaly or systemic disease, and with ventilation tubes inserted in the previous 6 months for chronic or recurrent middle ear effusion, were eligible for the study. Children who met the above criteria and whose parents gave informed consent were enrolled in this study.

Study 1:
Randomized Controlled Study of Effect of Adenoidectomy on ET Function

Subjects underwent ET function testing at three separate times. The classical inflation-deflation test, forced response test [8], and tubal compliance test [9] were performed each time when possible and the mean values were used as the prerandomization ET function test results. The subjects were randomly assigned to two groups (surgical and control) on the basis of mean closing pressure in the prerandomization period (< 50 mm H_2O, 50–100 mm H_2O, > 150 mm H_2O) and presence or absence of nasal obstruction due to obstructive adenoids. For subjects with bilateral tympanostomy tubes, randomization was based on the ear with the higher mean closing pressure. Children assigned to the surgical group underwent adenoidectomy under general anesthesia.

After assigned treatment, subjects were followed monthly, and ET function tests were performed every 2 months. The prerandomization ET function tests were compared with those at 2 and 6 months after assigned treatment.

Study 2:
Effect of Adenoidectomy on ET Function during URI

During the posttreatment period, the differences of ET function between the baseline (i.e., non-URI) condition and when a URI was present were compared between the two groups. The ET function data at the time nearest to (usually before) testing during a URI were taken as the baseline data.

Results

Population Characteristics

Seventy-four children were randomly assigned to the two treatment groups. Seventy-six percent of subjects were between 4 and 8 years of age; 57% were male. Only 4 (5.4%) were considered to have moderate or severe nasal obstruction. The percentages of subjects with mean closing pressures of > 150, 50–150, < 50 mm H_2O in the surgical group were 18.9, 73.0 and 8.1%, respectively. The corresponding percentages in the control group were 21.6, 70.3 and 8.1%.

Table 1. Results of ET function testing in surgical group

Parameter	n	Prerand	2M post	n	Prerand	6M post
OP	29	405 ± 174	393 ± 152	19	401 ± 134	378 ± 186
CL	29	122 ± 64	112 ± 61	18	123 ± 46	109 ± 94
PR-12	19	16.7 ± 14.4	17.3 ± 10.9	13	16.9 ± 7.2	16.5 ± 9.7
PR-24	24	10.6 ± 8.2	10.2 ± 5.7	12	8.5 ± 3.9	7.4 ± 3.0
PR-48	20	6.3 ± 4.3	5.7 ± 2.4	11	5.8 ± 1.8	4.5 ± 1.3
Tubal compliance	16	2.7 ± 0.8	3.1 ± 0.8	7	3.2 ± 0.9	3.0 ± 1.1

Prerand, 2M post, and 6M post = values at prerandomization period, 2 months and 6 months after randomization, respectively; OP = opening pressure (mm H_2O); CL = closing pressure (mm H_2O); PR-12, PR-24, PR-48 = values of passive resistance (mm H_2O/cc/min) at flow rates of 12, 24 and 48; n = number of subjects analyzed.

Study 1:
Effect of Adenoidectomy on ET Function

A total of 56 children (56 ears) were available for this study. The other 18 children either underwent spontaneous extubation (and therefore were unable to be tested) or were lost to follow-up. As shown in table 1, slight decreases in opening and closing pressures were observed both at 2 and 6 months after randomization in the adenoidectomized group, but they were not statistically significant (paired t tests, t = 0.59, 0.74). Improvements in positive pressure equalization and active behavior during swallowing both at 2 and 6 months after randomization were noted, but they were not statistically significant (χ^2 tests, χ^2 = 0.77, 3.47). No significant changes were observed in any other parameter. No significant changes were noted in the control group.

Study 2:
Effect of Adenoidectomy on ET Function during URI

There were 13 and 18 children in the surgical and control group, respectively, whose ET functions could be examined both at baseline and with URI. Although opening and closing pressures tended to increase more during URI in the control group than in the surgical group, none of the differences were statistically significant (χ^2 tests, $\chi^2 = 2.42, 1.32$). No differences were noted in any other parameters.

Discussion

Bluestone et al. [10] reported improvement of ET function in some children after adenoidectomy, and Honjo [11] found a significant improvement in ET active function following adenoidectomy. In the present study, no significant change was observed in ET function after adenoidectomy with or without a URI. The clinical effects of adenoidectomy on OM status in this population has not yet been analyzed, but from these results, if a beneficial effect of adenoidectomy on OM is found it cannot be attributed to improvement in the ET function parameters we measured. One important point is that very few of our subjects had large obstructive adenoids. It is quite possible that, in children with large adenoids that can obstruct the ET or the posterior nasal choanae or both, adenoidectomy would show an effect on ET function. On the other hand, Takahashi et al. [5] reported no improvement in active or passive resistance 1 month after adenoidectomy. The present results may have confirmed this with a larger sample size.

The questions remaining are how we can predict preoperatively which children will benefit from adenoidectomy, and whether children with non-obstructive adenoids should be candidates for adenoidectomy as the initial procedure. More detailed examinations of the adenoid and the ET by nasopharyngeal endoscopy or magnetic resonance imaging seem to be desirable to further investigate this issue.

References

1   Maw AR: Chronic otitis media with effusion (glue ear) and adenotonsillectomy: prospective randomized controlled study. Br Med J 1983;287:1586–1588.
2   Gates GA, Avery CA, Prihoda TJ: Effect of adenoidectomy upon children with chronic otitis media with effusion. Laryngoscope 1988;98:58–63.
3   Paradise JL, Bluestone CD, Rogers KD, Tailor FH, Colborn DK, Bachman RZ, Bernard BS, Schwarzbach RH: Efficacy of adenoidectomy for recurrent otitis media in children previously treated with tympanostomy-tube placement. JAMA 1990; 263:2066–2073.

4   Bulman CH, Brook SJ, Berry MG: A prospective randomized trial of adenoidec-
    tomy vs. grommet insertion in the treatment of glue ear. Clin Otolaryngol 1984;9:
    67–75.
5   Takahashi H, Fujita A, Honjo I: Effect of adenoidectomy on otitis media with effu-
    sion, tubal function, and sinusitis. Am J Otolaryngol 1989;10:208–213.
6   Fiellau-Nikolajsen M: Tympanometry and secretory otitis media – observations on
    diagnosis, epidemiology, treatment, and prevention in prospective cohort studies of
    three-year-old children. Acta Otolaryngol (Stockh) 1983(suppl 394):1–73.
7   Bluestone CD, Cantekin EI, Beery QC: Effect of inflammation on the ventilatory
    function of the eustachian tube. Ann Otol Rhinol Laryngol 1977;87:493–507.
8   Cantekin EI, Saez CA, Bluestone CD, Bern SA: Airflow through the eustachian tube.
    Ann Otol Rhinol Laryngol 1979;88:603–612.
9   Takahashi H, Hayashi M, Honjo I: Compliance of the eustachian tube in patients
    with otitis media with effusion. Am J Otolaryngol 1987;8:154–156.
10 Bluestone CD, Cantekin EI, Beery QC: Certain effects of adenoidectomy on eusta-
    chian tube ventilatory function. Laryngoscope 1975;85:113–127.
11 Honjo I: Adenoid vegetation and otitis media with effusion; in Eustachian Tube and
    Middle Ear Diseases. Tokyo, Springer, 1988.

Ellen M. Mandel, MD, Children's Hospital of Pittsburgh,
Department of Pediatric Otolaryngology, 3705 Fifth Avenue at DeSoto Street,
Pittsburgh, PA 15213 (USA)

Galioto GB (ed): Tonsils: A Clinically Oriented Update.
Adv Otorhinolaryngol. Basel, Karger, 1992, vol 47, pp 232–240

Hypertrophy of Adenoids and Tubal Functionality

Desiderio Passali

Università degli Studi di L'Aquila, Cattedra di Clinica Otorinolaringoiatrica,
L'Aquila, Italia

The hypothesis of a relationship between hypertrophy of adenoids and
tubal functionality dates back to over a century ago and was put in con-
crete form with the proposal to remove the adenoids to the purpose of
restoring an adequate tubal functionality and consequently of solving the
middle ear affection [1]. In fact it is well known that during the period of
the maximum growth, between 4 and 7 years of age, and in the condition of
hypertrophy, the pharyngeal tonsil can take up all the roof of the rhinopharyngeal cavity. In these conditions the lymphoepithelial tissue can mechan-
ically obstruct the pharyngeal ostium of the eustachian tube preventing the
normal course of ventilation and drainage functions. On the basis of these
anatomical and physiopathological remarks, the adenoidectomy has been
carried out for several years not only to restore an adequate nasal perviousness, getting rid of the dangerous oral breathing, but also to allow the
recovery of the secretory otitis media (SOM).

In recent years this therapeutical attitude has been subjected to careful critical examinations starting from the observation that many cases of
endotympanic effusions could not be attributed to an extrinsic mechanical obstruction of the eustachian tube, but had to be ascribed to disorders
of its normal functionality. In fact, even in the most favorable statistics
[2] adenoidectomy shows the 'ability' to solve SOM in 33–47% of cases.
However apart from different data, many authors agree upon considering
the hypertrophy of adenoids one of the possible causes, but not the only
one involved in giving rise to tubal disorders. Moreover, it is common
experience to point out the persistence of type B or C tympanograms in

young patients who underwent correctly performed operations of adenoidectomy.

In our experience adenoidectomy is necessary in the 25% of the children suffering from SOM, that is to say only in those cases in which subjective symptomatology, objective examination, rhinomanometry with decongestion test and measurement of mucociliary transport time demonstrate the real need and allow to foresee reasonably a positive result.

Therefore, in our opinion the problem of the relationship between hypertrophy of adenoids and tubal functionality must be framed within the wider ambit of the correlations between eustachian tube and nose, as organs integrated by anatomical and physiological connections in the nose-pharynx-tube unit. In fact, the tube is also named tympanic-pharyngeal channel just to underline its role of connecting the middle ear to the nasopharynx and therefore the middle ear's physiopathological dependence on the nasal fossae.

Really a direct relation is set up between the nose and the fibrocartilaginous portion of the eustachian tube, which has anatomical and histological characteristics suitable for performing the ventilation, drainage and defence functions in favor of the middle ear. Particularly the continuity of the nasal and rhinopharyngeal epithelium with that of the tube, the vascular, lymphatic and neurovegetative connections, linking up the different elements of the nose-pharynx-tube district create the conditions so that the tube can be affected by every inflammation, infection or obstruction which primarily involves the nose and the rhinopharynx. In other words the impairment of the main nasal functions (ventilation, conditioning and clearance) affects the physiological course of the tubal functions. In fact, for example, when there is nasal respiratory obstruction the air flow cannot follow its normal routes, but it is concentrated on small areas of the pharyngeal mucosa causing locally overevaporation and increase of mucus viscosity. Besides the absence of adequate filtration and conditioning and the impairment or the block of the mucociliary streams favor the invasion by pathogenic agents. In a previous study [3] the role played by nasal obstruction in the pathogenesis of tympanic effusion in 10 rabbits has been demonstrated. In fact, some days after the closure of one nostril with cotton wool and fibrin glue we pointed out the flattening of the tympanometric curves, previously normal, in the middle ears corresponding to the obstructed nostril.

In the light of these data and of the significant correlation between mucociliary transport and tympanometric pictures in children [3], we decided to analyze the relation between the middle ear condition and the efficiency of the main nasal functions during the period of passing from childhood to adolescence. To this aim we started from the demonstration of the nasal cycle [4] and of an inversely proportional relation between mucociliary velocity and local production of secretory immunoglobulins [5] in adults.

On the contrary, childhood is characterized by the immaturity of the whole nose-pharynx-tube district [6] and in particular by the absence of an alternate nasal cycle [7] and by deep anatomical, physiological and immunological differences of the eustachian tube compared to the adult age. Therefore, we have hypothesized that being absent in extrinsic mechanical obstruction the tubal impairment could be correlated to an incomplete maturation of ventilation, specific defence and mucociliary clearance nasal functions.

Materials and Methods

To this aim we examined 26 children aged from 11 to 14 years, suffering from SOM and previously subjected to adenoidectomy between 5 and 8 years of life. A careful ENT examination allowed to exclude mechanical obstructive causes, including the eventual relapse for hypertrophy of residual adenoids. During the first visit the tympanometric examination showed type B or C2 curves, which mean (following the commonly used classification): type B, absent peak, and type C2, peak placed on negative values higher than -150 mm H_2O.

The study of the nasal respiratory function was performed with a Markos NR6 rhinomanometer with anterior active test and taking into consideration as reference parameter the resistances of each side and the total nasal one, measured in pascal·s/l, at 1 h interval from 10 a.m. to 10 p.m. for 3 days. The examination of the specific nasal defence activity was referred to the nasal secretory IgA dosage. To this end the nasal secretion was drawn placing two pieces of cotton wool of known weight in each nasal fossa between the lower and middle turbinates and the septum using anterior rhinoscopy. After a 30-min interval these were removed, slipped into an insulin syringe and squeezed into a small test tube, where the secretion can eventually be frozen, and kept up until the analysis, that is to say the dosage of SIgA by ELISA (anti-SC antibodies; Dakopatts). Finally, for the evaluation of the mucociliary transport (MCT) we used the mixture of charcoal and saccharin 3% powder. This is deposited on the head of the lower turbinate by means of a tent made of cotton wool in the anterior rhinoscopy. The times elapsing from the deposition and the observation of the charcoal on the pharyngeal mucosa and from the same deposition and the onset of a sweet taste reported by the patient were measured [8].

Being easy to perform, this method gives the same results as the techniques that use radioactive indicators. In children the MCT times are considered normal if they are 10 ±

Table 1. Values of nasal resistance (Pa·s/l)

Time	Study subject			Control subject		
	right	left	total	right	left	total
10.00 a.m.	1.1	1.3	0.55	1.6	0.4	0.32
11.00	0.9	1.1	0.49	0.5	0.5	0.25
12.00	0.6	1.0	0.37	1.2	0.3	0.24
1.00 p.m.	0.8	2.6	0.61	0.5	0.8	0.30
2.00	1.4	0.5	0.41	0.8	0.4	0.26
3.00	1.5	0.6	0.46	1.3	0.4	0.30
4.00	1.8	0.6	0.47	0.4	1.1	0.29
5.00	1.1	1.3	0.59	0.4	0.7	0.25
6.00	1.2	1.3	0.48	1.2	0.5	0.35
7.00	1.6	0.8	0.53	0.7	0.3	0.21
8.00	1.3	0.7	0.47	0.3	1.1	0.23
9.00	1.2	0.6	0.40	0.5	0.7	0.29
10.00	0.8	0.5	0.30	0.6	0.4	0.24

3 min, delayed if ranging from 13 to 30 min, and the mucociliary function is blocked if the time is over 30 min. The MCT time was measured indifferently on the right or on the left side if the resistance values were the same or on the side with the lowest respiratory perviousness.

Both nasal secretion drawings and MCT test were repeated every 3 h from 10 a.m. to 10 p.m. of the same day and for the following 2 days. As a control group, 26 children, homogeneous for sex and age, were chosen. They were also subjected to adenoidectomy, but completely recovered and had type A tympanograms (peak at 0). The control group was subjected to the same tests at the same times.

Results

Table 1 shows the values of partial and total nasal resistance pertaining to a subject from the study group compared to a control subject. Drawing two graphs with those values relative to the 10 a.m.–10 p.m. interval, a different behavior of the respiratory function in the two groups is pointed out (fig. 1, 2). In fact, children suffering from tubal impairment show high fluctuations of total nasal resistance due to the absence of an alternate nasal cycle, typical of the adult free from nasal diseases. The pattern of partial and total nasal perviousness is different in the control group, which shows a constant alternation of congestion and decongestion in each nasal

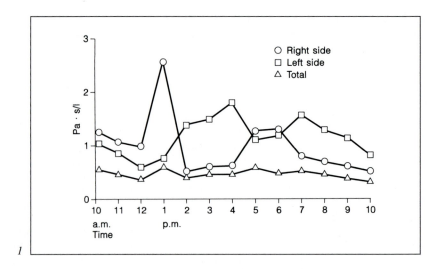

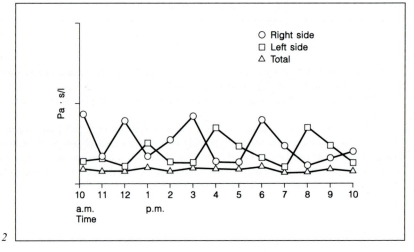

Fig. 1. Fluctuations of nasal resistance in a study subject (no nasal cycle).
Fig. 2. Nasal cycle in a child of the control group (type A tympanogram).

fossa, with a reciprocal coordination which guarantees a total resistance almost constant during the whole day. The mean values and SD of MCT times and SIgA concentrations in nasal secretion of the study subjects are presented in table 2, referring to the tests' performing times.

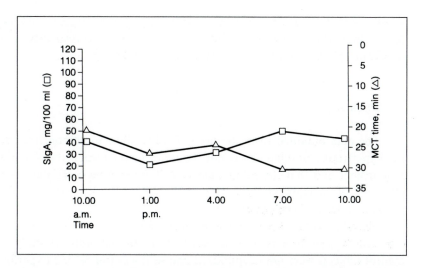

Fig. 3. Fluctuations of MCT times and SIgA concentrations in the study subjects (26 children had previously undergone adenoidectomy with type B and C2 tympanograms).

Table 2. Mean values and standard deviation (SD) of MCT times and secretory IgA (SIgA) concentrations in nasal secretion of the study subjects

Time	MCT, min	SD	SIgA, mg/100 ml	SD
10.00 a.m.	21	±9	43	±5
1.00 p.m.	27	±5	23	±10
4.00	25	±7	35	±12
7.00	30	±4	47	±4
10.00	30	±6	41	±7

The immaturity of clearance and specific defence nasal functions is clearly showed by the lengthening of MCT times compared to the normal values and by a low dosage of SIgA. The graphic pattern of these values allows to point out the absence of reciprocal coordination (fig. 3). On the contrary, the latter is present in the control group, whose normal clearance times and SIgA rates (table 3) follow a circadian rhythm similar to the adult's one [5]. In fact in the children with type A tympanogram the lowest MCT efficiency, within the ambit of normal values, corresponds to the maximum SIgA local production and vice versa (fig. 4).

Discussion

The data obtained from the present study allow to demonstrate that the hypertrophy of adenoids is not the main factor responsible for tubal impairment and that the middle ear conditions can be correlated to the efficiency of the main nasal functions, although the mechanism which controls this relation is still unknown.

The observation interval has been limited to the range between 10 a.m. and 10 p.m. because of practical reasons. In fact both the study and control subjects were not hospitalized and so it was impossible to perform the tests during the night. However, the homogeneity of the values obtained makes us sure of the significance of the available data. As regards the study group, a relationship between a middle ear pathological condition, sign of tubal impairment (type B or C2 tympanograms), and the immaturity of the main nasal functions is well evident. In fact as far as the respiratory function is concerned the absence of a true nasal cycle has been pointed out and as regards defence activities pathological values of MCT times and SIgA dosage have been obtained. Besides, the subjects belonging to this group turned out to be lacking in the reciprocally coordinated circadian pattern between aspecific (MCT) and specific (secretory immunoglobulins) defence, which guarantees a continuous compensation during the phases of relative functional impairment. On the contrary, in the control group a normal tubotympanic condition (type A tympanogram) is well correlated to an efficient nasal condition, characterized by an alternate nasal cycle and a coordinated cyclic pattern of MCT times and SIgA values, which are always in the normal range.

In the light of the previous observations, some conclusions are possible. First of all the importance of an adequate nasal functionality cannot be denied, not only for the higher airways, but also for the efficiency of the eustachian tube. Trying to analyze the several factors involved in these relations, it is necessary to recognize in the study group the influence exerted by the periodical alteration of the nasal ventilation, due to the same phases of the 'solidary' cycle. During these phases the swallowing acts, which are responsible for the air exchange in the middle ear, are performed

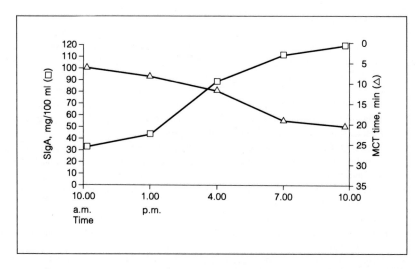

Fig. 4. Pattern of fluctuations of MCT times and SIgA concentrations in the control group (26 children had previously undergone adenoidectomy with type A tympanograms).

Table 3. Mean values and standard deviation (SD) of MCT times and secretory IgA (SIgA) concentrations in nasal secretion of the control group

Time	MCT, min	SD	SIgA, mg/100 ml	SD
10.00 a.m.	12	±3	35	±14
1.00 p.m.	13	±4	45	±7
4.00	16	±4	75	±11
7.00	20	±9	91	±12
10.00	22	±5	111	±9

in the presence of a nasal subobstructive condition. As a consequence a rhinopharyngeal overpressure is created which can cause difficulties in the tubal drainage and eventually aspiration of the secretions. Therefore, it is possible to conclude that hypertrophy of the adenoids is not the only cause of tubal impairment; on the other hand, when it is, it can act both as a mechanical extrinsic obstacle at the tubal ostium and as a cause of nasal respiratory obstruction, with deviation of the nasal mucociliary streams.

References

1   Meyer W: On adenoid vegetations in the naso-pharyngeal cavity: their pathology, diagnosis and treatment; in Paradise JL, Bluestone CD, Rogers KD, Taylor FH (eds): Efficacy of Adenoidectomy in Recurrent Otitis Media. Recent Advances in Otitis Media with Effusion. Ann Otol Rhinol Laryngol 1980(suppl 68):89.

2   Maw AR: The long-term effect of adenoidectomy on established otitis media with effusion in children; in Abstracts of Extraordinary International Symposium in Recent Advances in Otitis Media with Effusion, Kyoto 1985.

3   Passali D, Bellussi L, Lauriello M: Nasal mucociliary transport time and tubal functionality; in Sade J (ed): The Eustachian Tube: Clinical Aspects. Amsterdam, Kugler & Ghedini Publications, 1991.

4   Stoksted P: The physiologic cycle of the nose under normal and pathological conditions. Acta Otolaryngol (Stockh) 1952;42:175–179.

5   Passali D, Bellussi L, Lauriello M: Diurnal activity of the nasal mucosa: relationship between mucociliary transport and local production of secretory immunoglobulins. Acta Otolaryngol (Stockh) 1990;110:437–442.

6   Bellussi L, Lauriello M, Passali D: Alcune considerazioni sulla maturazione dell'unità rino-faringotubarica. Riv Ital Otorinolar Audiol Foniatr 1988;8:211–214.

7   Van Cauwenberge PB, Deleye L: Nasal cycle in children. Acta Otolaryngol 1984; 110:108–111.

8   Passali D, Bellussi L, Bianchini-Ciampoli M, De Seta E: Experiences in the determination of nasal mucociliary transport time. Acta Otolaryngol 1984;97:319–323.

Prof. D. Passali, Via Po 102, I–00198 Roma (Italy)

Galioto GB (ed): Tonsils: A Clinically Oriented Update.
Adv Otorhinolaryngol. Basel, Karger, 1992, vol 47, pp 241–245

Tonsillar Hypertrophy and Middle Ear Diseases

Paul B. Van Cauwenberge

Department of Otorhinolaryngology, University Hospital, Ghent, Belgium

Although acute and chronic tonsillitis are very common diseases and although many otorhinolaryngologists include tonsillectomy in the treatment of secretory otitis media (SOM) and acute otitis media (AOM), little is known about the role of the tonsils as possible predisposing factor in various middle ear diseases. The role of the adenoids is much more frequently studied, although also here there still exists a lot of controversy.

At the end of the 19th century chronic tonsillitis was considered as a focal infection responsible for SOM [1], and till now this unproven theory is still accepted by some. Others suggest that an infection of the tonsils may cause an ascending infection of the eustachian tube and middle ear or that the volume of the tonsils may have a mass effect thus impairing the eustachian tube dysfunction [2].

Arguments against the role of the tonsils in SOM are the absence of enlarged or chronically infected tonsils in the majority of cases of SOM and the observation of the appearance of SOM in children who already underwent a tonsillectomy [3, 4]. In addition, Tos et al. [5] did not find a correlation between the tonsillar status and the tympanometrical findings. Also, Stewart et al. [6] could not demonstrate a relationship between a history of tonsillitis, the volume of the tonsils and the presence of cervical adenopathy on the one hand, and the presence of SOM on the other.

In order to investigate the role of tonsillar pathology in AOM and SOM, we conducted a cross-sectional epidemiological and clinical study in a large population of apparently healthy preschool children.

Material

The study group consisted of 2,065 healthy preschool children (2.5–6 years), who attended kindergarten. The study of the role of the children was a part of a larger study in which the role of various possible predisposing factors was investigated.

Methods

The parents completed a questionnaire with 65 questions on the personal and family history. We also performed a general physical examination and a full ENT examination. The technical examinations included tympanometry, and also pure tone audiometry and rhinomanometry wherever possible.

The statistical analysis included the multiple linear regression analysis (MLRA), to exclude any false and indirect correlation because many factors were studied at the same time, the χ^2 for the analysis of individual parameters, and the analysis of variation (Anova) for the statistical analysis of mean values.

Results

With the MLRA we found a highly statistical significant correlation between the tonsillar status and the tympanometrical findings (p = 0.003); there was, however, no correlation between the annual frequency of acute tonsillitis and the tympanometrical findings (p = 0.5). There was, with the MLRA, also a highly significant correlation between the annual frequency of acute tonsillitis and that of acute otitis (p = 0.004), but not really between the tonsillar status and the annual frequency of acute otitis (p = 0.09) (table 1). We will further elaborate these positive correlations.

Table 1. Results of the MLRA

	χ^2	MLRA
Tympanometrical findings		
Annual frequency of acute tonsillitis	0.07	0.5
Tonsillar status	<0.0001	0.003
Tonsillectomy before	0.3	0.7
Annual frequency of AOM		
Annual frequency of acute tonsillitis	0.0001	0.003
Tonsillar status	0.4	0.09
Tonsillectomy before	0.5	0.8

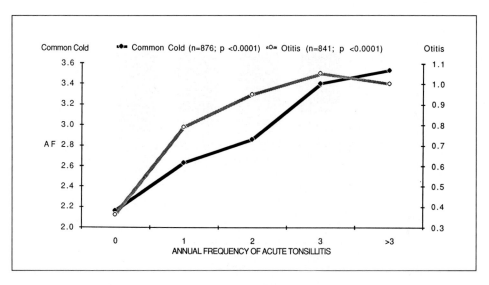

Fig. 1. Relationship between the annual frequency (AF) of acute tonsillitis and that of AOM. n = Number of children studied; p = according to Anova.

Annual Frequency of Acute Tonsillitis

Not only with the MLRA but also with the Anova ($p < 0.0001$) there was a clear correlation between the annual frequency of acute tonsillitis and that of acute otitis (fig. 1). The mean annual frequency of acute otitis was, e.g., 0.4 for children without acute tonsillitis while it was 1.1 for children with more than 3 annual episodes of acute tonsillitis.

Tonsillar Status

When plotting the tonsillar status with the homolateral tympanometrical findings, we found that a pronounced hypertrophy of the tonsils was significantly correlated with a higher prevalence of SOM (fig. 2). When adding the left and right findings there is a high statistical significance ($p = 0.0001$, χ^2; $p = 0.003$, MLRA). We examined the children with SOM 6 weeks later so we could identify a group with persisting SOM. When examining the role of the tonsils in this group by comparing it with the tonsillar status in children with normal tympanograms, the role of pronounced hypertrophy of the tonsils as a predisposing factor to persisting SOM became more obvious although the number of children was smaller (left side: $p = 0.007$; right side: $p = 0.02$, χ^2) (fig. 3).

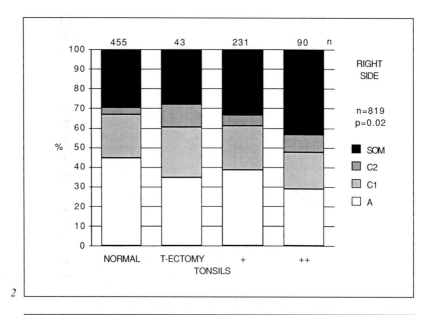

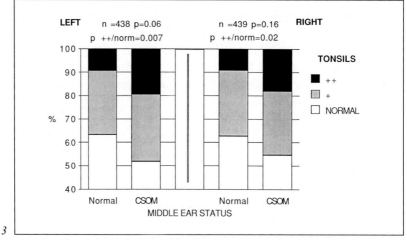

Fig. 2. Relationship between the right tonsillar status and the homolateral tympa-nometrical findings. n = Number of children studied; p = according to χ^2 test; T-ectomy = tonsillectomy; + = moderate hypertrophy of the tonsil; ++ = pronounced hypertrophy of the tonsil.

Fig. 3. The tonsillar status in children with normal tympanograms (A or C1) and in children with persisting SOM (CSOM). n = Number of children studied; p = according to χ^2 test; p ++/norm = statistical significance of the differences between children with pro-nounced tonsillar hypertrophy and children with normal tonsils.

Discussion and Conclusion

It was not a surprise to find that there existed a strong correlation between the annual frequency of acute tonsillitis and that of AOM. In cases of acute infection of the upper respiratory tract in children, very often more than one part of this tract is involved [7].

Contrary to the findings of other authors [5, 6], we could demonstrate a significant correlation between the tonsillar status and the tympanometrical findings. Children with pronounced hypertrophy of the tonsils had a higher incidence of SOM. Probably we could demonstrate this because the number of studied children in our study was higher. The most interesting finding was that the role of tonsillar hypertrophy was most obvious in children with persisting SOM.

This epidemiological and clinical study does not tell us anything about the underlying mechanisms. Further studies are needed to investigate if the correlation between tonsillar hypertrophy and SOM is due to an ascending infection via the eustachian tube or to a functional obstruction of the eustachian tube or to a coexistence of adenoid and tonsillar pathology, or perhaps by a lymphatic obstruction due to the tonsillar mass.

References

1   Black N: Causes of glue ear. J Laryngol Otol 1985;99:953–963.
2   Van Cauwenberge P: Sécrétoire otitis media; thesis Ghent 1989.
3   Dawes JDK: The aetiology and sequelae of exudative otitis media. J Laryngol Otol 1970;84:583–588.
4   Mawson SR, Fagan P: Tympanic effusions in children. J Laryngol Otol 1972;86: 105–109.
5   Tos M, Poulsen G, Borch J: Etiologic factors in secretory otitis. Arch Otolaryngol 1979;105:582–588.
6   Stewart I, Kirkland C, Simpson A, Silva P, Williams S: Some factors of possible etiologic significance related to otitis media with effusion; in Lim DJ, Bluestone CD, Klein JO, Nelson JD (eds): Recent Advances in Otitis media with Effusion. Philadelphia, Decker, 1984, pp 25–28.
7   Van Cauwenberge P: Otitis media in relation to other upper respiratory tract infections; in Sadé J (ed): Acute and Secretory Otitis media. Amsterdam, Kugler Publ, 1986, pp 129–134.

Prof. Dr. P. Van Cauwenberge, Department of Otorhinolaryngology,
University Hospital, B-9000 Ghent (Belgium)

Galioto GB (ed): Tonsils: A Clinically Oriented Update.
Adv Otorhinolaryngol. Basel, Karger, 1992, vol 47, pp 246–250

Significance of Adenoidectomy in the Treatment of Secretory Otitis media

I. Honjo, A. Fujita, K. Kurata, H. Takahashi

Department of Otolaryngology, Faculty of Medicine, Kyoto University,
Kyoto, Japan

The favorable effects of adenoidectomy on otitis media with effusion (OME) have been established by various findings [1, 2], e.g. decreases in recurrence rate of OME, improvements in hearing, and decreases in negative middle ear pressure. However, the follow-up periods after the surgery were at most 2 years in those studies, and the long-term benefits of adenoidectomy have not yet been fully discussed.

In this report, the long-term effects of adenoidectomy were investigated, and the factors which prevented a full OME cure after adenoidectomy were analyzed.

Materials and Methods

Participants in this study were 130 children (244 ears) with chronic OME aged 4–8 years. They were divided into two groups: the adenoidectomized group (57 children, 103 ears) which was treated both by adenoidectomy and ventilation tube insertion and the nonadenoidectomized group (73 children, 141 ears) which was treated by ventilation tube insertion only. We found no significant difference between the two groups in any of the factors which may affect the prognosis of OME, indicating that the subjects were randomly distributed (table 1).

After surgery, children were followed up periodically for up to 3 years. A full cure of OME was defined as the absence of ME effusion for 3 successive months, as scored by pneumatic otoscopy, audiometry and tympanometry.

The ears which were not cured during the period of observation were defined to be refractory OME cases, and they were examined with respect to their mastoid pneumatization, eustachian tube function and nasal condition, since these factors have been considered to be the most important in the pathogenesis of OME. Mastoid pneumatization was judged to be good when its area on Schüller's roentgen view was > 7.5 cm^2, and to be

Table 1. Characteristics of the two groups

	Sex (M/F)	Mean age	Initial hearing level, dB
Adenoidectomized group (57 cases, 103 ears)	1.71	6.1	29.8
Nonadenoidectomized group (73 cases, 141 ears)	1.52	6.1	27.4

No results were significant ($p < 0.05$).

poor when it was < 7.5 cm^2. Eustachian tube function was examined with the passive opening test and the positive and negative ME pressure equalizing function test. We also performed a sniffing test to discover any possible tubal closing failure. As an indicator of any inflammation of the upper respiratory tract, we examined the paranasal sinuses by nasal roentgenograms.

Results

The increases in the cure rates of OME over the 3 years is summarized in figure 1. In the adenoidectomized group, the cure rates were 44 and 67% in the first and second years, respectively, whereas those in the nonadenoidectomized group were 16 and 49%, respectively. This indicates a significantly better cure rate for the adenoidectomized group in the first 2 years (χ^2 test, $p < 0.01$). By the third year, however, the cure rates were 74 and 75% in the adenoidectomized and nonadenoidectomized group, respectively; there is no significant difference between the two groups. The frequency of refractory cases was, therefore, quite similar between them: 26% in the adenoidectomized group and 25% in the nonadenoidectomized group.

Among the 62 refractory OME ears (27 ears from the adenoidectomized group and 35 ears from the nonadenoidectomized), 87% of them (54 ears) showed poor mastoid pneumatization. On the other hand, 56% of the 182 ears of successfully treated cases showed good mastoid pneumatization (significant difference $p < 0.01$).

Eustachian tube function test of the 46 refractory OME cases indicated that 35% had a higher tubal opening pressure than the normal upper limit, 48% were within the normal range and 17% of lower pressures

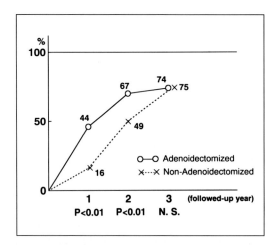

Fig. 1. Cure rate of OME.

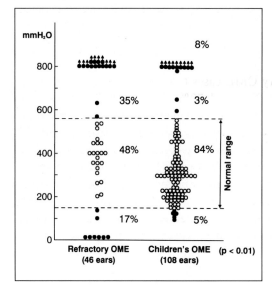

Fig. 2. Opening pressure of the E-tube.

(fig. 2). Thus, more than half of these refractory cases were accompanied by abnormal patency of the E-tube. Compared with the ordinary OME cases in childhood, the incidence of abnormal opening pressure cases was significantly higher (χ^2 test, significant difference $p < 0.01$) in the refractory group.

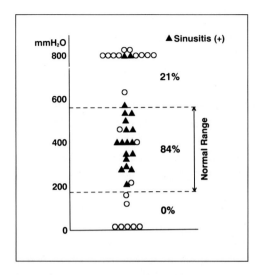

Fig. 3. Frequency of nasal sinusitis in relation to the tubal patency.

In 30% of the refractory OME cases (14/46), a negative middle ear
pressure was induced by sniffing and 79% of them (11/14) showed an
opening failure of the tube after sniffing (lock phenomenon). Thus, it is
possible that in the treatment failure ears, there may be some cases of
sniffing-induced OME.

Paranasal sinusitis was documented in 52% of the refractory OME
cases (17/23 cases), which was significantly lower (χ^2 test, significant difference p = 0.01) than the children's OME cases. However, 84% of the
refractory cases with normal patency of the tube were accompanied by
nasal sinusitis, while only 14% of those with abnormal opening pressures
had sinusitis (fig. 3).

Discussion

One of the most remarkable findings in this study was that the cure
rate from OME became quite similar between the adenoidectomized and
nonadenoidectomized groups by the third year, though it was better in the
adenoidectomized group for first 2 years. This may indicate that adenoidectomy merely shortens the time required for a cure from OME in
under 3 years. However, this does not mean that adenoidectomy has no

additional merit to ventilation tube insertion. To bring about a more rapid cure of OME in these children means they may be released from their ventilation tube earlier, reducing the possibility of sequelae such as atelectatic ears or cholesteatomas. The indication of adenoidectomy for OME should be based on individual factors.

Another notable finding was a higher incidence of poor mastoid pneumatization in the refractory OME group. Several experimental studies have demonstrated that poor mastoid pneumatization can be induced by inflammation of the middle ear in early infancy. This may indicate that many of the refractory OME cases actually had a history of otitis media from infancy.

The ETs of the refractory OME cases showed a tendency to have abnormally high or low opening pressures, indicating excessive or poor tubal patency. Therefore, some unknown organic disorder of the ET in the refractory ears could be one of the causes of OME occurring in early infancy and becoming refractory later on. On the other hand, the treatment failure ears were accompanied by upper respiratory inflammation much less frequently than the children's OME cases. Most of the refractory OME cases with normal tubal patency, however, are accompanied by paranasal sinusitis. Thus, they would appear to have the same characteristics as ordinary children's OME: ventilatory dysfunction of the eustachian tube plus inflammation of the upper respiratory tract. In these cases, complications resulting from upper respiratory infection should also play an important role as a cause of persistent OME.

In summary, (1) adenoidectomy has some curative effect on OME in children under 3 years of age, and (2) the causes of refractory cases are due to other etiological factors, such as a highly affected E-tube and/or recurrent URI.

References

1   Gates CA, Avery CA, Cooper JC, Prinoda TJ: Chronic secretory otitis media: Effect of surgical management. Ann Otol Rhinol Laryngol 1989(suppl 138):2–32.
2   Maw AR, Jean WD, Cable HR: Adenoidectomy: a prospective study to show clinical and radiological changes two years after operation. J Laryngol Otol 1983;97:511–518.

Iwao Honjo, MD, Department of Otolaryngology, Faculty of Medicine,
Kyoto University, 54 Kawahara-cho, Shogoin, Sakyo-ku, Kyoto 606 (Japan)

Galioto GB (ed): Tonsils: A Clinically Oriented Update.
Adv Otorhinolaryngol. Basel, Karger, 1992, vol 47, pp 251–259

Tonsil Surgery in Heavy Snoring Young Children

G. Pestalozza[a], *E. Tessitore*[a], *R. Bellotto*[a], *M. Zucconi*[b]

[a] ENT Division, Children's Hospital 'V. Buzzi', Milan, and
[b] Center for Sleep Disorders, Neurologic Clinic, University of Milan, Italy

Noisy nocturnal breathing in young children is often associated with increased upper airways resistance, and such a condition may lead to clinical symptoms. Eventually, episodes of hypopnea may be present that are characteristic of obstructive sleep apnea syndrome (OSAS).

Adult OSAS has been defined as a state in which airflow stops for at least 10 s more than 5 times per hour, or at least 30 times in 7 h night sleep [1]. In children aged 6 months to 6 years the majority of authors agree that apneas and hypopneas are characterized by a duration longer than 5 s [2].

Repeated apnea and hypopnea episodes in severe OSAS cases cause oxygen desaturation, hypoventilation and alveolar hypoxia, and these, with time, can lead to blood hypertension and chronic pulmonary heart syndrome (cor pulmonale); hypoxia may induce vagal reflexes and consequent bradyrhythmia; in extreme cases sudden infant death syndrome (SIDS) may intervene.

However, it has been demonstrated that children differ from adult subjects in that clinical symptoms of increased upper airways resistance may appear without complete apnea and without significant drops in oxygen saturation, probably because increased negative intrathoracic pressure induces significant mechanical changes in children's cardiorespiratory function [3].

Moreover, other physiopathologic consequences of upper airways obstruction may be present in heavy snoring children: (a) diurnal somnolence and behavioral troubles affecting learning capabilities; (b) reduced growth rate, due to impaired swallowing and to altered growth hormone incretion during specific sleep stages [4]; (c) disproportional development of the maxilla – retrognathia and open bites – following excessive molar tooth eruption and low tongue posture [5]; (d) higher occurrence of intrinsic asthma due to impaired respiratory nasal function [6].

In the child below 6 years of age, hypertrophy of tonsils and adenoids is the most frequent cause of heavy snoring and respiratory troubles during sleep. In cases with associated malformations of the nasal septum and palate, the clinical picture is more severe.

Adenotonsillectomy is the treatment of choice to relieve obstruction of upper airways in most pediatric cases, preventing the development of OSAS and other complications listed before. In our experience adenoidectomy alone is not enough to relieve OSAS, inasmuch as improvement of respiratory troubles is partial and temporary (regrowth of lymphoid tissue in young children). The operation of adenotonsillectomy must be performed before irreversible cardiocirculatory disease and craniofacial growth anomalies appear.

Although no specific immune deficiency, systemic or local, consequent to ablation of palatine and pharyngeal tonsils was ever demonstrated in healthy subjects, the following results from immunological research should be considered [7, 8]: (a) It is commonly thought that 'immunological competence' is reached by 8 years of age, and that lymphatic tissue of Waldeyer's ring has a role in the elaboration of humoral immune responses; as a matter of fact, immunohistochemical studies have demonstrated that all subtypes of Ig-positive cells in palatine tonsils show age-related statistically significant differences. (b) Moreover, the identification at tonsillar level of a subpopulation of cells expressing simultaneously OKT4 and OKT8 markers (probably immature cells) suggests that tonsillar tissue share some characteristic features of central lymphatic organs.

Indications to the intervention of adenotonsillectomy have changed: the problem of obstruction is getting prominent over that of infection. We performed therefore the present study with two main purposes: (1) identification of a reliable diagnostic method to assess the severity of OSAS in very young children, and (2) identification of a surgical procedure to relieve upper airways obstruction with minimal interference with the maturation of the child's immune response.

Material and Methods

We included in our study 95 consecutive children aged 16–72 months, submitted to surgery for obstruction of upper airways, in whom the prominent symptom was loud snoring during sleep.

Children had a clinical evaluation before surgery and were controlled after surgery by means of an ENT visit and a questionnaire filled by parents. The follow-up period ran from 6 to 18 months.

A homogeneous subgroup of 43 children were referred to the Sleep Disorders Center and underwent a polysomnographic (diurnal or nocturnal) examination before surgery; postsurgical recordings were obtained in 14 cases at 6–12 months after surgery.

Polysomnography (PSG) included recording of EEG and eye movements, electromyography of mylohyoid and intercostal muscles, registration of oronasal, thoracic and abdominal breathing and measurement of heart rate and blood O_2 saturation during sleep.

PSG was used to define the severity of OSAS since it permits: (a) good control of sleep efficiency and stages distribution; (b) identification of sleep stage shifts; (c) evaluation of respiratory efficiency (apnea/hypopnea index); (d) measurement of blood oxygen saturation during the whole period under observation.

Since it was our intention to respect as much as possible the maturation of immune responses of our little patients, two different surgical procedures were used: 50 children were submitted to adenoidectomy and monotonsillectomy (AMT), and 45 were submitted to adenoidectomy and bilateral tonsillectomy (ABT). Children's age distribution and type of operation in the whole group (95 cases) and in the PSG subgroup (43 cases) are illustrated in figures 1 and 2. As shown in figure 1, the type of operation was not selected at random: according to clinical and ethical considerations, AMT was preferred in young children with heavy snoring not associated with repeated tonsillitis.

Results

Clinical Follow-Up

Sixty-two subjects (representing 65% of the total group) were controlled after surgery by means of PSG and/or ENT visit and questionnaire. Fifty-one questionnaires were filled out by children's parents (32 AMT and 19 ABT cases). We checked 40 out of 50 (80%) children submitted to AMT, and 22 out of 45 (48.8%) children submitted to ABT. Duration of follow-up is indicated in table 1.

Table 1. Children controlled after surgery

Follow-up	Cases
⩾ 6 months	62
⩾ 12 months	27
⩾ 18 months	4

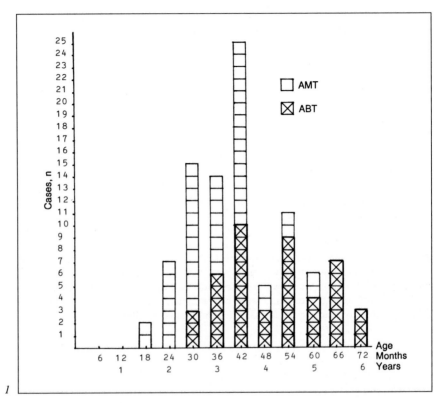

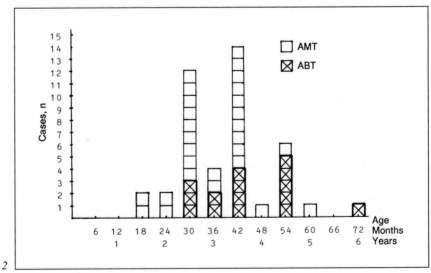

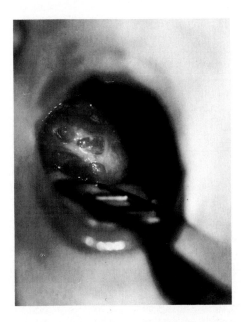

Fig. 3. Marked hypertrophy of residual tonsil, 1 year after AMT operation.

Clinical results after surgery are summarized by the following items: (a) All children had an immediate improvement of breathing during sleep, no matter what surgery (AMT or ABT) had been performed. (b) The improvement was still present at the end of the follow-up period in 94% of the checked cases; the 3 children who did not keep on breathing well had been treated with 2 AMT and 1 ABT operations. (c) Parents were not satisfied with the postoperative course of their child in only 12% of the cases (4 submitted to AMT and 2 submitted to ABT). In the same cases a significant number of fever episodes due to upper airways infections were reported. (d) In 38/40 (95%) children submitted to AMT and controlled postoperatively, the residual tonsil was not affected by phlogistic episodes in the follow-up period. (e) The 2 children who had repeated tonsillitis in the residual tonsil developed a marked hypertrophy of residual lymphoid tissue and consequently lost their respiratory improvement (fig. 3).

Fig. 1. Age distribution of 95 heavy snoring children submitted to tonsil surgery.
Fig. 2. Age distribution of 43 heavy snoring children submitted to tonsil surgery, studied with preoperative PSG.

Table 2. Results of PSG before surgery in 43 children: stages classification according to Lugaresi et al. [9]

	Cases	AMT	ABT
Stage 00 (neg)	2	1	1
0	14	10	4
1	22	11	11
2	5	5	–

Table 3. PSG parameters of 14 AMT children

	Before surgery		After surgery		p (t test)
	mean	SD	mean	SD	
SE, %	96.05	2.71	91.79	7.83	NS
St. 1 NREM, %	6.79	3.79	5.99	2.70	NS
St. 2 NREM, %	47.59	9.92	44.36	8.30	NS
St. 3–4 NREM, %	25.25	6.60	28.43	7.55	NS
St. REM, %	20.36	5.44	21.23	4.21	NS
WASO, min	8.13	7.28	21.75	18.74	NS
SHIFT	54.38	16.28	52.38	9.41	NS
A + H I	14.78	11.94	3.64	1.90	0.01
Min SaO$_2$, %	81.63	3.81	88.25	4.56	0.05

SE = Sleep efficiency; WASO = waking time after sleep onset; SHIFT = sleep disruptions; A + H I = apnea/hypopnea index; Min SaO$_2$ = minimal O$_2$ saturation during sleep.

PSG Study

PSG results before surgery in 43 children are listed in table 2. Figures 4 and 5 represent, respectively, mean apnea/hypopnea index and mean minimal blood O$_2$ saturation during sleep in 14 children submitted to adenomonotonsillectomy, studied before and after surgery. It appears that a clear difference exists between pre- and postsurgical values, the latter being normal. Table 3 shows pre/postsurgical changes of several sleep efficiency and respiratory efficiency parameters, and their statistical significance (paired t test).

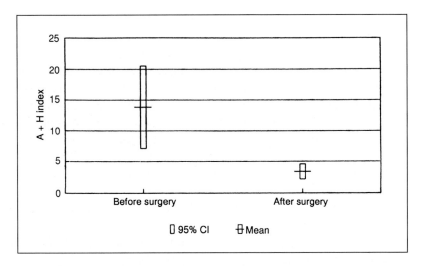

Fig. 4. Apnea/hypopnea index, before and after surgery, in 14 children submitted to AMT. A + H index = Apnea/hypopnea index; CI = confidence interval.

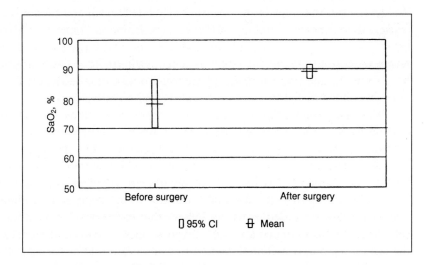

Fig. 5. Minimal blood O_2 saturation during sleep, before and after surgery, in 14 children submitted to AMT. SaO_2, % = Minimal blood O_2 saturation during sleep; CI = confidence interval.

Discussion

On the basis of the results of this study we can draw the following conclusions: (1) PSG is a reliable technique to evaluate sleep disruption and cardiopulmonary impairment produced by OSAS. In fact, results of PSG are in agreement with clinical findings, and they enable us to visualize significant changes after surgery (namely O_2 saturation and apnea index). (2) In the short period (6–12 months) monotonsillectomy associated with adenoidectomy is as good as bilateral tonsillectomy to resolve OSAS. At present we cannot compare the results of the two surgical procedures in the long period. We must consider, however, that 2 children submitted to AMT at the age of 2 years underwent the ablation of the other tonsil 1 year later because of relapsing phlogistic episodes: the consequence of inflammatory processes was a marked enlargement of the residual tonsil and a relapse of sleep apneas.

Up to now, clinical investigations did not demonstrate any definite damage to the immune system of very young children produced by tonsillectomy [10]. The lack of such a demonstration may result from the following facts: (a) children submitted to tonsillectomy are not comparable with 'normal' children, just because of reasons which required the intervention (OSAS or recurrent inflammatory processes); (b) residual lymphoid tissue of Waldeyer's ring may replace the functions of ablated tonsils and adenoids. A conservative surgical technique, however, is welcome in younger children below 3 years of age, since there is no doubt that maturation of immune responses is still in progress in such patients; furthermore, palatine tonsils have some unique characteristics [7, 8] which make them different from other lymphoepithelial tissues of respiratory and digestive tracts.

When polysomnographic findings show severe alterations, indications to deobstructive surgery on the pharyngeal lymphoid tissue is absolute and pressing, even in very young children (16–18 months in some cases). If surgery is performed at this age, however, the child sometimes needs a further intervention 1–2 years later because of regrowth of adenoids and/or marked hypertrophy of the residual tonsil due to relapsing acute inflammatory processes. Consequently, we believe that monotonsillectomy has a role in the treatment of pediatric OSAS as first operation in children below the age of 3 years. If a child comes to our observation after the age of 3 years with indication to surgery for severe OSAS, adenoidectomy associated with bilateral tonsillectomy should be held as a safer and definitive procedure.

References

1 Puckett CL, Pickens J, Reinsch JF: Sleep apnea in mandibular hypoplasia. Plast Reconstr Surg 1983;70:213.
2 Gaultier C, Prand JP, Canet E, Delaperche F, D'Allet AM, Nedelco H: Respiratory adaptation during sleep in healthy infants. Bull Eur Physiopathol Resp 1986;22: 54.
3 Guilleminaut C, Winkle R, Korobkin R, Simmons B: Children and nocturnal snoring: evaluation of the effects of sleep-related respiratory resistive load and daytime functioning. Eur J Pediatr 1982;139:165.
4 Stradling JR, Thomas G, Warley ARH, Williams P, Freeland A: Effect of adenotonsillectomy on nocturnal hypoxaemia, sleep disturbance and symptoms in snoring children. Lancet 1990;335:249.
5 Tevens WJ, Vermerire PA, Van Schil L: Bronchial hyperreactivity in rhinitis. Eur J Resp Dis 1983;64(suppl 128):72.
6 Principato JJ: Upper airway obstruction and craniofacial morphology. Otolaryngol Head Neck Surg 1991;104:881.
7 Surjan L: Lymphoepithelial structures in the pharynx immunobarriers. Acta Otolaryngol (Stockh) 1987;103:396.
8 Korsrud FR, Brandetzaeg P: Immunohistochemical evaluation of J-chain expression by intra- and extra-follicular immunoglobulin-producing human tonsillar cells. Scand J Immunol 1981;13:271.
9 Lugaresi E, Mondini S, Zucconi M, Montagna P, Cirignotta F: Staging of heavy snorers disease: a proposal. Bull Eur Physiopathol Resp 1983;19:590.
10 Bussi M, Carlevato MT, Zoppo M, Roncarolo MG: Phenotype expression and production of IL-2 tonsillar and blood lymphocytes in patients with tonsil pathology. Acta Otorhinolaryngol Ital 1989;9:149.

Dr. G. Pestalozza, ENT Division, Children's Hospital 'V. Buzzi',
Via F. Albani 11, I–20149 Milan (Italy)

Galioto GB (eds): Tonsils: A Clinically Oriented Update.
Adv Otorhinolaryngol. Basel, Karger, 1992, vol 47, pp 260–266

Measurement of Mesopharyngeal Pressure in Patients with Obstructive Sleep Apnea

Yasuo Koike, Kayoko Takeichi, Tatsuya Ishida, Mikio Yamaguchi, Shin-ya Ohtsu

Department of Otolaryngology, University of Tokushima School of Medicine, Tokushima, Japan

Many methods and techniques have been proposed for diagnosis of upper airway obstruction during sleep since Guilleminault et al. [1] reported the existence of sleep apnea syndrome due to airway obstruction in infants and children. These methods include the measurement of respiratory motion of the thorax, the registration of electroencephalogram, recording of O_2 and CO_2 levels in the blood flow, and many others. Since the results of measurement with these methods have been considerably variable, however, it has not been easy to precisely assess the degree of airway constriction, or obstruction, from the results of measurement with these methods.

Also, no definite means of determining the exact site of obstruction within the airway has so far been available. Although lateral X-ray films have been widely adopted for this purpose, it has been often difficult to pinpoint the virtual location of obstruction inside the upper respiratory system on these films. There is no need of lengthy explanation for the need of establishing an objective and reliable method for evaluating the degree of, and the site of, upper airway obstruction.

On the other hand, close observation of the infants and children with sleep apnea syndrome suggested the existence of a strong negative pressure within the respiratory system of these patients. The measurement of air pressure inside the respiratory system has thus been undertaken, in the hope that this pressure may serve as an indicator of the degree of constriction, or obstruction, in the upper respiratory system. This pressure infor-

Table 1. Classification of the subjects based on clinical symptoms and signs

Group	Sex, m:f (total)	Symptom		
		snoring	retracting respiration	sleep apnea
A	36:12 (48)	(−)	(−)	(−)
B	38:22 (60)	(+)	(−)	(−)
C	41:16 (57)	(+)	(+)	(−)
D	27:9 (36)	(+)	(+)	(+)

mation was thought to be useful to elucidate the site of obstruction also if it could be measured at multiple locations inside the respiratory system.

Materials and Methods

The subjects of the present study consisted of 201 patients with adenotonsillar hypertrophy. The ages of the patients ranged from 7 months to 14 years. Otolaryngological examinations were made on these children while they were awake, and lateral X-ray pictures were taken to assess the degree of adenotonsillar hypertrophy. These subjects were classified into 4 groups on the basis of clinical symptoms and signs, as depicted in table 1. Group A consisted of the patients without evidence of upper airway obstruction. The cases in group B had snoring in common, without retracting respiration and sleep apnea episode. The children in group C had snoring and retracting respiration, but they had no episode of sleep apnea. The subjects in group D had sleep apnea, along with snoring and retracting respiration.

An all-night polysomnography including mesopharyngeal pressure recording was performed on these subjects. Figure 1 shows the block diagram of the polysomnography employed. A miniaturized pressure transducer (Gaeltec S7b) was inserted into the mesopharynx through the nostril of the subject, and placed just below the palatine tonsils (fig. 2). The absolute value of the maximum amplitude of the pressure wave recorded during expiration and inspiration (mesopharyngeal pressure amplitude: MPA) was measured from the recorded data, and was adopted as an indicator of the negative pressure inside the respiratory system.

Other parameters of the polysomnography included the breath stream sensed by a thermistor, the thorax movement picked up with a strain gauge, and the sound of snoring. In 46 cases the level of oxygen saturation was also registered with an oxygen saturation monitor (Criticare Systems 501), as shown in figure 1. The polysomnography was repeated 1 week after adenotonsillectomy on 59 patients, in order to observe the effect of surgery on the recorded parameters. Various quantitative indices including apnea index (AI) and arterial oxygen saturation (SaO_2) were calculated from the recorded polysomnograms and were compared with the severity of clinical symptoms and signs.

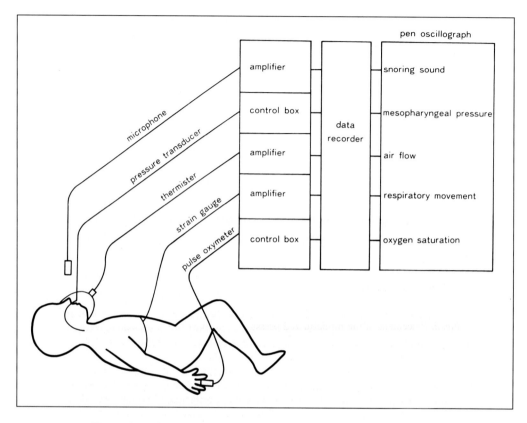

Fig. 1. Block diagram of polysomnography.

Results

Figure 3 shows the MPA values during sleep for the 4 subject groups. The MPA values for the patients in groups B, C, and D were significantly higher than those for the children in group A. The cases in group D, with obstructive sleep apnea, revealed evidently high MPA values. The children in group C, with retracting respiration and snoring, showed moderately high MPA values. The subjects in group B, with snoring only, demonstrated slightly high MPA values. It is apparent that the MPA value is closely associated with the severity of clinical symptoms and signs.

The symptoms and signs of upper airway obstruction, such as obstructive sleep apnea, retracting respiration, and snoring, were apparently

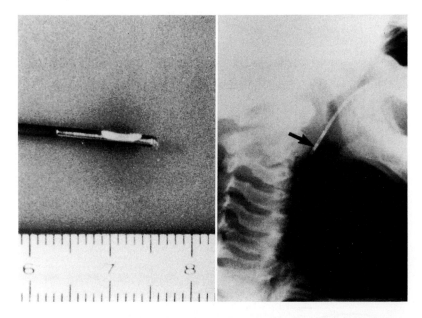

Fig. 2. Placement of the miniaturized pressure transducer in the mesopharynx.

improved after adenotonsillectomy. Figure 4 discloses the MPA values for each subject group after the surgery. The MPA values are seen to be remarkably reduced after the operation, and the difference in the mean MPA value among different subject groups was not significant any more. The close relationship between the MPA value and the degree of airway constriction can be known from this fact also.

Figure 5 illustrates polysomnograms for 3 representative cases. The tracings on the left side (case 1) show the data for a boy with retracting respiration and snoring. The AI value for this patient was 0.7, which was within the normal limits, and the SaO_2 was also within the normal range. The downward deviation of the mesopharyngeal pressure wave increased with time, however, and the MPA reached 63 cm H_2O, indicating the exis- tence of a strong negative pressure. The tracings in the middle (case 2) demonstrates the data for a patient with retracting respiration and snoring. This patient could not be diagnosed as obstructive sleep apnea syndrome (OSAS) on the conventional standard, since the AI value for this case was 2.8 (within normal limits). This case, nevertheless, revealed an MPA value

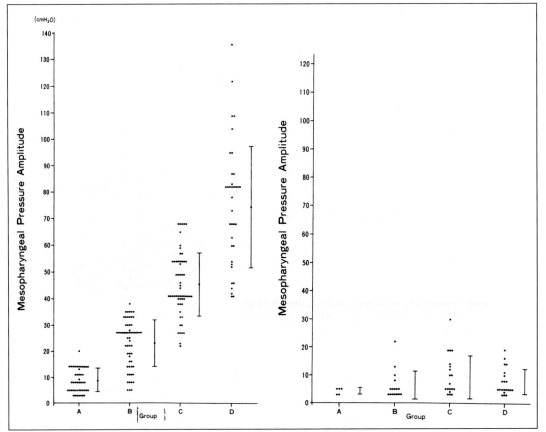

Fig. 3. Preoperative MPA values for subject groups A–D.
Fig. 4. Postoperative MPA values for subject groups A–D.

of 71 cm H_2O, implying the existence of a strong negative pressure inside the respiratory system. These two cases were judged to have obstructive hypopnea, secondary to adenotonsillar hypertrophy.

The tracings on the right side of figure 5 (case 3) display the data for a case with OSAS, with an AI value of 22.4. The lowest level of SaO_2 of this patient decreased to 70% during sleep, though the SaO_2 while awake was 98%. The MPA value was quite high (88 cm H_2O), and agreed well with other index values as well as with clinical findings.

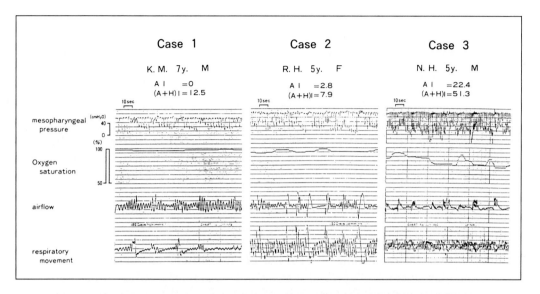

Fig. 5. Polysomnograms for representative cases. The amplitude of MPA wave for case 1 remarkably increases with time, though AI and SaO_2 remain within normal limits. The MPA for case 2 also reaches a high value, independent of AI and SaO_2. The data for case 3, with obstructive sleep apnea, show an apparent abnormality in MPA, as well as in AI and SaO_2.

Discussion

It seems justifiable to mention that the MPA is a useful index revealing the pathologic status in the pharynx of the patients with upper airway obstruction, on the basis of the data presented above. It is clear that the MPA value can demonstrate abnormality in the cases with OSAS, as good as the AI does. It seems to be particularly important here, however, that the MPA could reveal pathologic status even when the AI did not indicate any abnormality, as demonstrated by the cases shown in figure 5.

It is well known that there exist many patients with upper airway obstruction, or constriction, who reveal considerable clinical symptoms and signs without having a high AI value. It may be considered, therefore, that the AI is not sufficient to detect mild cases of upper airway obstruction, even though it may be suited for the description of severe cases such as OSAS. This may be due to the fact that the AI is based on the time characteristics of the prominent apnea episodes only. On the one hand, therefore, improvement of the AI may be needed. Since an improved AI [(A+H)I], which takes hypopnea events also into account, has already been proposed [2], the efficiency of this index in revealing abnormality may be worth studying.

On the other hand, many more factors associated with sleep disturbances should be considered to assess the degree of upper airway obstruction. The MPA proposed here may be regarded as one of such attempts. It is known that an MPA value of up to 10 cm H_2O is within the normal limits [3]. The MPA seems to be quite sensitive to the hypopnea status, or mild cases of upper airway obstruction, as have been discussed above. It should be added here also that the behavior of the MPA is closely associated with the rise and fall of clinical symptoms and signs such as retracting respiration and snoring over a wide range of the MPA values.

The determination of the site of obstruction, or constriction, is another important aspect of diagnosis. As mentioned earlier, it has not been easy to decide the virtual site of obstruction in the respiratory system with the conventional methods for diagnosis. By measuring the MPA at multiple locations inside the respiratory system, however, it is feasible to determine the virtual position of obstruction inside the respiratory system [4]. This procedure should provide with a quite useful information for deciding surgical indication and for selecting the mode of surgery. Although not much emphasis was placed on this point in the present article, the technique of MPA measurement at multiple locations should be further developed to improve the diagnosis and treatment of upper airway obstruction.

References

1   Guilleminault C, Tilkian A, Dement W: The sleep apnea syndromes. Annu Rev Med 1976;27:465–484.
2   Guilleminault C: Sleeping and Waking Disorders: Indications and Techniques. Menlo Park, Addison-Wesley, 1982.
3   Ishida T: The measurement of mesopharyngeal pressure in patients with upper airway obstruction. Pract Otol (Kyoto) 1985;78:411–432.
4   Takeichi K: Evaluation of sleep respiratory disorders in children with adeno-tonsillar hypertrophy. Jpn J Otol (Tokyo) 1988;91:88–100.

Yasuo Koike, MD, Department of Otolaryngology, University of Tokushima School of Medicine, 3 Kuramoto, Tokushima 770 (Japan)

Galioto GB (ed): Tonsils: A Clinically Oriented Update.
Adv Otorhinolaryngol. Basel, Karger, 1992, vol 47, pp 267–270

Obstructive Sleep Apnea in Children

Tomoko Shintani, Kohji Asakura, Akikatsu Kataura

Department of Otorhinolaryngology, Sapporo Medical College, Japan

Upper airway obstruction during sleep induces obstructive sleep apnea syndrome (OSAS). OSAS patients usually complain of heavy snoring, daytime sleepiness and, in severe cases, cardiovascular disorders. Furthermore, OSAS in children may affect facial growth and also cause chest deformities. The most important cause of OSAS in children is thought to be adenoid and tonsillar hypertrophy. However, abnormalities in maxillofacial developments may also contribute to OSAS by narrowing the skeletal structure of the upper airway. In order to evaluate the contributions of these factors, we performed cephalometric analysis in OSAS children.

Material and Methods

One hundred and eleven OSAS children (75 boys and 36 girls, mean age 4.5 ± 1.7 years) were evaluated with a sleep study using respiratory inductive plethysmography (Respigraph, Nims, USA) and cephalometric analysis. Eighty-three patients were treated surgically (adenotomy only 8, tonsillectomy only 3, and adenotonsillectomy 66 cases) and the above evaluations were performed before and 2 months after treatment. The severity of OSAS was determined by apnea-hypopnea index (AHI). The children who showed more than 50% improvement in apnea index after treatment were divided into the good responders group and those with less than 50% improvement into the poor responders group. The cephalometric analysis was performed by using a lateral maxillofacial roentgenogram, which was taken at upright position with the mouth closed. The distance between the source of radiation and the film was 150 cm. Figure 1 shows the methods for evaluation of adenoidal hypertrophy. AA′ represents an absolute value of adenoidal hypertrophy expressed as a perpendicular distance at maximum convexity [1]. AN ratio [2] is a relative value of a width of adenoidal shadow to a depth of nasopharyngeal space. It represents a relative contribution of adenoidal hypertrophy in nasopharyngeal stenosis. PNS-A [3] is a distance from the posterior nasal spine to the nearest adenoid tissue measured along the line posterior nasal spine–basion, and it represents the width of the airway. Figure 2 shows a method of cephalometric analysis for evaluation of maxilloman-

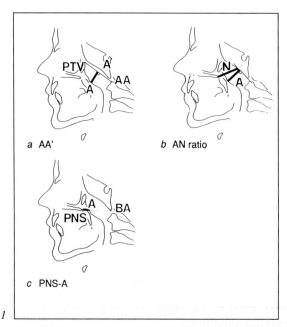
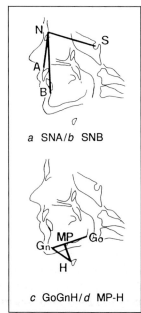

Fig. 1. a–c Methods for evaluation of adenoidal hypertrophy. PTV = Pterygoid vertical; AA = anterior of atlas; N = nasopharyngeal measurement; A = adenoidal measurement; PNS = postnasal spine; BA = basion.
Fig. 2. Method of cephalometric analysis for evaluation. *a/b* S = Sella point; N = nasion; A = subspinale; B = supraspinale. *c/d* Go = Gonion; Gn = gnathion; H = hyoid bone; MP = mandibular plane.

dibular developments and hyoid bone position. SNA angle reveals the protrusion of the maxilla and SNB reveals the protrusion of the mandible. A position of hyoid bone was evaluated by GoGnH angle and MP-H distance.

Results and Discussion

Relationships between Cephalometric Values and OSAS Severity

As a result, severe OSAS children (AHI ≥ 20) tended to have larger adenoids and smaller airspace than mild OSAS children (AHI < 20) (AN ratio: mild/0.68, severe/0.72, p < 0.01; PNS-A: mild/9.4 mm, severe/ 10.0 mm). There were no differences in SNA and SNB angles with maxillomandibular developments (SNA; mild/78.6, severe/79.5, SNB; mild/75.6, severe/75.3). However, compared with adult OSAS patients, SNA and SNB angles in OSAS children were significantly smaller than those in adult OSAS patients. Thus, compared with adult's airway space, adenoid or adenotonsillar hypertrophy can easily affect children's airspace.

Relationship between Cephalometric Values and Treatment

In adult OSAS patients, the most popular surgical treatment, UPPP, is effective in only 50–60% of the patients. However, in OSAS children it is thought that the majority of patients were successfully treated with adenotonsillectomy. Seventy-seven patients were treated surgically and we divided them into two groups: in good responders the adenoids tended to be larger and the epipharyngeal airspace tended to be smaller than those in poor responders (AN ratio: good R./69.0, poor R./64.2; PNS-A: good R./8.8 mm, poor R./10.1 mm). GoGnH and MP-H represented the position of the hyoid bone. In the two parameters, good responder's values were significantly larger than poor responder's values (GoGnH: good R./22.9, poor R./17.9; MP-H: good R./12.5 mm, poor R./9.4 mm). There were no differences in maxillomandibular developments measured by SNA and SNB angles between these two groups. As a result, good responders for adenotonsillectomy tended to have larger adenoids and tonsils, and low set hyoid bones. From these studies it was determined that OSAS children with adenotonsillar hypertrophy can successfully be treated with adenotonsillectomy.

Reports of Difficult Cases in Treatments

In OSAS children with adenotonsillar hypertrophy the relation of treatment results and protrusion of maxilla and mandible has not been clarified. We also studied 5 severe OSAS children who showed no signs of adenotonsillar hypertrophy. All of these cases had some other congenital malformations and general associated disorders. In relation to upper airway obstruction, micrognathia was noted in 4 cases, anterior dislocation of the atlas in 1 case and cerebral palsy in 2 cases. In each patient, apnea occurred from birth. In the results of cephalometric analysis, as indicated in AA', AN ratio and PNA-A values, no signs of adenotonsillar hypertrophy were noted in 4 children except for the second case. However, no adenoidal hypertrophy was noted in precise examination under general anesthesia in the second case. There were no massive changes at the epipharynx except for a slight fibrous sclerosis at the veropharyngeal space. As indicated in SNA and SNB values, a poor prognathism of the maxilla and mandible was noted. Lower positioned hyoid bone was noted in all cases examined. In these cases, skeletal morphology was thought to contribute to upper airway obstruction. As a treatment, tracheostomy was performed in 3 cases, and UPPP was effective in the third case. If no adenotonsillar hypertrophy was apparent, UPPP with or without adenotonsillectomy could improve in selected children [4, 5].

Conclusion

Adenotonsillar hypertrophy is the most common cause of OSAS in children, in which adenotonsillectomy is an effective treatment. Because maxillomandibular development in children is significantly poorer than that of adults, it is suspected that the skeletal morphology contributes to OSAS in children. Some OSAS children without adenotonsillar hypertrophy can be successfully treated with UPPP.

References

1   Koizumi T, Furuhata T: X-ray observations on pharyngeal tonsils: Second report on the changes seen before and after adenotomy. Jiko 1958;30:637–641.
2   Fujioka M, Young LW, Leftridge GM, Cassisi NJ: Upper airway obstruction during sleep in children. Am J Roentgenol 1979;133:213–216.
3   Linder-Aronson S, Stockholm L: Adenoids: Their effect on mode of breathing and nasal airflow and their relationship to characteristics of the facial skeleton and the dentition. Acta Otolaryngol 1970(suppl):265.
4   Allan B, Seid LCDR, Peter J, Martin USN, Seth M, Pransky D, Kearns B: Surgical therapy of obstructive sleep apnea in children with severe mental insufficiency. Laryngoscope 1990;100:507–510.
5   Mufid H, Abudu J, Feghali G: Uvulopalatopharyngoplasty in a child with obstructive sleep apnea. J Laryngol Otol 1988;102:546–548.

Dr. Tomoko Shintani, Department of Otolaryngology, Sapporo Medical College, S.1, W.1b, Chuo-ku, Sapporo (Japan)

Galioto GB (ed): Tonsils: A Clinically Oriented Update.
Adv Otorhinolaryngol. Basel, Karger, 1992, vol 47, pp 271–275

Obstructive Sleep Apnea Syndrome and A&T Surgery

M. De Benedetto, D. Cuda, M. Leante

ORL Department, S. Caterina Novella Hospital, Galatina, Lecce, Italy

Obstructive sleep apnea syndrome (OSAS) can occur frequently in children with adenoid and tonsillar hypertrophy (ATH) [1–3]. It is well known that A&T surgery is a very effective treatment when obstructive symptoms are unequivocally attributable to ATH, affording complete relief [4–6]. For these reasons, OSAS represents a definite indication for A&T operation [4, 5].

OSAS is a disease potentially severe in children and it is characterized by a wide range of symptoms: sleep disturbances, diurnal manifestations (behavioral disturbance, excessive daytime somnolence) and in some cases severe cardiopulmonary sequelae [7–13]. It appears likely that OSAS may be more common than it is generally appreciated.

The identification of children affected by OSAS is a difficult task because of poor knowledge of epidemiology and the difficulties in the diagnosis of disease.

We consider three different levels of diagnostic definition of OSAS: 'suspect', 'likely' and 'definite'. 'Definite OSAS' is a diagnosis based on polysomnographic recordings. However, the poor availability of sleep laboratories, the costs and the possible nonacceptance preclude a large use of polysomnography in the pediatric population. 'Likely OSAS' is based on a simplified test that monitors tissular O_2 saturation during sleep. The evidence of several phasic drops in O_2 saturation is strongly suggestive of OSAS in children with ATH [14]. Several clinical oximeters are now available and regular usage is also possible at the child's home. 'Suspect OSAS' is based on clinical data such as habitual snoring and/or direct parental observation of apneas during sleep in a child with significant ATH.

In order to quantify the problem of OSAS in relation to A&T surgery, in this paper we refer epidemiological data of 'suspect OSAS' and 'likely OSAS' in some clinical pediatric populations. We refer also about current A&T surgical trends at our Department.

'Suspect' OSAS

A questionnaire concerning sleep disturbances and related problems was submitted to parents of 307 children aged 0–10 years (mean 4.7, SD 2.4) referred consecutively to their pediatrician for various clinical problems. 141 were girls and 166 were boys. In 101 cases (32.9%) snoring was referred to as occasional ('sometimes' or 'often') or habitual ('always'). Habitual snoring was described in only 17 cases (5.5%). Sleep apnea was referred to in 6.9% of cases. It is important to remember, however, that an answer to this question was difficult to obtain in 17.3% of cases due to the parents' lack of awareness about this sleep disorder. Significant ATH was mentioned by pediatricians in 30.2% of the cases in question. Percentage data concerning the total prevalence of snoring and prevalence of habitual snoring alone, of apnea and of ATH per age groups, are shown in table 1; the close link between ATH and snoring is also emphasized. They present an overlapping age trend and similar prevalence. Prevalence reaches its peak between 5 and 7 years of age. Despite a few discrepancies in the upper age groups probably due to the low number of patients, habitual snoring and apnea also show a similar trend.

In summary, from the gathered data we can conclude that about 30% of the children of the general pediatric practice have ATH strictly correlated to some sort of snoring. Cases with major obstruction (habitual snoring and apnea) were pinpointed in 5–7% with a maximum peak at the age of 5–7 years. These data are in accord with Corbo et al. [15], who report a mean prevalence of habitual snorers of 7.3% in a large sample of children aged 6–13 years.

'Likely' OSAS

As an indicator of the likely presence of OSAS in children, we recorded O_2 tissular saturation during sleep with a transcutaneous electrode in 36 children (average age 4.6, SD 2.6) with obstructive and/or

Table 1. Prevalence of snoring, apnea and A&T hypertrophy in a pediatric sample

Age	Patients	Snoring %	Hab. snoring %	Apnea %	A&T hypertrophy %
1	18	0	0	0	0
2	43	4.7	0	0	5
3	45	24.4	6.7	8.0	22.7
4	52	32.7	5.8	8.7	30.6
5	38	52.6	7.9	5.9	48.6
6	36	47.2	11.1	15.8	45.5
7	30	50.0	13.3	11.1	41.4
8	17	47.1	0	12.5	40.0
9	17	41.2	0	11.1	35.3
10	11	36.4	0	0	36.4

infectious symptoms of the upper airways referred for A&T surgery evaluation. On the basis of our usual clinical approach, derived from Pittsburgh criteria [5], 16 cases were indicated to surgical intervention (12 A&T, 1 T, 3 A), whilst the remaining 20 cases were not; the latter were considered as a 'control group'. The 'Event Index' (EI) was considered as the oximetric index. It was defined by the average number of 'respiratory events' per hour of sleep. In other words, EI was the number of times in which O_2 tissular saturation drops below 4%, that is to basal values. The average EI in the operated group (presurgical values) was 27.7 (SD 28.8) against 11.9 (SD 12.7) of the control group; this difference was statistically significative ($t = -2.21$, $p = 0.03$).

A second recording carried out after an average of 18 days after surgical intervention (range 1–85) showed an average EI of 9.8 (SD 8.5). This data was statistically different from the presurgical values (EI 27.7) and similar to that of the control group (EI 11.9). Considering a normality criterion of 15 events per hour of sleep, 15 children out of 36 (41.6%) had oximetric data suggestive of OSAS: 10 in the surgically treated group (10/16 = 62.5%) and 5 in the non operated group (5/20 = 25%). Out of the 10 surgically treated children with a presurgical EI > 15,8 had a normal index when recorded after the operation; the 2 remaining cases approached the extreme value of normality (EI 16.2, 18).

Table 2. A&T operations performed at ENT Department, Galatina

Year	A, %	A&T, %	T, %	Age
1986	86	1	13	6.1
1987	76	11	13	5.8
1988	55	31	14	5.3
1989	37	52	11	5.4
1990	32	59	9	5.3

These data indicate a high prevalence of OSAS (probability diagnoses) in subjects with A&T diseases, estimated at about 40%. By referring to the usual ENT clinical indications for A&T surgery, the prevalence seems to be higher than 60% (sensitivity 60%) for surgically treated children and only 25% for nonsurgically treated children (specificity 75%). Moreover, it is quite likely that sensitivity data are underestimated since they also include cases that are prevailingly infectious within the group in question. Low specificity rate indicates that the current clinical approach must be revised in order to include cases of possible mild OSAS in treated group. A larger clinical criteria and/or a simple test such as oximetry need to be further evaluated in this respect.

Surgical Trends

During the 5 years from 1986 to 1990, 834 A&T surgical interventions were carried out at our Department. The percentages of the single operations per year as well as the average age of the patients with regards to the 1- to 10-year age group are shown in table 2. Operations of tonsillectomy alone are quite constant though there is a slight decrease in the last 2 years, whilst adenoidectomies have constantly decreased in favor of a growing number of A&T operations. The average age of intervention has decreased gradually to a steady age of about 5.3 years. This trend reveals an increasing number of surgical indications for obstructive problems with suspect OSAS; in fact, A&T operation represents at our Department the choice treatment for obstructive cases in this age group. A similar trend is referred to by Rosenfeld and Green [16].

References

1   Bradley TD, Brown IG, Grossman RF: Pharyngeal size in snorers, nonsnorers and patients with obstructive sleep apnea. N Engl J Med 1986;315:1327–1331.

2   Brouillette RT, Fernbach SK, Hunt CE: Obstructive sleep apnea in infant and children. J Pediatr 1982;100:31–40.

3   Guilleminault C, Korobkin R, Winkle R: A review of 50 children with obstructive sleep apnea syndrome. Lung 1981;159:275–287.

4   Eliasker I, Lovie P, Halperin E, Gordon C, Alroy G: Sleep apnea episodes as indications for adenotonsillectomy. Arch Otolaryngol 1980;106:492–496.

5   Paradise JL: Tonsillectomy and adenoidectomy; in Bluestone CD, Stool SE, Arjona SK (eds): Pediatric Otolaryngology. Philadelphia, Saunders, 1983, pp 992–1006.

6   Potsic WP, Pasquariello PS, Baranak CC: Relief of upper airway obstruction by adenotonsillectomy. Otolaryngol Head Neck Surg 1986;4:476–480.

7   Grundfast KM, Wittich DJ: Adenotonsillar hypertrophy and upper airway obstruction in evolutionary perspective. Laryngoscope 1982;92:650–656.

8   Mauer KW, Staats BA, Olsen KD: Upper airway obstruction and disordered nocturnal breathing in children. Mayo Clin Proc 1983;58:349–353.

9   Sidman JD, Fry TL: Exacerbation of sickle cell disease by obstructive sleep apnea. Arch Otolaryngol Head Neck Surg 1988;114:916–917.

10 Levy AM, Tabakin BS, Harrison JS: Hypertrophied adenoids causing pulmonary hypertension and severe congestive failure. N Engl J Med 1967;277:506–511.

11 Menashe VD, Fearron C, Miller M: Hypoventilation and cor pulmonale due to chronic upper airway obstruction. J Pediatr 1965;67:198–203.

12 Noonan JA: Reversible cor pulmonale due to hypertrophied tonsil and adenoids. Circulation 1965;32(suppl 2):164.

13 Talbot AR, Robertson LW: Cardiac failure with tonsil and adenoid hypertrophy. Arch Otolaryngol 1973;98:272–281.

14 Cuda D, Graziuso M, Leante M, Mauro N, Vitale S: Utilità della SaO$_2$ nella diagnostica dell'apnea ostruttiva nel sonno in età pediatrica. Atti III Incontro Interdisciplinare su: Le infezioni delle vie respiratorie – I disturbi respiratori nel sonno, Lecce 1990, pp 291–298.

15 Corbo G, Fuciarelli F, Foresi A, De Benedetto F: Snoring in children: association with respiratory symptoms and passive smoking. Br Med J 1990;299:1491–1494.

16 Rosenfeld RM, Green RP: Tonsillectomy and adenoidectomy: changing trends. Ann Otol Rhinol Laryngol 1990;99:187–191.

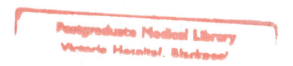
Dr. Michele De Benedetto, Via Pascoli, 19, I-73013 Galatina, Lecce (Italy)

Galioto GB (ed): Tonsils: A Clinically Oriented Update.
Adv Otorhinolaryngol. Basel, Karger, 1992, vol 47, pp 276–280

Alveolar Hypoventilation due to Adenoid and Tonsillar Hypertrophy

A. Battistini[a], *G. Pisi*[a], *T. Ferri*[b]

Departments of [a]Pediatrics and [b]Otolaryngology, University of Parma, Italy

It took 20 years to single out all the secondary clinical expressions of an obstructive adenotonsillar (A&T) hypertrophy. In fact, we go back to 1965 when the very first cases of cardiocirculatory insufficiency from A&T hypertrophy [1] were described up until 1986 when we realized that snoring [2] represents the initial sign of nasal-pharyngeal obstruction. By taking into consideration the various clinical pictures, we are also able today to trace in a precise manner the natural history of the obstructive A&T hypertrophy (fig. 1). It is however simple to imagine how the various clinical expressions do not represent something very irreversible: a common viral infection may be enough to momentarily worsen the obstruction and therefore lead temporarily from snore to hypoventilation or from this to a series of apnea during sleep. This temporary, intraindividual variability is certainly one of the factors which may cause a more difficult diagnosis, especially during the initial phases when the patient begins to hypoventilate.

The aim of the study was to facilitate the diagnosis by pointing out the anamnestic and clinical medical data which better characterize the beginning of a hypoventilation due to A&T hypertrophy.

Materials and Methods

119 patients (82 males) were studied. Median age was 1 year and 9 months; median age at the beginning of the symptom was 9 months. They all had a suggestive history for an obstructive A&T hypertrophy but only 74 were hypercapnic. Out of the latter, 38 were less than 2 years old.

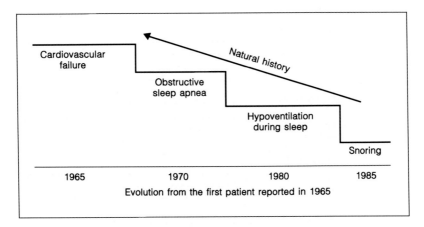

Fig. 1. The evolution of the medical literature compared with the natural history of the obstructive A&T hypertrophy.

The anamnestic data available were: (a) *while awake:* oral respiration, heavy breathing, dysphagia, vomiting, otitis, chronic rhinorrhea, sleepiness, aggressiveness, inappetence; (b) *during sleep:* snoring, oral respiration, respiratory pauses, agitated sleep, frequent awakenings, profuse sweat.

The clinical data available were: (a) *while awake:* heavy breathing, adenoidal facies, pectus excavatum, lung sounds, tonsillar hypertrophy; (b) *during sleep:* snoring, oral respiration, respiratory pauses and/or apnea, agitated sleep, Müller maneuver, chest wall retractions.

The capnography was performed during night sleep. The highest normal limit of the end-tidal CO_2 (or $PACO_2$) was considered equal to 42 mm Hg. The incidence of the anamnestic and clinical data was examined in the following groups: (A) patients with a history of an obstructive A&T hypertrophy divided into two subgroups: hypercapnic versus normocapnic, and (B) patients suffering from obstructive A&T hypertrophy and hypercapnia divided into two groups: patients < 2 years of age versus patients > 2 years of age.

Statistical analyses were carried out with the χ^2 test.

Results

The anamnesis does not present any significant difference between hypercapnic and normocapnic patients. Three clinical parameters during wake (underweight, tonsillar hypertrophy, loud respiration) and four during sleep (snoring, oral respiration, inspiratory retractions, respiratory pauses) are more frequent in the hypercapnic patient than in the normo-

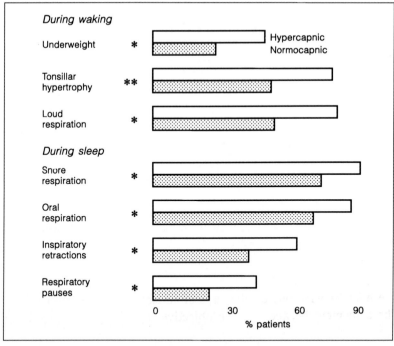

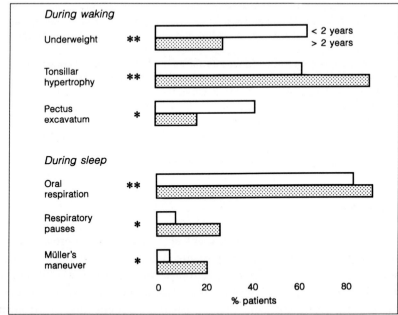

capnic patient (fig. 2). Younger children present less frequently otitis, sinusitis, and oral respiration. Moreover, the younger child more often presents pectus excavatum and is underweight while instead he rarely presents tonsillar hypertrophy, oral respiration, apnea, and Müller maneuver (fig. 3).

Discussion

Normocapnic Patients versus Hypercapnic Patients

The fact that hypercapnic patients have an overlapping anamnesis to that of normocapnic patients, confirms the hypothesis that the obstructive situation undergoes many swingings in time. Normocapnic patients are in fact most probably subjects who in the past have had an obstruction and therefore a symptomatology from acute phlogosis which at the moment of $PACO_2$ determination was resolved. When facing a suggestive history it would therefore be a serious mistake to put aside the diagnosis of obstructive A&T hypertrophy on the basis of an isolated result of normocapnia. The agreement between certain objective reports and the presence of a hypercapnia not only confirms the importance of the clinical exam, particularly the one performed during sleep, but it points out many qualifying reports for a hypoventilation and precisely: loud respiration whilst awake, snoring, respiratory pauses, and inspiratory retractions. Tonsillar hypertrophy and open mouth respiration are also important, even though these reports may be missing in the youngest child (see below).

Patients < 2 Years Old versus > 2 Years Old

The major incidence of pectus excavatum during the first 2 years of life is most probably referable to the major malleability of the sternum which becomes therefore more easily deformed by the abnormal intrathoracic depressions during the inspiration. The minor incidence of tonsillar hypertrophy in younger children is referable to the fact that during the first 2 years the development of the lymphatic tissue has not yet reached its

---

Fig. 2. Hypercapnic versus normocapnic patients. Only items with a significant difference are reported: ** $p < 0.01$; * $p < 0.05$.

Fig. 3. Hypercapnic patients < 2 years old versus older hypercapnic patients. ** $p < 0.01$; * $p < 0.05$.

highest point. The advantage of a minor tonsil obstruction nevertheless is cancelled in the youngest child by the difficulty of oral respiration not only because of a more restricted oropharynx (epiglottis closer to the palate) but also because in front of a nasal obstruction an opening of the mouth reflex may be missing [3]. We explain in this way the less frequent oral respiration in the youngest child as far as the anamnestic and objective data is concerned. Even apnea and/or respiratory pauses during sleep and the consequent Müller maneuver are less frequent in the youngest child: this probably is to reconduct to the minor duration in time (months) of the hypoventilation and therefore to a minor increase of the awakening threshold.

The anatomical and functional peculiarities of the first 2 years of life on the one hand make the clinical picture less rich, on the other hand they do not reduce the hypoventilation and its consequences. In fact, the average value of $PACO_2$ in the youngest child overlaps that of the oldest child while the percentage of underweight children is greater in the group of children under 2 years of age. If to all of this we add that the number of children diagnosed during the first 2 years of life is greater than the number of oldest children and that the median age of the beginning of the symptoms in our population globally considered is 9 months, we can understand why the diagnosis of obstructive A&T has to be performed during the very first years of life. However, the diagnosis may offer more difficulty during the first years of life because of a minor frequency of signs as important as tonsillar hypertrophy, open mouth respiration and apnea during sleep.

References

1   Menashe VD, Farrehi C, Miller M: Hypoventilation and cor pulmonale due to chronic upper airway obstruction. J Pediatr 1965;67:198–203.
2   Battistini A: Apnea e ipoventilazione notturna da ostruzione delle prime vie aeree. Atti 8° Convegno di Neurologia Neonatale 'Le Apnee del Neonato e del Lattante', Modena 1986, pp 51–58.
3   Mautone AJ, Cataletto MB: Mechanical defense mechanisms of the lung; in Scarpelli EM (ed): Pulmonary Physiology: Fetus, Newborn, Child, and Adolescent. Philadelphia, Lea & Febiger, 1990, pp 192–208.

Dr. A. Battistini, Centro Fisiopatologia Respiratoria Infantile, Università, Via Gramsci 14, I–43100 Parma (Italy)

Galioto GB (ed): Tonsils: A Clinically Oriented Update.
Adv Otorhinolaryngol. Basel, Karger, 1992, vol 47, pp 281–283

Natural History of Otitis media with Effusion in Children under Six Years of Age

G. Bartolozzi, A. Sacchetti, P. Scarane, P. Becherucci

Pediatric Clinic I, University of Florence, Italy

Otitis media with effusion (OME) is defined [1] as an inflammation of the middle ear, with fluid present, without symptoms or signals of intense infection as otalgia and fever: OME can present itself after an acute otitis or strike at any given moment [2]. The incidence of OME has been predominantly studied by Anglo-Saxon authors [3–5]. It seemed worthwhile considering the behavior of this pathology in Italian children.

Materials and Methods

441 children were examined (221 males, 220 females; infants to 6 years of age) who attended six nursery schools or four kindergartens in Florence. Children with a tympanostomic tube were excluded and so were those with an acute otitis as well as those who were known to have a hearing deficiency.

The subjects studied were categorized as follows: (a) 71 subjects (16.1%) up to 2 years of age; (b) 177 subjects (40.1%) from 2 to 4 years of age, and (c) 193 subjects (43.8%) from 4 to 6 years of age. The children's parents were asked to sign a letter of consent in order to proceed with the study. A group of medical practitioners (two pediatrician experts for tympanometer screening and the otoscopy exam and one nurse) visited the children once a month between February and June with another visit in September of the same year. The instrument used was a portable computerized tympanometer (Welch Allin). Every child's nose, ears and throat were examined. The visit included otoscopy and tympanometry of the ear. The clinical history was asked for possible infections in these regions. Possible absences, their causes and possible treatment were also noted. If tympanometry was pathological for one practitioner, the other one would repeat the test: we noted a constant compatibility of the results. 4,008 tympanograms were done with an average of 4.5 exams/child. The tympanograms were classified according to Paradise et al. [6]. The length of OME duration was calculated on the basis of the time in which the pathologic exam was taken and the resolution, after a continuous period of study. Chil-

Table 1. Percentage of the various results of all subjects studied in that month: the frequency of distribution in each category (χ^2) is very significant (p < 0.001)

	Normal ears	One pathologic	Two pathologic
February	30.2	26.0	43.8
March	41.7	26.4	31.9
April	46.6	19.2	34.2
May	65.8	14.1	20.1
June	64.4	15.5	20.1
September	83.0	8.5	8.5

dren affected by OME were those who had pathological otoscopy and tympanogram, mono- or bilaterally. Children affected by chronic OME were those who had a pathological tympanogram within three recurrent visits (about 3 months). No matter what the results were, no treatment was suggested.

Results

The percentage of the results of all subjects studied is listed in table 1. The frequency of distribution in each category is very significant (p < 0.001). A progressive decrease of pathology is evident, both mono- and bilaterally, in the spring and summer months. If we consider categorization according to age (0–2, 2–4, >4) the result is the same, even if in younger subjects pathology decreases more slowly. Looking at the overall study, 313 subjects (70.9%) had at least one OME, while 215 (48.8%) had one in the right and one in the left ear. This confirms the extreme frequency of this pathology in preschool children: moreover, 71 children under 2 years of age had at least one OME (84.5%). The average duration of OME was 1.91 ± 1.23 months. 18.4% of the children had chronic OME, while 15.4% had at least one relapse. These percentages are considerably increased if we only consider cases under 2 years of age (chronicity 28.2%, relapses 30.9%). Furthermore, the average age of the subjects with chronic OME is 2.9 ± 1.2 years, with 4.0 ± 1.3 of healthy subjects or with occasional OME (p < 0.0001); those with relapses are considerably younger (3.4 ± 1.6 years; p < 0.0001). In subjects with monolateral OME, the relapse almost always attacks the ear that was previously infected: of the 136 subjects with right OME in February, 58 experienced a recurrence in April, but only 8 recovered and had it in the left ear.

Conclusions

From the above data we can formulate certain conclusions. (1) OME has a seasonal incidence (winter) and is very frequent in subjects who go to kindergarten, often with spontaneous recovery, especially for children over 4 years of age. (2) Chronicity and relapses are present, especially in young subjects: usually occurring for brief periods (2 months on average). (3) There are (anatomical, functional) factors that predetermine the incidence of OME. This is clearly obvious as subjects with monolateral pathology are always affected in the same ear.

References

1   Bluestone CD: State of the art: definitions and classifications; in Lim DJ (ed): Recent Advances in Otitis media with Effusion. Philadelphia, Decker, 1984, pp 34–36.
2   Paparella MM, Schachern PA, Toon TH, et al: Otopathologic correlates of the continuum of otitis media. Ann Otol Rhinol Laryngol 1990;15:147–153.
3   Casselbrant ML, Brostoff LM, Cantekin EI, et al: Otitis media with effusion in preschool children. Laryngoscope 1985;95:428–436.
4   Tos M, Holm-Jensen S, Sorensen CH: Changes in prevalence of secretory otitis from summer to winter in four-year-old children. Am J Otol 1981;2:324–327.
5   Lous J, Fiellau-Nicholajsen M: Epidemiology of middle ear effusion and tubal dysfunction. A one-year prospective study comprising monthly tympanometry in 387 non-selected seven-year-old children. Int J Pediatr Otorhinolaryngol 1981;3:303–317.
6   Paradise JL, Smith CG, Bluestone CD: Tympanometric detection of middle ear effusion in infant and young children. Pediatrics 1976;58:198–210.

Prof. Giorgio Bartolozzi, Ospedale A. Meyer, via Luca Giordano 13, I–50132 Florence (Italy)

Galioto GB (ed): Tonsils: A Clinically Oriented Update.
Adv Otorhinolaryngol. Basel, Karger, 1992, vol 47, pp 284–289

Aspects of Prevention of Obstructive Sleep Apnea Syndrome in Developing Children

Enrico Viva[a], *S. Stefini*[a], *G. Annibale*[a], *R. Pedercini*[a], *M. Zucconi*[b], *L. Ferini Strambi*[b]

[a]City Hospital, Children's Hospital, Brescia, and
[b]Neurology Clinic, Milan University, Milan, Italy

Snoring is what we call the noise made, during sleep, by the respiratory airflow against the soft redundant pharyngeal membranes in the course of a partial restriction of the upper airways. It is to be considered an early stage of the obstructive sleep apnea syndrome (OSAS). For OSAS we mean a syndrome characterized by episodes of arrest in the nose-mouth respiratory airflow with a minimum duration of 10 s. The OSAS can, in origin, be *central,* thus being caused by the lack of stimulation of the respiratory muscles and especially of the diaphragm muscle which is immobile, or, more often, *peripheral* or more appropriately, obstructive [1, 2].

Mechanical obstructions and/or negative genetic implications at the oronasopharyngeal crossroad level increase the resistance to the passage of air in the upper airways, the strain on the diaphragm, the negative intrapharyngeal pressure, the collapse of the pharyngeal membranes and, as a consequence, also increase the probabilities that the OSAS may occur.

Let us now see which are the various points of obstruction at an anatomical level which can explain the cause of snoring and the OSAS.

At the nasal level, there may be respiratory stenosis with a double component, which can be fixed (deviated septum, low crests, etc., in a context of narrow nasal cavities and hypoplasia of the relative jawbones) and variable, related to the vascularity of the erectile submembranous tissue – especially in the turbinates – influenced both by reflex phenomena and by the prone position in bed, in short, by the contents and the shape of the nasal chambers. At the nose/throat level, the importance of the adenoids must not be forgotten. At the oropharyngeal level, it is important to consider the tonsils and the tongue (macroglossia and position). The tongue must be examined section by section: the tip, the main body and the base. Most authors agree on the major importance of the alteration of the position of the tongue in determining incorrect development of the maxillary, facial and oral structure (see Infantile Deglutition in Adults).

The force of gravity acts differently on the various segments of the bone and muscle structure in relation to the position of the subject (orthostatic or clinostatic). The fall of the tongue is counterbalanced by the holding capacity of the antagonistic muscles, that is, the genioglossus muscle and the geniohyoideus muscle starting from the upper apophysis genian of the mandible. The former supports the tongue and the second supports the hyoid bone and the epiglottis in a clinostatic position. This is provided that such muscles work physiologically and that there are no alterations to the bone structure, for example, micrognathia, or functional disorders like infantile deglutition. Lastly, due importance must also be given to anatomical and spatial alterations to the upper and lower jawbones because it is obvious that a maxillary or mandibular micrognathia, or a backward position compared to the norm, reduce the volume of the oronasopharyngeal cavity and can favor the fall of the tongue into the oropharynx.

General Diagnostic and Therapeutical Aspects of Snoring and OSAS

Modern diagnostics has at its disposal sophisticated means of testing (polysomnography, cephalometric analysis, kinematography, CAT, RMN, both at rest and in movement, nasopharyngeal endoscope with or without the Müller maneuver) [3–6].

The *medical therapy* is limited to the indication of slimming diets (obesity is a factor closely related to snoring and to the OSAS), the discouragement from the use of tranquillizers, and the treatment of metabolic defects – especially that regarding oxygen – with CPAP (continuous positive airway pressure).

The *surgical therapy* proposes – in the most serious cases where there is an acute arising of the phenomenon, especially in obese subjects with short necks – a tracheotomy, which consents the bypassing, in one go, of all the possible sites of obstruction above the trachea. In other cases, surgery is used simply to remove the presumed next cause of the obstruction without mentioning that it may, in itself, be an effect.

Thus the proposal of the various operations on the nose and on the soft palate, which go from simple uvulectomy to the UPPP with or without tonsillectomy, to the partial resection of the palate according to, as yet, not unequivocal criteria, to the partial glossectomy on the median line of the tongue base, to the glossoplasty associated with hyoidplasty, etc. Such operations are not immune from risks, so much so that, as a rule, it is advisable to effect a preventive tracheotomy and/or have an intensive care unit at disposal for the immediate postoperative period.

Facial-maxillary surgical operations like the bringing forward of the upper or lower jawbone, resolve all round not only the snoring problem and the OSAS, but also the masticatory, phonatory and swallowing functions as well [7, 8].

Considerations

(1) The number of unsatisfactory results obtained through surgery on the soft tissues induces us to reconsider not only the multiple sites of anatomical obstruction but also, and above all, the primary and/or secondary functional alterations, as well as the related muscular and bone structure alterations. For example, a snorer who breathes through his mouth also during the day, due to a skeletal open bite, will not gain any advantage from nasal surgery, though correctly carried out, and will continue to use the shorter mouth-lungs bypass instead of the longer nose-lungs breathing, and this, in itself, is the cause of the snoring because of the abnormal falling backwards of the tongue during sleep.

(2) Modern means of diagnosis, radiographic or otherwise, only show the various anatomical situations in a static or dynamic situation or during the Müller maneuver (which is the reverse of a Valsalva maneuver) but they do not show the different levels of muscular relaxation within the physiology or pathology of the region, and/or the importance of the alteration of pathological functions (deglutition, respiration, phonation, mastication) in determining breathing difficulties during sleep. Form and function must go side by side on parallel lines both from a radiological-diagnostic and a clinical point of view.

(3) The proposed operations to be effected on the base of the tongue, apart from being risky, are – in our opinion – too scholastic. The tongue, in fact, should be considered anatomically as a whole and not as an assembly of base, tip and body. It is thus necessary to distinguish between a true or absolute macroglossia and a relative macroglossia due to a restricted oral cavity. In both cases, surgery to narrow or shorten the edges and tip of the

tongue – carried out using sufficiently experimented techniques – apart from being easier and surer, can give the same result. Bearing in mind the above, it remains that the position of the tongue is much more important than the macroglossia in itself (the former depends on the extrinsic tongue muscles and the latter on the intrinsic muscles).

(4) The available data in our hands refer exclusively to adult patients whose only symptom seems to be snoring or the OSAS. We do not know: whether this snoring started a month or a year ago, suddenly or gradually; whether the patient has always snored right from childhood; whether the patient is a compelled daytime mouth breather and why; whether, during the day, he is still affected with infantile deglutition; whether the patient has, from childhood, malformations of the bone structure and dental-orofacial-maxillary malformations. In brief, do primary breathing problems exist only during sleep and in adults, or do these problems imply that there are anatomical or functional alterations *which effect daytime breathing as well and which already existed in childhood?* Is snoring a symptom or an illness of adulthood? Is it the whole of the iceberg, or only the tip?

Prevention

Snoring and/or OSAS are not pathologies which arise all at once during adulthood, rather they imply that orofacial-maxillary anatomical alterations existed previously, together with functional disorders which need to be rehabilitated in any case, if pathological, inasmuch as the restoring of correct functions is, in itself, a morpho-corrector.

The oronasopharyngeal region is in conformity with the facial morphology of the patient (long, narrow face: tall, narrow oronasopharynx; wide, low face: low, wide oro-nasopharyngx). It is also necessary to consider both the uniqueness of the oronasopharyngeal crossroad as a whole, genetically conformed, in which various functions join normally or pathologically, and the coaxial of the structures contained therein [9].

These latter considerations tend to extend the indication for an adenotonsillectomy operation not only in cases of hypertrophy but also in cases where there is no tonsillar hypertrophy or hyperplasia but where growth disorders of the orofacial-maxillary structure exist, whether genetic [see Asburgo], anatomical or functional.

Small tonsils, even though not hypertrophic, in a small oropharynx can produce serious consequences. The concept of straightforward adenotonsillar hypertrophy must be overcome and the concept container/contents must prevail. All the authors relate, in a directly proportional sense, the oronasopharyngeal restriction to the degree of seriousness of OSAS.

Tonsillectomy and/or adenotonsillectomy (never monotonsillectomy) in childhood certainly have a favorable effect on the anatomy of the oronasopharyngeal crossroad and, therefore, a favorable effect on the snoring. The backward counterpoised movement of the tongue also improves the *function and the position* of the tongue. Surgery, however, should not be limited to this exiguous ambit of snoring but can and should, if necessary, be a first, preparatory, step towards improving the growth of the oronasofacial-maxillary structure. This growth can be guided, stimulated, slowed down both by removing mechanical anatomical obstacles (adenotonsillectomy, extraction of the first permanent molars, frenectomy, partial glossectomy) and, above all, by proceeding with the rehabilitation of the pathological functions of the tongue, lips, deglutition, respiration, etc. The operation must cover the whole cervical-facial maxillary ambit (respiration, deglutition, craniocervical posture and their correlations) [10–12].

Conclusions

Snoring is a symptom and a snorer is a person who suffers from chronic asphyxiation which, in the future, will lead to serious damage (chronic pulmonary heart, heart attack).

In childhood it is possible to prevent snoring by improving facial growth through myofunctional, orthopedic or surgical treatment (which can avoid or reduce the possibility – in adulthood – of merely surgical facial-maxillary operations, with undoubted economic and social advantages).

The anatomical growth must be studied as a whole, through objective examinations – both static (in orthostatism) and dynamic (in clinostatism) – and also from a functional point of view (functional diagnosis) with cephalometric analysis support.

If correctly prescribed, the adenotonsillectomy for mechanical reasons in patients at risk – and snoring is a risk for the general health of an individual – if associated with orthopedic-orthodontic therapy and with myofunctional therapy, can do a lot for snoring (the correlation between the degree of seriousness of the snoring, OSAS and oronasopharyngeal restriction) but also, and above all, for the anatomical and functional improvement of the entire region.

The treatment of children who snore, therefore, means not only improving their facial growth but also avoiding future general damage of a more serious nature.

The parents' contribution is vital not only at case history level but also and above all in the rehabilitation to eliminate bad habits.

In the diagnostic-therapeutic team there must necessarily be, together with a neurologist and an ENT specialist, also an expert in general and oronasofacial-maxillary auxology.

References

1   Chouard CH, Valty J, Meyer B, Chabolle F, Fleury B, Vericel R, Laccoureye O, Josset P: La roncopathie chronique ou ronflement. Ann Otolaryngol 1986;103:319–327.
2   Maurizi M, Modica V, Pezzuto RV: La roncopatia cronica (Lo stato dell'arte). Otorinolaringologia 1989;39:409–432.
3   Brodsky L, Adler E, Stanievich IF: Nose and oropharyngeal dimensions in children with obstructive sleep apnea. Int J Pediatr Otorhinolaryngol 1989;17:1–11.
4   Cavallo F: La sindrome da apnea ostruttiva durante il sonno: aspetti radiologici. Atti del terzo incontro interdisciplinare sui disturbi respiratori nel sonno, Lecce, 10–12 Maggio, 1990.
5   De Berry Borowiecki B, Kukwa A, Blanks RHI: Cephalometric analysis for diagnosis and treatment of obstructive sleep apnea. Laryngoscope 1988;98:226–234.
6   Riley R, Guilleminault C, Hermann J, Powell N: Cephalometric analysis and flow volume loops in obstructive sleep apnea patients. Sleep 1983;6:303–311.
7   Chabolle F, Fleury B, Riu B, Meyer B, Chouard CH: Résultats de UPPP dans le syndrome d'apnée du sommeil. Ann Otolaryngol 1988;105:283–289.
8   Curioni C, Baciliero U, Meneghini F: Il ruolo della chirurgia maxillo-facciale nei disturbi respiratori nel sonno. Atti del terzo incontro interdisciplinare sui disturbi respiratori nel sonno, Lecce, 10–12 Maggio, 1990.
9   Cassano P: Sindrome apnoica ostruttiva del sonno nel bambino. Diagnosi e trattamento. Acta Otorhinolaryngol Ital 1989;9:271–280.
10 Viva E: Biomeccanica masticatoria e protesi applicata oro-maxillo-facciale. Roma, Ed Universitaria, 1989.
11 Viva E, Stefini S, Annibale G, Pedercini R: Crescita oro-maxillo-facciale e adenotonsillectomia. Lecce, Ed Milella, 1989.
12 Viva E: Appunti di patologia maxillo-facciale. Milano, Ed Casa dello Studente, 1986.

Dr. Enrico Viva, Senior Maxillary-Facial Consultant Surgeon,
The City Hospital of Brescia, Via Garzetta 28, I-25060 Brescia (Italy)

Galioto GB (ed): Tonsils: A Clinically Oriented Update.
Adv Otorhinolaryngol. Basel, Karger, 1992, vol 47, pp 290–296

Adenoids and Otitis media with Effusion in Children

Tetsuo Watanabe, Tatsuya Fujiyoshi, Kazuhiro Tomonaga,
Goro Mogi

Department of Otolaryngology, Oita Medical University, Oita, Japan

Adenoids have long been recognized as an important factor in the pathogenesis of otitis media with effusion (OME). There have been some reports that adenoidectomy was a useful procedure for correction of medically resistant OME. However, there is still much debate about whether the adenoids play an important role in the etiology of OME, and there have been no detailed investigations of the adenoids of patients both with OME and without OME. The purpose of this study is to compare adenoids both with OME and without OME, and to determine whether adenoids may be a cause of OME.

Materials and Methods

Over the past 10 years, 171 patients have undergone adenoidectomy under general anesthesia at the Oita Medical University (Japan). Their ages ranged from 0 to 35 years (mean age, 6 years). One hundred and sixty-five of the 171 patients (96%) were from 2 to 15 years old. One hundred and six of those 171 patients had OME; the other 65 did not. In this study, we compared adenoids both with OME and without OME, clinically, histologically, and bacteriologically.

Clinical Study

In the clinical study, we selected 88 patients from 5 to 7 years of age. Fifty-nine of those 88 patients had OME; the other 29 did not have OME.

We evaluated the size of adenoids from two perspectives: macroscopic size and relative size. The macroscopic size of the adenoid was examined using an indirect mirror or flexible fiberscope. They were graded from 0 to IV, defined as follows [1]: grade 0, no obvious lymphoid tissue on the posterior wall, including the roof of the nasopharynx, or no enlargement below the level of the superior margin of the choanae; grade I, enlargement reaching the superior margin of the choanae; grade II, enlargement covering one third to one half of the choanae; grade III, enlargement covering one half to two thirds of the choanae; and grade IV, enlargement covering the choanae by more than two thirds. The relative size of adenoids was measured by lateral skull radiography as an adenoidal-nasopharyngeal ratio (A/N ratio) obtained by dividing the adenoidal thickness by the nasopharyngeal distance [2]. Also, we examined the incidence of patients who had sinusitis and nasal allergy.

Histological Study

In the histological study, we selected the same patients as in the clinical study mentioned above for light microscopy. Patients whose ages ranged from 2 to 15 years were selected for scanning electron microscopy (SEM).

For light microscopy, adenoids from patients were examined by the standard method: embedded in paraffin and stained with hematoxylin and eosin. The specimens were also placed in Karnovsky's fixative (2.5% glutaraldehyde and 2% paraformaldehyde in 0.2 M cacodylate buffer pH 7.4) for 2–3 h. Standard methods were used for SEM. Also for SEM, the prefixed tissue specimens were postfixed in buffered 2% osmium tetraoxide for 2 h, dehydrated through graded concentrations of ethanol, and dried with t-butyl alcohol. The specimens were coated with gold and examined with a scanning electron microscope (S-800; Hitachi, Tokyo, Japan).

Light microscopy was centered on the development of the germinal centers and the reticular formation of the epithelium. To evaluate the development of the germinal centers, we measured the area of the germinal center with a Nexus 6800 image processor (Kashiwagi Research Co., Tokyo, Japan). To semiquantitate the reticular formation of the epithelium, we measured a more than 10 mm length of the epithelium with a Nexus 6800. The reticular formation was expressed as a percentage of the epithelium without lymphocyte infiltration (normal epithelium). SEM were centered on the ratio of ciliated and nonciliated epithelium. The findings were graded from 0 to 3, defined as follows: grade 0, no ciliated cell; grade 1, the area of ciliated cells was under 30%; grade 2, the area of ciliated cells was over 30%; grade 3, the area of ciliated cells was over 70%.

Bacteriological Study

We selected 165 patients from 2 to 15 years of age. Adenoid tissues were cultured immediately after adenoidectomy, and bacterial isolates were identified by aerobic and anaerobic cultures in the bacterial laboratory of the Oita Medical University Hospital (Japan). The bacteriologic findings of middle ear effusions were noted in our previous report [3].

Results

Clinical Study (fig. 1)

There was no significant difference between patients with OME and without OME regarding size of the adenoids examined by indirect mirror or flexible fiberscope. The mean A/N ratio was 0.67 ± 0.09 in the patients

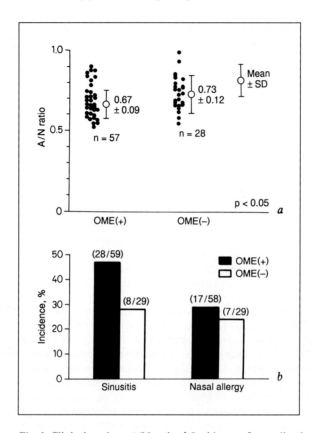

Fig. 1. Clinical study. *a* A/N ratio. *b* Incidence of complications.

with OME (n = 57), and 0.73 ± 0.12 in the patients without OME (n = 28).
The A/N ratio was significantly lower in the patients with OME than in the
patients without OME (p < 0.05). The incidence of sinusitis was 47% in
the patients with OME (n = 59), and 28% in the patients without OME (n =
29). The incidence of sinusitis tended to increase in the patients with OME
(p < 0.1). The incidence of nasal allergy was 29% in the patients with
OME (n = 58), and 24% in the patients without OME (n = 29). There was
no significant difference regarding the incidence of nasal allergy.

Histological Study (fig. 2)
    The mean area of the germinal center was 0.23 ± 0.08 mm² in the
patients with OME (n = 33), and 0.27 ± 0.1 mm² in the patients without

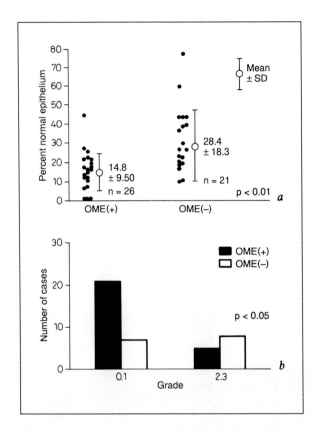

Fig. 2. Histological study. *a* Reticular formation. *b* Ciliated epithelium.

OME (n = 22). There was no significant difference regarding area of germinal center. The mean percentage of normal epithelium was 14.8 ± 9.5% in the patients with OME (n = 26), and 28.4 ± 18.3% in the patients without OME (n = 21). The percentage of normal epithelium was significantly lower in the patients with OME than in those without it (p < 0.01). That is, reticular epithelium formation was extended in the patients with OME. In the 26 patients with OME, 21 were graded 0 or 1, and 5 were graded 2 or 3, by SEM observation. In the 15 patients without OME, 7 were graded 0 or 1, and 8 were 2 or 3. There was a significant difference between these two groups (p < 0.05). A tendency toward increased stratified squamous epithelium and decreased ciliated epithelium was apparent in patients with OME.

Table 1. Bacteriological study: bacterial isolates from (*A*) adenoid and from (*B*) middle ear effusion

A

Species	OME (+) (n = 65)		OME (–) (n = 31)	
	n	%	n	%
H. influenzae	41	63.1	12	38.7
S. pneumoniae	18	27.7	4	12.9
S. aureus	15	23.1	11	35.5
B. catarrhalis	9	13.8	1	3.2
S. pyogenes	7	10.8	3	9.7
Others	54	83.1	24	77.4
Positive culture	60 (50[1])/65 = 92.3% (76.9%)		27 (21[1])/31 = 87.1% (67.7%)	

B

Species	Adenoidectomy (+) (n = 26)		Adenoidectomy (–) (n = 264)	
	n	%	n	%
H. influenzae	5	19.2	24	9.1
S. pneumoniae	3	11.5	17	6.4
S. epidermidis	2	7.7	17	6.4
S. aureus	2	7.7	9	3.5
B. catarrhalis	2	7.7	2	0.8
Others	3	11.5	11	4.1
Positive culture	16 (12[1])/26 = 61.5% (46.2%)		80 (52[1])/264 = 30.3% (19.7%)	

[1] Number of ears from which *H. influenzae, S. pneumoniae, B. catarrhalis,* and *S. aureus* were isolated.

Bacteriological Study (table 1)

Haemophilus influenzae were cultured in 41 adenoid specimens from 65 patients with OME, while 12 of 31 patients without OME were found to have *H. influenzae* in their adenoid specimens. There was a significant difference between the patients with OME and without OME (p < 0.05).

On the other hand, *Streptococcus pneumoniae* were cultured in 13 adenoid specimens from 47 patients with OME, while 4 of 23 patients without OME were found to have *S. pneumoniae* in their adenoid specimens. There was no significant difference between patients with OME and those without OME regarding *S. pneumoniae* and other species. In the bacteriologic findings of middle ear effusion, the combined number of positive *H. influenzae, S. pneumoniae, Staphylococcus aureus,* and *Branhamella catarrhalis* cultures from OME patients with adenoidectomy was significantly greater than from OME patients without adenoidectmoy ($p <$ 0.01).

Discussion

In the present study, the adenoid size was somewhat smaller in the patients with OME than in the patients without OME. Roydehouse [4] and Gates et al. [5] could not demonstrate any clinically significant differences in outcome by adenoid size. Our results were the same as those reports. In the histological study, extension of reticular epithelium formation and decreased ciliated epithelium were apparent in patients with OME. These findings suggest an increase of inflammation in the patients with OME. The incidence of sinusitis was higher in the patients with OME than in the patients without OME, and this also supports the increase of inflammation finding. Roukonen et al. [6] emphasized the importance of adenoiditis as a causative agent of OME. Considering these findings, our study suggests that not only adenoid hypertrophy, but also inflammation of the adenoids plays an important role in the pathogenesis of OME.

Infection of the nasopharynx and adenoid tissue has been considered a causative factor of OME. It is known that *H. influenzae* is an important factor in OME. In our bacteriological study, the incidence of *H. influenzae* cultured from adenoids was significantly greater in patients with OME than in patients without OME. And, the incidence of *H. influenzae* and other species from the middle ear effusion was significantly greater in patients with adenoidectomy than in patients without adenoidectomy.

Our findings suggest that the adenoids play an important role in the etiology of OME by being a reservoir for pathogenic bacteria, and that infection of the adenoid is an important factor in the inflammation of adenoids.

References

1   Fujiyoshi T, Watanabe T, Ichimiya I, Mogi G: Functional architecture of the naso-
    pharyngeal tonsil. Am J Otolarygol 1989;10:124–131.
2   Fujioka M, Young LW, Girdany BR: Radiographic evaluation of adenoidal size in
    children: Adenoidal-nasopharyngeal ratio. AJR 1979;133:401–404.
3   Tomonaga K, Kurono Y, Chaen T, Mogi G: Adenoids and otitis media with effu-
    sion: Nasopharyngeal flora. Am J Otolaryngol 1989;10:204–207.
4   Roydehouse N: A controlled study of adenotonsillectomy. Arch Otolaryngol 1970;
    92:611–616.
5   Gates GA, Avery CA, Cooper JC, Prihoda TJ: Chronic secretory otitis media:
    Effects of surgical management. Ann Otol Rhinol Laryngol 1989;98(suppl 138):1–
    32.
6   Roukonen J, Sandelin K, Makinen J: Adenoids and otitis media with effusion. Ann
    Otol Rhinol Laryngol 1979;88:166–171.

Goro Mogi, MD, Department of Otolaryngology, Oita Medical University,
Hasama-machi, Oita 879–55 (Japan)

Medical and Surgical Therapy

Galioto GB (ed): Tonsils: A Clinically Oriented Update.
Adv Otorhinolaryngol. Basel, Karger, 1992, vol 47, pp 297–301

Effects of Tonsillectomy

Kyozo Kikuchi

Department of Otolaryngology, Nihon University, School of Medicine,
Tokyo, Japan

Habitual Tonsillitis

It is commonly acknowledged that habitual tonsillitis is the most typical disorder for which tonsillectomy is conducted. When a patient is diagnosed as having habitual tonsillitis, most cases indicate tonsillectomy. The condition of the patients improves after tonsillectomy at a rate of 90–99%. On the contrary, however, there are rare cases that do not get well but rather suffer from diverse reactions after surgical operation [1, 2]. Among the secondary reactions that occur after tonsillectomy are sensory disorders such as sensations of sticking, tickling, hoarseness and others.

Focal Infection due to Chronic Tonsillitis

When a tonsil is suspected of causing focal infection, however, opinions differ among physicians of otolaryngology, pediatrics, internal medicine and dermatology on whether or not the tonsil should be removed. In many cases the sequence of cause and effects is proven only when the systematic disease is improved by the removal of the tonsil.

Therapeutic Effects of Tonsillectomy on Acute Nephritis

In cases of acute nephritis triggered by tonsillitis, any otolaryngologist would agree to an early removal of the tonsil [3]. It is an established fact that the earlier the tonsils are removed, the better the prognosis. However, some pediatricians and internists believe that an operation is not necessary for acute nephritis, because it may possibly be cured through conservative treatment. Even though early operations are known to result in favorable prognosis, it is advisable to conduct internal medical treatment for 2–6 months after the occurrence of the disease and to consider the possibility of an operation, through consultations with internists or pediatricians, only when the symptoms are prolonged thereafter with no improvement in test results.

Effects of Tonsillectomy on Chronic Nephritis

The effects of tonsillectomy on chronic nephritis are significant for its ability to prevent expanded inflammation [4]. There are some reported cases in which urinary observation following tonsillectomy indicated some improvement in chronic nephritis that had not been cured by internal medical treatment. These findings suggest that tonsillectomy could be more widely applied to treatment of chronic nephritis.

Extensive studies have been made by Japanese researchers on the effects of tonsillectomy on nephritis. The results have demonstrated many diversified views. Summarized here are some of the typical views that have been expressed.

Otolaryngologists

For patients with acute nephritis, it is important to initially examine with caution the progress of their disease while providing them with internal medical treatment. If, after 2 months, the disease is not cured and no improvement is observed in examinations, tonsillectomy is necessary.

Internists and Pediatricians

Tonsillectomy is very effective for nephritis which evidently occurred immediately after tonsillitis. The therapeutic effects of tonsillectomy are small for progressive chronic nephritis, even if nephritis was caused by focal tonsil. However, tonsillectomy is still considered applicable for cases of worsening nephritis symptoms triggered by repeated acute exacerbation caused by chronic tonsillitis.

Therapeutic Effects of Tonsillectomy on Slight Fever

Some internists and pediatricians recommend tonsillectomy for cases of slight fever with unidentified causes. Indeed, many textbooks of internal medicine, pediatrics and otolaryngology state that there is a correlation between the two. The idea is presumably based on the accumulated clinical experiences of physicians since it has been in existence even before the popularization of the concept of focal infection. Although the relationship between slight fever and the tonsil has not yet been fully elucidated, some physicians believe tonsillitis is caused by focal infection. There are also reports that many of the tonsil tissues of patients with slight fever show chronic inflammation. The therapeutic effects of tonsillectomy on slight fever emerge early. Improvement is shown in more than 50% of the cases within 1 week after tonsillectomy, and those who will be cured are cured within 1 month. On the other hand, no significant effect of the operation can be expected for patients who are still suffering from slight fever 3 months or more after the operation.

Therapeutic Effects of Tonsillectomy on Dermatological Diseases

A wide range of dermatological disorders are considered to be triggered by chronic tonsillitis. Among them, palmoplantar pustulosis is the most popular subject of research in Japan [5–7]. It is interesting to note that some common factors were found among cases who exhibited improvement after the operation and had actually been cured by tonsillectomy. Specially, a study on the cases for which tonsillectomy proved effective revealed that the patients with the following clinical observation results can be expected to improve as a result of the operation: (1) Patients who have previously suffered from tonsillitis. (2) Late occurrence of the symptom and early removal of the tonsil. In other words, the older the age of occurrence and the shorter the period from occurrence to operation (within 1 year after occurrence) the better the prognosis. (3) Slight tonsillar hypertrophy with pus seeping out when the tonsil is depressed. (4) Close relation between the occurrence of tonsillitis and exacerbation of the exanthema.

Some dermatologists believe that the therapeutic effects of tonsillectomy on dermatological disorders may be good in the short term but not in the long term. Nevertheless, long-term observations on palmoplantar pustulosis, which has a high probability of being cured by removal of the focus, demonstrated that patients who had had their infected focus removed clearly had a much higher chance of being cured (94%), compared with patients who had not (55%).

Therapeutic Effects of Tonsillectomy on Sleep Apnea Syndrome

Application of tonsillectomy for the treatment of sleep apnea syndrome is attracting much attention in Japan today [8]. The definition of sleep apnea syndrome is that 30 or more apnea lasting for 10 s or more are observed during a 7-hour sleep. Symptoms of the syndrome consist of excessive or insufficient sleep, apnea during sleep, heavy snoring, hypertrophy of the heart. Disorders caused in the otolaryngology areas are those triggered by hypertrophy of the tonsils and other abnormalities of the upper airway.

Diagnosis of sleep apnea syndrome in infants is difficult: it is rare for infants to complain of snoring or apnea during sleep as subjective symptoms and hence they seldom seek clinical advice unless their family notices the symptoms. Clinical symptoms for determining the therapeutic effects of tonsillectomy on the syndrome include snoring, breathing difficulties during sleep, daytime sleepiness, early morning headache, loss of concentration and decline of memory. Some researchers are studying polysomnography and/or the condition of oxygen and carbonic acid gas in the blood as a means of objectively determining respiratory disorders. The results of tonsillectomy and/or adenotomy on sleep apnea syndrome patients have proved prominently effective for infants but not for adults. As a whole, they exhibit the limitations of applying tonsillectomy as a treatment for the syndrome.

Medical Accidents after Tonsillectomy

During 23 years from 1948 to 1974, there were 418 deaths due to medical accidents in Japan, including 61 otolaryngological cases. Accidents after tonsillectomy occurred in 20 cases. The causes of death were bleeding and anesthesia. Accidents after tonsillectomy were investigated by a questionnaire during 10 years from 1974 to 1983. There were 270 cases, including 13 deaths. Postoperative bleeding was found in 221 cases, and medical toxication was found in 19 cases. The causes of death were 5 postoperative bleeding, 4 medical toxication, 2 malignant high fever, 1 shock, and 1 unknown [9].

Table 1. Improvements of symptoms after tonsillectomy

Pharyngeal pain	86–96%
Hard of hearing	46–79%
Nasal obstruction	45–48%
Snoring	74–80%

Table 2. Postoperative improvement on focal infection

Slight fever	77–91%
Skin diseases	64–91%
Kidney diseases	18–78%

Conclusion

Effects of tonsillectomy are summarized in tables 1 and 2. Tonsillectomy is a useful treatment for tonsillar diseases and its complications when the indication is correct.

References

Each of the nine papers listed below was written in Japanese with an English summary.

1   Kojima M, et al: Long-term observation of postoperative course of tonsillectomy. Jpn J Tonsil 1987;26:173–179.
2   Yoshida A, Okamoto K: The clinical study for chronic tonsillits. Jpn J Tonsil 1989; 28:181–188.
3   Suzuki M: Studies of prognosis of tonsillectomy of kidney diseases, Jpn J Tonsil 1977;16:141–147.
4   Sugiyama N, Masuda Y: Immunological study of IgA nephropathy after tonsillectomy. Jpn J Tonsil 1986;25:77–82.
5   Noda Y, Ura M: Pustulosis palmaris et plantaris possibly due to tonsillogenic focal infection. Jpn J Tonsil 1982;21:189–210.
6   Yamanaka N, Sambe S, Kataura A: Tonsil and pustulosis palmoplantaris. Jpn J Tonsil 1982;21:202–210.
7   Kimura T, Tabata T, et al: A retrospective survey of tonsillectomy for pustulosis palmaris et plantaris. Jpn J Tonsil 1986;25:86–91.
8   Uruma Y, Nishimura T, et al: Sleep apnea syndrome caused by adenotonsillar hypertrophy. Jpn J Tonsil 1990;29:289–295.
9   Takeyama I: On the medical accidents after tonsillectomy. Jpn J Tonsil 1985;24: 283–287.

Dr. Kyozo Kikuchi, Department of Otolaryngology, Nihon University Hospital, 1-8, Kanda-Surugadai, Chiyoda, Tokyo (Japan)

Galioto GB (ed): Tonsils: A Clinically Oriented Update.
Adv Otorhinolaryngol. Basel, Karger, 1992, vol 47, pp 302–310

The Family Physician and Pathologies of the Tonsils: Therapeutic Practices

A. Marinoni[a], *G.B. Galioto*[b], *E. Mevio*[a], *M. Curti*[a], *V. Camerini*[c]

[a] Department of Biometrics, University of Pavia;
[b] Department of Otorhinolaryngology, University of Pavia,
and IRCCS Policlinico S. Matteo, Pavia;
[c] LPB Industria Farmaceutica, Milano, Italy

It is well known that family physicians hold an important role in the health care system not only because they are often the initial point of reference within the system for the patient but also because as such they determine the patient's health care needs which, in turn, become demands upon the health care system.

The explosion of health care costs and the necessity of holding these down has brought family physicians to the forefront in the discussion of these problems as they mobilize an important part of the health care resources and are those who 'order' the first expenditures according to modalities completely unknown.

The aim of the present study is to analyze the diagnostic and therapeutic practices of family physicians regarding inflammatory diseases of the tonsils. This type of pathology was chosen as it is of special interest for otorhinolaryngology clinics since it is a very common type of disease. Also, an understanding of the practices of the family physicians and the reasons why they consulted a specialist seemed particularly interesting [1–4].

Materials and Methods

This cross-sectional epidemiologic investigation involved approximately 1,700 Italian family physicians who were given a questionnaire to complete. Consultants from a pharmaceutical company which operates throughout Italy, who were suitably prepared, were asked to distribute the prepared questionnaire ad hoc for a prearranged period of time (3 months) to all physicians with whom they have contact. The information gathered

by means of the questionnaire concerned: personal data of the physician including educational background; most prevalent types of pathologies of the tonsils seen by the physician, and medical practices and therapeutic choices of the physicians.

Results

1,207 physicians, approximately 70% of those contacted, participated
in the study. 84.32% were males; the average age was 40; the average
number of years of postgraduate practice was 14 years.

Our study had a greater representation of physicians from northern
Italy with respect to the other regions of Italy. More than half of the family
physicians declared that the majority of their patients who presented tonsillar pathologies were children, especially between the ages of 6 and 13
years; less than 10% were older than 20 years.

While the family physicians of northern and central Italy reported that
spring and winter were the two seasons in which tonsillar pathologies most
often occurred, those of southern Italy reported an equal distribution
among the various seasons with the exception of summer when its occurrence is negligible. In 90% of the cases in which a patient presented a
tonsillar pathology the physicians administered a medical therapy independently of age of the patient. A more thorough examination (hematologic and blood chemistry exams, pharyngeal culture) was done more frequently with children, while a visit to a specialist was more frequently
suggested for elderly patients.

It is interesting to note that older physicians had a tendency to ask
more often for more thorough exams and, especially, to send their patients
more frequently to a specialist (table 1). Tonsillar plaques and tonsillar
ulcers were the morphologic lesions that more often induced physicians to
ask for more thorough examinations. Again, this was more frequent among
older physicians (table 2). Those patients who had a history of recurrent
tonsillitis were those who underwent more often more extensive examinations (table 3).

The analysis of the medical practices of family physicians, according
to the region in which they practised, revealed that general practitioners in
southern Italy and the islands tend to ask more often for more thorough
exams and for visits to a specialist with respect to their northern colleagues
while having the same trends mentioned above, i.e. more frequent exams
for patients with a history of recurrent tonsillitis and those having tonsillar
plaques and tonsillar ulcers. Having a specialization did not influence the

practices of the family physicians, while the years of practice did not influence those trends seen according to the age of the physician.

The types of drugs most often prescribed for bacterial tonsillitis were antibiotics and antiphlogistic agents and, limited to younger physicians, antipyretic agents. For viral tonsillitis, antiphlogistic and antipyretic agents were prescribed more often among younger physicians, while antiphlogistic and immunostimulating agents were prescribed by older physicians. More than 30% of older physicians also prescribed antibiotics (fig. 1).

Table 1. Different approach to the patient with a tonsils disease according to the patient's age

| Age of patient | 0–13 | | 14–20 | | 21–59 | | ≥ 60 | |
Age of physician	<45	>45	<45	>45	<45	>45	<45	>45
Medical therapy	*92*	*96*	87	*95*	82	*91*	82	86
Hematological exams	34	*50*	26	*45*	18	28	22	29
Pharyngeal swab	*43*	35	24	25	13	17	11	13
ENT visit	12	23	8	21	10	24	15	*28*
Hospital recovery	0.3	0.0	0.3	0.7	0.3	0.7	0.4	0.7

Italicized values indicate the most significant results.

Table 2. Different approach to the patient, in relation to the physician's age, according to their tonsillar morphologic allerations

| | Tonsillar hypertrophy | | Erythema | | Plaques | | Ulcers | |
Age of physician	<45	>45	<45	>45	<45	>45	<45	>45
Medical therapy	24	42	48	61	97	98	*89*	*94*
Hematological exams	22	39	16	27	42	*61*	*67*	*80*
Pharyngeal swab	19	23	19	24	52	55	*64*	*71*
ENT visit	12	29	*61*	20	14	29	*52*	*69*
Hospital recovery	0.3	0.0	0.1	0.0	0.5	0.7	*5*	*4*

Italicized values indicate the most significant results.

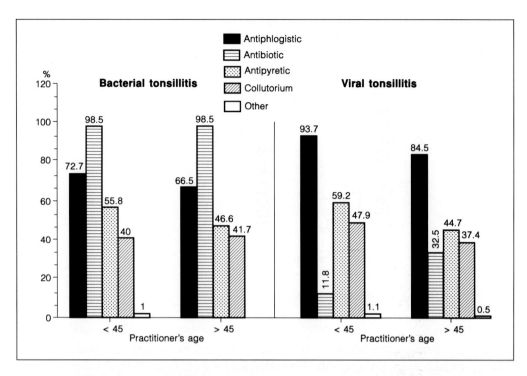

Fig. 1. Therapy versus etiology of tonsillitis.

Table 3. Different approach to the patient with the pathologic tonsils according to the clinical course of the disease (in relation to the age of the physician)

	First episode		Previous tonsillitis		Recurrent tonsillitis		Recent tonsillitis	
Age of physician	<45	>45	<45	>45	<45	>45	<45	>45
Medical therapy	63	*80*	63	76	*88*	*88*	*92*	*92*
Hematological exams	22	*32*	24	43	*70*	*80*	*79*	*84*
Pharyngeal swab	25	24	25	28	*70*	*67*	*79*	*72*
ENT visit	6	17	8	23	*53*	*50*	*50*	*55*
Hospital recovery	0.1	0.0	0.3	0.7	0.5	0.7	*2*	*3*

Italicized values indicate the most significant results.

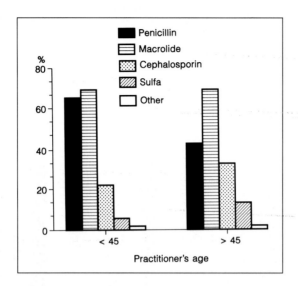

Fig. 2. Antibiotic therapy versus practitioner's age.

Family physicians in southern Italy prescribed antiphlogistic and immunostimulating agents more often for viral tonsillitis than did those of northern and cental Italy. No difference was seen between the therapies prescribed by family physicians who had a specialization and those who did not. Macrolides and penicillin were usually the antibiotics more frequently prescribed, especially by younger physicians. The prescription of cephalosporins and sulfonamides was also widespread among older physicians (fig. 2).

Parenteral administration was considered the most appropriate means of introducing the drug, especially by older physicians. It is surprising that only 36% of physicians asked for an antibiogram before starting antibiotic therapy. Among physicians who had a specialization the percentage was 40%, while among those without one it was 32%. When pharyngeal cultures were negative, only 18.3% would suspend antibiotic therapy while the remaining 92% would still recommend taking the drug for 5–10 days.

Approximately 60% of physicians prescribed prolonged acting penicillin, 1 vial every 15 days for a variable number of times, if a patient had an elevated antistreptolysin 0 titer (250 U). Among the antiphlogistic agents, the ones most often prescibed (61.1%) were the FANS with no difference between younger and older physicians (fig. 3).

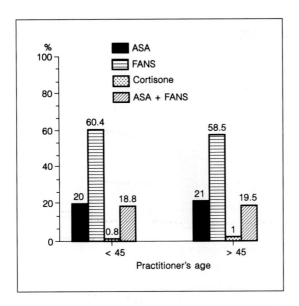

Fig. 3. Antiphlogistic therapy versus practitioner's age.

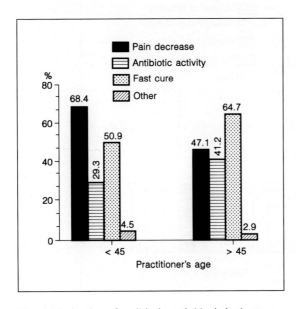

Fig. 4. Motivation of antibiotic-antiphlogistic therapy versus practitioner's age.

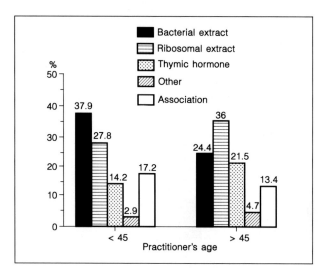

Fig. 5. Immunotherapy versus practitioner's age.

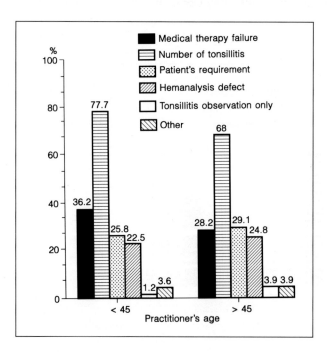

Fig. 6. Motivation of ENT visit.

The reason for which an antiphlogistic agent was associated with the antibiotic dependent on the age of the physician: among young physicians the reduction of pain prevailed while among older physicians the reduction of recovery time carried weight (fig. 4). Among the immunostimulating drugs those most often prescribed were either bacterial or ribosomal extracts (fig. 5). The frequent number of episodes of tonsillitis was the principal reason why a patient was sent to a specialist (fig. 6).

Discussion

The aims of this study on inflammation of the tonsils, other than analyzing the characteristics of its diffusion, were to study the medical practices of family physicians and their relationship with the specialist. We were able to obtain a well-defined picture of its diffusion in the different regions of Italy which have very different climatic and environmental conditions. For example, the frequency of tonsillar diseases according to seasons were very different when comparing northern and central Italy with southern Italy.

The family physicians were asked to decribe their therapeutic practices as well as to explain the reasons for consulting an otorhinolaryngologist. As far as their therapeutic practices are concerned, we found that the general practitioners were well prepared in choosing a therapy for acute pathologies as well as selecting supplementary examinations (hematologic and blood chemistry exams, bacterial cultures, etc.) in cases of recurrent inflammations.

Although only 30% of those physicians who participated in the study did an antibiogram before prescribing an antibiotic, the selection of the drug and the period of administration seemed nonetheless adequate. It should not be overlooked, however, that a family physician often finds himself confronting a situation of acute inflammation (statistically believed to be of a well-defined etiology) so that awaiting the results of this exam would be questionable. The request for an antibiogram was more frequent for cases of recurrent inflammations.

As far as the choice of the antibiotic is concerned, it is interesting to note that macrolides were preferred, thus allowing coverage also against emerging pathogens and β-lactamase-producing strains that are becoming increasingly common. Penicillin and its derivatives were the antibiotics most often used while benzathine penicillin remained the antibiotic of first choice in the prevention of recurrent forms of inflammation. Among the other types of therapies chosen, the association of an antibiotic with an antiphlogistic agent seemed well justified. The immunostimulating drugs were generally bacterial extracts and, more recently, ribosomal extracts which were commonly used in the prevention of recurrent forms of inflammation.

The older physicians, especially those of southern Italy, were the ones who most frequently asked for a specialist consultation. The motives were for the most part justified. Consultation was asked especially for younger patients and for patients who had a recurrent form or who were resistant to therapy prescribed previously.

In conclusion, we were extremely pleased with the preparation and the up-to-dateness of the family physicians and their collaboration with the specialists of otorhinolaryngology.

References

1   Gehanno P, Pangon B, Moisy N, Dournon E, Akoun P: Les angines actuellement. Enquête épidémiologique. Corrélations cliniques. Incidences thérapeutiques. Ann Otolaryngol Chir Cervicofac 1987;2:137–141.
2   Bredahal C, Ovesen L: Otorhinolaryngologic diseases in general practice. Ugeskr Laeger 1989;151:1237–1240.
3   Timon CI, Cafferkey MT: Management of tonsillitis by the general practitioner. Ir Med J 1990;83:70–71.
4   Griffiths E: Incidence of ENT problems in general practice. J R Soc Med 1979;72: 740–742.

Prof. G.B. Galioto, Clinica Otorinolaryngoiatrica, Policlinico S. Matteo, Piazzale Golgi, I–27100 Pavia (Italy)

Galioto GB (ed): Tonsils: A Clinically Oriented Update.
Adv Otorhinolaryngol. Basel, Karger, 1992, vol 47, pp 311–318

A Modern Medical Therapy Approach to Streptococcal Pharyngotonsillitis

Nicola Principi, Paola Marchisio

Pediatric Department IV, Milano University Medical School, Milano, Italy

Resurgence of rheumatic fever in some areas of the United States and in some European countries in the mid-1980s clearly underlines the importance of a diligent pursuit and treatment of streptococcal pharyngitis [1, 2]. Penicillin, and particularly penicillin V and benzathine penicillin G, have been the agents of choice for the therapy of this disease for the past four decades, while macrolides have been considered alternative drugs to be used in penicillin-allergic children [3]. Studies carried out before 1964 [4, 5] have demonstrated that the eradication rate of group A β-hemolytic Streptococcus from the pharynx, evaluated at 60 days of follow-up, has generally been over 90% for benzathine penicillin G and usually over 80% for penicillin V. However, more recent studies seem to demonstrate that the efficacy of penicillin is progressively decreasing and that nearly 30% of apparent group A β-hemolytic streptococcal pharyngitis are not cured with such therapy [6] (fig. 1).

In order to explain these differences in the efficacy of oral or intramuscular penicillin, four major hypotheses have been advanced: (1) decreased patient compliance; (2) increased number of β-lactamase-producing oropharyngeal flora which are causing synergistic infection with group A streptococcus; (3) penicillin tolerance, and (4) suppression of host immunity with early antibiotic use.

Decreased Patient Compliance

As far as compliance is concerned it is possible that problems in this regard may be more significant today than in the past. The reason may be that in recent years many long-acting antibiotics have been marketed and for many diseases simplified schemes of therapy have been suggested and

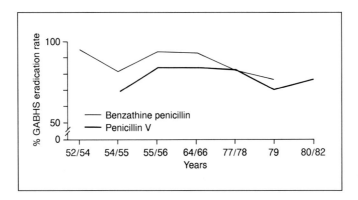

Fig. 1. Changes over time of efficacy of penicillin for the treatment of group A β-hemolytic streptococcal (GABHS) pharyngitis.

proved effective. So, many parents and some physicians may be led to believe that also for streptococcal pharyngitis oral penicillin may be administered with a total daily dosage and/or with a fractioning lower than those usually recommended. However, if this may be true for some of the newest antibiotics, such as clarithromycin, this is not entirely applicable to penicillin V, which, to be certainly effective, must be administered according to previous recommendations, i.e. in three or four daily doses on an empty stomach. Moreover, Gerber et al. [7] have recently shown that once-daily penicillin V therapy is highly unsuccessful despite the fact that the total dosage was not lower than that usually employed. However, we do not believe that differences in compliance may have a major role in explaining the reduction of efficacy of penicillin V in recent years. Studies which included a comparison arm with intramuscular penicillin have demonstrated that a decrease in efficacy was present also in this case. Gastanaduy et al. [8], for example, found the same 19% failure rate among patients treated with oral or intramuscular penicillin.

Indirect Pathogenicity

The problem of indirect pathogenicity is probably more relevant. Several investigations have suggested that β-lactamase production by normal flora in the upper respiratory tract may be responsible for the greater

	Penicillin						
	80	84	87	94	30	17	72
Cefalexin	91						
Cefatrizine		96					
Cefaclor			93				
Cefadroxil				98			
Amoxicillin + Clavulanic acid					91		
Dicloxacillin						50	
Penicillin + Rifampin							100

Fig. 2. Bacteriologic eradication (%) of group A β-hemolytic streptococcal pharyngitis in acute and recurrent pharyngitis penicillin versus other antibiotics.

occurrence of treatment failure with penicillin therapy [9, 10]. The proposed mechanism of action involves elaboration of β-lactamase by indigenous flora, including *Staphylococcus aureus, Haemophilus influenzae, Moraxella catarrhalis* and a variety of anaerobic species, which thereby provide 'protection' of the Streptococcus from penicillin by inactivation of the antibiotic.

Starting from these premises it was hypothesized that an antibiotic active against both β-lactamase-producing bacteria and β-hemolytic Streptococcus would be successful in patients with acute streptococcal pharyngitis. Most of the clinical studies have demonstrated that this hypothesis could be considered really consistent because an improved bacteriological eradication compared with that observed with penicillin has been found with a lot of oral cephalosporins [6] and with dicloxacillin [11], amoxicillin-clavulanic acid [12], lincomycin [13], clindamycin [14] and the combination of penicillin and rifampin [15] (fig. 2).

However, it is probable that not all the failures after penicillin treatment are to be ascribed to indirect pathogenicity. Because a shift in the oral microbial population with selection of β-lactamase-producing strains takes place especially in subjects who received repeated penicillin administrations [16], it is probable that indirect pathogenicity may play an important role only in recurrent pharyngitis, previously treated with repeated courses of penicillin. On the contrary, in sporadic cases β-lactamase production does not seem to have any significant importance.

Penicillin Tolerance

The third hypothesis regards a change in the degree of sensitivity of hemolytic Streptococcus to penicillin. In this regard it must be underlined that, in vitro, all β-hemolytic streptococci are susceptible to penicillin. However, Streptococcus strains recovered from children with pharyngitis can show variations in degrees of tolerance to penicillin [17]. The role of tolerance in conditioning treatment failures is controversial. In 1985, Kim and Kaplan [18] reported that tolerance could be identified in 25% of isolates in penicillin treatment failures in contrast to none of the strains isolated from patients successfully treated with penicillin. However, 2 years later a second study by the same authors [11] indicated that tolerant strains of β-hemolytic streptococci were not more frequently isolated from children in whom initial penicillin treatment failed than from those who were successfully treated. The importance of penicillin tolerance could be also demonstrated by a study from Israel which reported a widespread epidemic of pharyngitis caused by penicillin-tolerant Streptococcus in a kibbutz with subsequent control by mass treatment with erythromycin [19]. On the other hand, cephalosporins have not been shown to eradicate penicillin-tolerant Streptococcus.

Early Antibiotic Use

The last point regards the possibility that penicillin failures may depend on the time of the beginning drug administration. It was suggested that an early antibiotic therapy might have a potential adverse effect inhibiting the development of time-specific immunity to the infecting bacteria. Recently, Pichichero et al. [20] found a significantly higher number of recurrences of β-hemolytic streptococcal pharyngitis in children who had the initial episode immediately treated with penicillin than in those who received this drug after 48–56 h. On the contrary, Gerber et al. [21] were not able to confirm these data and concluded that there was no adverse effect of immediate penicillin therapy for streptococcal pharyngitis with respect to an increased incidence of recurrences. As a consequence they do not recommend, contrarily to what was suggested by Pichichero et al. [20], to wait 48 h to initiate penicillin therapy for a patient with documented streptococcal infection.

These conflicting experiences do not permit to draw definite conclusions on the real role of the time of the beginning penicillin therapy on its efficacy in treating pharyngitis. However, it must be underlined that both these studies present a methodologic design that can be discussed. The first one, by Pichichero, can be criticized for the absence of serotyping data on the isolated Streptococcus strains, so that it is impossible to distinguish between patients who really had a relapse and those who had a reinfection. The second one includes both symptomatic and asymptomatic recurrences and probably considers not only children with true streptococcal infection but also streptococcal carriers, whose sterilization is much more difficult. Anyway, even if present, this problem cannot concern only penicillin but must regard all the bactericidal antibiotics, so it cannot explain the reduction of efficacy of penicillin administration. On the other hand, we think that an early beginning of antibiotic administration can be always justified by some other advantages clearly demonstrated by several different studies: a more certain improvement and more rapid relief of symptoms in treated than in untreated patients, although the difference is not dramatic, usually in the range of 24–36 h. Moreover, there is the likelihood that with treatment we can prevent various local suppurative complications, particularly peritonsillar or retropharyngeal abscess, or cervical adenitis, cellulitis or abscess. Finally, an early treatment reduces the risk of intrafamilial spread of hemolytic streptococci.

In conclusion, even if several data demonstrate that penicillin preparation have in time reduced their efficacy and many hypotheses have been suggested to explain this phenomenon, today we do not know its real origin. However, it is clear that while in the last 40 years the antibiotic therapy for streptococcal pharyngitis was essentially based on penicillin, with macrolides to be used in penicillin-allergic patients, today we may find several cases in which a different therapeutic choice may be rational. Among them must be included children who fail to respond to penicillin or who continue to become reinfected after a correctly administered penicillin therapy. In these cases the drugs of choice are to be considered oral cephalosporins and macrolides, especially those recently synthesized like clarithromycin, which has better pharmacokinetic characteristics, a higher tolerability and a more rapid activity than the old erythromycin.

Speaking on the treatment of streptococcal pharyngitis we cannot keep silent on the problem of the duration of the therapy to assure the highest degree of efficacy. Since 1953 it was stated that oral treatment with penicillin or macrolides had to be given for 10 days because a reduction of this time was clearly associated to a higher persistence of the infecting bacteria. However, some attempts to reduce the duration of the antibiotic therapy using oral cephalosporins carried out in the early 70s seemed to demonstrate the

Table 1. Etiology of acute pharyngitis in 865 Italian children [data from 26]

		n	%
Bacterial pharyngitis		276	31.9
Nonbacterial pharyngitis		589	68.1
Streptococcal pharyngitis	Group A	230	26.6
	Group B	3	0.3
	Group C	13	1.5
	Group D	26	3.0
	Group F	4	0.5

possibility to reduce the treatment to 7 days. However, these studies are debatable and were not subsequently confirmed. On the contrary, two different researches [22, 23], carried out in 1981 and 1987 respectively, have without any doubt shown that a reduction under 10 days of penicillin administration is associated with a higher bacteriologic failure rate (31 vs. 18% and 18 vs. 6%, respectively). These data, in a period of resurgence of rheumatic fever, support the old recommendation for a full 10 days of any oral antibiotic therapy for the treatment of streptococcal pharyngitis.

The last problem is the importance of non-group A streptococci as etiological agents of bacterial pharyngitis and the need of treatment of those children in whom these germs are isolated during acute pharyngitis. Some studies using anaerobic culture method have demonstrated that these bacteria are frequently present in the pharynx of children with symptomatic pharyngitis suggesting their possible causative role in determining the acute disease. Especially group B, C, F and G streptococci were isolated [24–26] (table 1). However, detection of an infectious agent in the throat of patients with pharyngitis is insufficient to prove its causative role in the disease. Such patients could be carriers of non-group A organisms with an illness caused by another agent, such as a respiratory virus. This hypothesis seems to be supported by the data reported in the paper by Hayden et al. [27] who demonstrated that the prevalence of non-group A organisms detected in patients with sporadic pharyngitis was essentially the same as the prevalence in age- and season-matched controls. On the other hand, groups C and G streptococci have been incriminated in several outbreaks [28, 29], so that many authors deem possible a causative role of these bacteria but not of group B and F streptococci. However, from a therapeutical point of view the lack of a definition of the importance of non-group A streptococci as causative agents of pharyngitis justifies the use of antibiotic therapy when these bacteria are cultured in a child with an acute sore throat.

References

1   Veasy LG, Wiedmeier SE, Orsmond GS, Ruttenberg HD, Boucek MM, Roth SJ, Tait VF, Thompson JA, Daly JA, Kaplan EL, Hill HR: Resurgence of acute rheumatic fever in the intermountain area of the United States. N Engl J Med 1987;316: 421–427.

2   Rogari P, Bonora G, Acerbi L, Frattini D, Martelli A, Perletti L: Ripresa della malattia reumatica nella provincia di Milano (area Melegnano). Riv Inf Ped 1989;4: 183–188.

3   Dillon HC: Streptococcal pharyngitis in the 1980s. Pediatr Infect Dis J 1987;6: 123–130.

4   Breese BB, Disney FA: The successful treatment of beta-hemolytic streptococcal infections in children with a single injection of respiratory penicillin (benzathine penicillin G). Pediatrics 1955;15:516–521.

5   Breese BB, Disney FA: Penicillin in the treatment of streptococcal infections: A comparison of five different oral and one parenteral form. N Engl J Med 1958;259: 57–62.

6   Pichichero ME, Margolis PA: A comparison of cephalosporins and penicillins in the treatment of group A beta-hemolytic streptococcal pharyngitis: a meta-analysis supporting the concept of microbial copathogenicity. Pediatr Infect Dis J 1991;10:275–281.

7   Gerber MA, Randolph MF, DeMeo K, Feder HM, Kaplan EL: Failure of once-daily penicillin V therapy for streptococcal pharyngitis. AJDC 1989;143:153–155.

8   Gastanaduy AS, Kaplan EL, Huwe BB, McKay C, Wannamaker LW: Failure of penicillin to eradicate group A streptococci during an outbreak of pharyngitis. Lancet 1980;ii:498–502.

9   Denny FW: Current problems in managing streptococcal pharyngitis. J Pediatr 1987;111:797–805.

10 Brook I: Role of anaerobic beta-lactamase-producing bacteria in upper respiratory tract infections. Pediatr Infect Dis J 1987;6:310–316.

11 Smith TD, Huskins WC, Kim KS, Kaplan EL: Efficacy of beta-lactamase resistant penicillin and influence of penicillin tolerance in eradicating streptococci from the pharynx after failure of penicillin therapy for group A streptococcal pharyngitis. J Pediatr 1987;110:777–782.

12 Kaplan EL, Johnson DR: Eradication of group A streptococci from the upper respiratory tract by amoxicillin with clavulanate after oral penicillin V treatment failure. J Pediatr 1988;113:400–403.

13 Breese BB, Disney FA, Talpey WB: Beta-hemolytic streptococcal illness: comparison of lincomycin, ampicillin, and potassium penicillin treatment. AJDC 1966;112: 21–27.

14 Randolph MF, Redys JJ, Hibbard EW: Streptococcal pharyngitis. III. Streptococcal recurrence rate following therapy with penicillin or with clindamycin (7-chlorolincomycin). Del Med J 1970;42:87–91.

15 Chaudhary S, Bilinsky SA, Hennessy JL, Soler SM, Wallaca SE, Schacht CM, Bisno AL: Penicillin V and rifampin for the treatment of group A streptococcal pharyngitis: a randomized trial of 10 days' penicillin vs. 10 days' penicillin with rifampin during the final 4 days of therapy. J Pediatr 1985;106:481–486.

16 Brook I, Gober AE: Emergence of beta-lactamase-producing aerobic and anaerobic bacteria in the oropharynx of children following penicillin. Clin Pediatr 1984;23: 338–339.

17 Kim KS: Clinical perspectives on penicillin tolerance. J Pediatr 1988;112:509–514.

18 Kim KS, Kaplan EL: Association of penicillin tolerance with failure to eradicate group A streptococci from patients with pharyngitis. J Pediatr 1985;107:681–684.

19 Dagan R, Ferne M, Sheinis M, Alkan M, Katzenelson E: An epidemic of penicillin-tolerant group A streptococcal pharyngitis in children living in a closed community: mass treatment with erythromycin. J Infect Dis 1987;156:514–516.

20 Pichichero ME, Disney FA, Talpey BS, Green JL, Francis AB, Roghmann KJ, Hoekelman RA: Adverse and beneficial effects of immediate treatment of group A, beta-hemolytic streptococcal pharyngitis with penicillin. Pediatr Infect Dis J 1987;6: 635–643.

21 Gerber MA, Randolph MF, DeMeo KK, Kaplan EL: Lack of impact of early antibiotic therapy for streptococcal pharyngitis on recurrence rates. J Pediatr 1990;117: 853–858.

22 Schwartz RH, Wientzen RL Jr, Pedreira F: Penicillin V for group A streptococcal pharyngitis: a randomized trial of seven vs. ten days' therapy. JAMA 1981;246: 1790–1795.

23 Gerber MA, Randolph MF, Chanatry J, Wright LL, DeMeo K, Kaplan EL: Five vs. ten days of penicillin V therapy for streptococcal pharyngitis. AJDC 1987;141:224–227.

24 Putto A: Febrile exudative tonsillitis: viral or streptococcal? Pediatrics 1987;80: 6–12.

25 Cimolai N, Elford RW, Bryan L, Anand C, Berger T: Do the beta-hemolytic non-group A streptococci cause pharyngitis? Rev Infect Dis 1988;10:587–601.

26 Principi N, Marchisio P, Onorato J: Streptococcal pharyngitis in Italian children: epidemiology and treatment with miocamycin. Drugs Exp Clin Res 1990;16:639–645.

27 Hayden GF, Murphy TF, Hendley JO: Non-group A streptococci in the pharynx. Pathogens or innocent bystanders? AJDC 1989;143:794–797.

28 Gerber MA, Randolph MF, Martin NJ, Rizkallah MF, Cleary PP, Kaplan EL, Ayoub EM: Community-wide outbreak of group G streptococcal pharyngitis. Pediatrics 1991;87:598–603.

29 Turner JC, Hayden GF, Kiselica D, Lohr J, Fishburne CF, Murren D: Association of group A beta-hemolytic streptococci with endemic pharyngitis among college students. JAMA 1990;264:2644–2647.

Prof. Nicola Principi, Pediatric Department IV, University of Milan,
Ospedale L. Sacco, Via GB Grassi 74, I–20157 Milano (Italy)

Galioto GB (ed): Tonsils: A Clinically Oriented Update.
Adv Otorhinolaryngol. Basel, Karger, 1992, vol 47, pp 319–324

Surgery for Otitis media:
Results of Randomized Clinical Trials as
Related to Clinical Practice

Charles D. Bluestone

Department of Otolaryngology, University of Pittsburgh,
School of Medicine, Division of Pediatric Otolaryngology,
Children's Hospital of Pittsburgh, Pa., USA

Myringotomy with tympanostomy tube insertion is the most common surgical procedure performed in children after the newborn period and tonsillectomy or adenoidectomy, or both procedures, are the most common *major* surgical operations performed in children, many of which are for prevention of otitis media. Thoughtful clinicians and parents question whether the potential benefits of these operations in the treatment and prevention of otitis media outweigh the potential risks and the known costs. Today, we now have the benefit of the results of large-scale randomized clinical trials reported during the last several years to guide physicians and parents in this decision-making process.

In this review I would like to present a method for the clinician to use when evaluating a child who many possibly benefit by a surgical procedure for treatment and prevention of otitis media. Figure 1 shows a three-by-three table in which each one of the nine blocks represents a nonsurgical or surgical recommendation. Related to surgery on the pharynx, the clinician is faced with either performing no surgery on the pharynx, an adenoidectomy, or an adenoidectomy with tonsillectomy. Related to surgery on the ear, the clinician may recommend no surgery, myringotomy, or myringotomy with tympanostomy tube insertion. Each one of the nine blocks represents one or more of these options. Now what evidence is there that myringotomy and tympanostomy tube insertion is effective in prevention of recurrent acute otitis media in infants and young children? Gebhart [1] and Gonzalez et al. [2] conducted randomized clinical trials, which showed that tympanostomy tube insertion was more effective than no surgery in infants who were otitis prone. However, prophylactic antimicrobial agents are also effective for prevention of recurrent acute otitis media in this age group [3, 4]. On the other hand, the clinician could recommend no method of prevention, if the episodes are not frequent, since the child probably will improve with advancing age. However, if prevention is desirable, a prophylactic antimicrobial agent, such as amoxicillin (20 mg/kg/day) would be an effective initial method of prevention. A trial with a prophylactic antimicrobial agent for 6–8 weeks is usually recommended, and for those who fail to have their recurrent attacks of otitis media prevented by antimicrobial prophylaxis, tympanostomy tubes can then be recommended. For those infants and young children who continue to have recurrent episodes of acute otitis media, despite the presence of functioning tympanostomy tubes, manifested by otorrhea, a daily prophylactic dose of an antibiotic is usually effective.

What evidence is there that myringotomy, with or without tympanostomy tube, is an effective surgical procedure for treatment and prevention of chronic otitis media with effusion? Mandel et al. [5] conducted a study of 109 Pittsburgh children who had chronic middle-ear effusion, which was unresponsive to antimicrobial therapy. This study revealed that myringotomy and tympanostomy tubes provided more otitis media free time and better hearing than myringotomy alone or nonsurgical control. However, otorrhea and persistent perforation occurred in a few patients with tympanostomy tubes. These children were followed for 3 years during the study, and during this time only one myringotomy and tympanostomy tube procedure was required in 50% of the subjects, but the remaining 50% required a second or third procedure; 30% required a second procedure while 20% had to have three operations. We also found that myringotomy without tympanostomy tubes provided no advantage over no surgery and both methods had a high incidence of treatment failures.

Adenoidectomy, with and without tonsillectomy, as a method of prevention of otitis media, has been evaluated in several clinical studies during the past 30 years, but only during the last few years have there been well-controlled randomized clinical trials reported. Adenoidectomy, with and without tonsillectomy, was evaluated by Maw [6] in 103 children from Bristol, England, all of whom had chronic middle-ear effusion. This investigator showed that adenoidectomy was more effective than no surgery and that adenotonsillectomy did not add substantially to the efficacy of adenoidectomy alone. A subsequent study reported by Gates et al. [7] of 578 four-

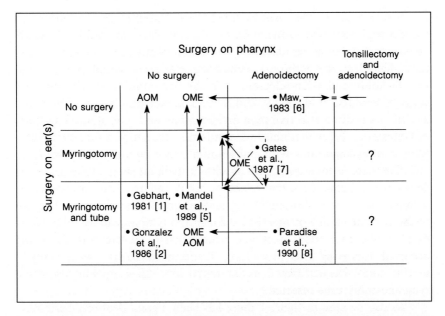

Fig. 1. Results of randomized clinical trials of the most common surgical procedures for treatment/prevention of recurrent acute otitis media (AOM) and chronic otitis media with effusion (OME) are graphically displayed in a three-by-three table. Each block represents either surgery on the ear or pharynx, or both, or neither. Direction of the arrows indicate which surgical procedures were reported to be more effective than others or no surgery. Equal sign indicates that there were no significant differences found between two procedures or combination of procedures. Question marks indicate insufficient data available. [Data from 12, with permission.]

to 8-year-old Texas children, all of whom had chronic middle-ear effusion, which was unresponsive to antimicrobial therapy, showed that adenoidectomy and myringotomy, with and without tympanostomy tube insertion, was more effective than myringotomy with or without tubes; myringotomy without tubes had the worst outcome. Paradise et al. [8] conducted a study of 99 Pittsburgh children who had had previous tympanostomy tubes inserted and who had recurrence of their otitis media after the tympanostomy tube spontaneously extruded. That clinical trial showed that for selected at-risk children, all with previous tubes, the efficacy of adenoidectomy was definite but limited over a 2-year period. The effect was greater for middle-ear effusion than for recurrent acute otitis media.

Figure 1 shows the three-by-three table related to these randomized clinical trials. Related to the efficacy of adenoidectomy, Maw's [6] study demonstrated that adenoidectomy was more effective than no surgery and that adenoidectomy without tonsillectomy was about equal in efficacy to tonsillectomy and adenoidectomy for chronic middle-ear effusion. The study of Paradise et al. [8] showed that adenoidectomy and myringotomy and tube was more effective than myringotomy and tube alone. The study of Gates et al. [7] which had four random arms, showed that adenoidectomy and myringotomy, with and without tympanostomy tube, was more effective than myringotomy with or without tympanostomy tube insertion. Gates et al. [7] concluded that adenoidectomy and myringotomy should be recommended over adenoidectomy and myringotomy with tube, because of the high incidence of otorrhea through the tympanostomy tube. However, in the two adenoidectomy groups, when recurrent otitis media occurred following the procedure, it occurred earlier when only a myringotomy was performed, as compared with the group who also had a tympanostomy tube inserted.

As can be seen in figure 1 there has been a great deal of information derived from randomized clinical trials during the last decade regarding the indications for surgery for otitis media. However, these clinical trials had very specific criteria for entry and many patients were excluded. Therefore, decisions for or against surgical intervention (myringotomy/tympanostomy tube/adenoidectomy/tonsillectomy) should be *individualized* [9].

Some of the factors in the decision-making process are the following: assessment of the frequency, duration, and severity of otitis media (including the degree of hearing loss), determining if the child received appropriate and adequate medical management, and determining if the child had been an antimicrobial prophylaxis failure. The age of the patient may be important, since in the usual operative setting, adenoidectomy and tonsilelctomy is of somewhat a greater risk in infants. Most clinicians would not recommend surgery on the pharynx (tonsillectomy or adenoidectomy, or both) for children who are an anesthetic risk, unless a child has severe upper respiratory tract obstruction. Likewise, the season of the year may be a determinant, since an older child with otitis media may want to engage in competitive swimming, which may make the insertion of tympanostomy tubes less desirable. Other indications for surgery on the ears or pharynx would make the decision for performing ear/pharyngeal surgery more compelling, such as deformation of the eardrum (e.g., a deep retraction pocket), presence of sleep apnea due to obstructive tonsils/adenoids, or frequently recurrent tonsillitis [10, 11]. Also, patients who are in special populations may be more benefitted by insertion of tympanostomy tubes, than by watchful waiting, such as those children with cleft palate or Down's syndrome.

In summary then, we now have evidence from randomized clinical trials that myringotomy with tympanostomy tube insertion can benefit some children who have had frequently recurrent acute otitis media and others with chronic otitis media with effusion, and adenoidectomy can reduce the morbidity of otitis media, but other clinical trials still in progress will have to be completed and reported and still others should be conducted to answer certain questions that remain. There is a need to improve our selection process of candidates for surgery when prevention of otitis media is a goal. Information derived from clinical trials can improve our decision-making process for or against surgical intervention, which in turn should enhance the quality of the health care of our patients who suffer from otitis media.

References

1   Gebhart DE: Tympanostomy tubes in the otitis media prone child. Laryngoscope 1981;91:849–866.
2   Gonzalez C, Arnold JE, Woody EA, et al: Prevention of recurrent acute otitis media: Chemoprophylaxis versus tympanostomy tubes. Laryngoscope 1986;96:1330–1334.
3   Maynard JE, Fleshman JK, Tschopp CF: Otitis media in Alaskan Eskimo children: Prospective evaluation of chemoprophylaxis. JAMA 1972;219:597–599.
4   Perrin JM, Charney E, MacWhinney JB Jr, et al: Sulfisoxazole as chemoprophylaxis for recurrent otitis media: A double-blind crossover study in pediatric practice. N Engl J Med 1974;291:664–667.
5   Mandel EM, Rockette HE, Bluestone CD, et al: Myringotomy with and without tympanostomy tubes for chronic otitis media with effusion. Arch Otolaryngol Head Neck Surg 1989;115:1217–1224.
6   Maw AR: Chronic otitis media with effusion (glue ear) and adenotonsillectomy: Prospective randomized controlled study. Br Med J 1983;287:1586–1588.
7   Gates GA, Avery CA, Prihoda TJ, et al: Effectiveness of adenoidectomy and tympanostomy tubes in the treatment of chronic otitis media with effusion. N Engl J Med 1987;317:1444–1451.
8   Paradise JL, Bluestone CD, Rogers KD, et al: Efficacy of adenoidectomy for recurrent otitis media in children previously treated with tympanostomy-tube placement: Results of parallel randomized and nonrandomized trials. JAMA 1990;263:2066–2073.

9 Bluestone CD, Klein JO: Otitis media, atelectasis and Eustachian tube dysfunction; in Bluestone CD, Stool SE (eds): Pediatric Otolaryngology. Philadelphia, Saunders, 1990, pp 408–415.

10 Paradise JL: Tonsillectomy and adenoidectomy; in Bluestone CD, Stool SE (eds): Pediatric Otolaryngology. Philadelphia, Saunders, 1990, pp 915–926.

11 Paradise JL, Bluestone CD, Bachman RZ, et al: Efficacy of tonsillectomy for recurrent throat infection in severely affected children: Results of parallel randomized and nonrandomized clinical trials. N Engl J Med 1984;310:674–683.

12 Bluestone CD: Indications for tonsillectomy, adenoidectomy and tympanostomy tube insertion: Results of randomized clinical trials as applied to clinical practice; in Myers EN, Bluestone CD, Brackmann DE, Krause CJ (eds): Advances in Otolaryngology-Head and Neck Surgery. Chicago, Mosby Year Book, vol 5, pp 193–208.

Prof. Charles D. Bluestone, MD, Division of Pediatric Otolaryngology,
Children's Hospital of Pittsburgh One Children's Place,
3705 Fifth Avenue at DeSoto Street, Pittsburgh, PA 15213 (USA)

Galioto GB (ed): Tonsils: A Clinically Oriented Update.
Adv Otorhinolaryngol. Basel, Karger, 1992, vol 47, pp 325–327

Adenotonsillectomy as Correction of Dentofacial Growth and Dysfunctions

R. Ghirardo[a], *I. Dus*[b]

[a]Department of Otorhinolaryngology, Vittorio Veneto Hospital, Vittorio Veneto;
[b]Orthodontic and TMJ Clinic, Brugnera, Italy

Tonsillectomy indications have been restricted in the last 10 years especially in consideration of the importance of tonsils as an immunological organ [1]. At present, indications for tonsillectomy are considered mainly when an important hypertrophy exists along with respiratory obstruction, snoring and microarousals during nighttime which cannot be controlled by conventional medical treatment. Other indications for tonsillectomy are determined by the so-called 'focal infections' (much controversy exists about this) or by many episodes of acute tonsilar inflammation [2]. Very rarely, tonsillectomy is taken into consideration for craniofacial growth alterations secondary to hypertrophy of the adenotonsillar system.

Neurophysiology

Over 20 years ago, Ricketts [3, 4] showed that the mouth breather in order to create space for the air column, moves forward the mandible, tongue, mouth floor, hyoid bone complex, altering in so doing the entire neuromuscular system of the neck and face involving as well all the vertebral column and therefore the body posture.

Recently new technologies have been available for the examination of the neuromuscular system. The instrumentation consists of sophisticated

EMG controlled by computer software which is able to monitor EMG signals at different frequencies either in a static position or during movement. The test is performed by monitoring two groups of muscles that are responsible for movement of the head; the movement is studied either in its symmetrical or asymmetrical portion. Using a spectral analysis (signal calculated using Fourier transformed FFT), it is possible to see the behaviors of the muscle involved and therefore determine if muscle fatigue is present by observing the shift of the frequency in the spectrum. The possibility to determine 'co-contraction' (co-contraction is the simultaneous contraction of an antagonist group of muscles during an asymmetrical movement) is very important for rehabilitation of muscle behavior to avoid neuromuscular problems over time.

The above procedure has allowed us to study the behavior of the face and neck muscles in the presence of respiratory obstruction: the findings show a muscular defect characterized by hypoxia and abnormal contractions performed in order to position the head in the typical position of the mouth breather. These muscle dysfunctions are known as dysponesis and co-contraction and lead to muscle fatigue.

Material and Methods

From 1985 to 1990, 37 children were treated with adenotonsillectomy in order to solve maxillofacial growth problems. More specifically, 23 cases were treated with bilateral adenotonsillectomy and 14 cases with adenoidectomy plus monotonsillectomy. The age of the patients was between 4 and 10 years. Concerning tonsillectomy, we preferred not to operate before the age of 4, and in small children monotonsillectomy was the preferred method. Partial or reducible tonsillectomy was never practiced, as suggested by different authors [5].

All patients showed a class 2 or class 3 growth skeletal pattern. There is evidence that hypertrophy of tonsils tends to produce more a class 3 pattern, while nasal adenoid obstruction tends to produce more a class 2 pattern. We are not in full agreement with this type of distinction since the type of growing pattern is very dependent upon the type of postural mechanism that the patient develops to compensate the obstruction of the airways.

As diagnostic procedure the patient underwent the following examinations: orthodontic checkup including lateral and frontal x-rays, cephalometric analysis and evalution, growth forecast, static and dynamic EMG, otorhinolaryngology checkup, rhinomanometry, chemical blood examination, immunological tests (immunoglobulin, complement, T lymphocytes, T-helper) and others in order to evaluate the immunological maturity of the patient. The adenotonsillectomy operation was performed at the Vittorio Veneto Hospital with an average hospitalization of 2 days.

Results

None of the patients suffered from any postoperative problems; only in 1 patient who had undergone adenoidectomy and monotonsillectomy was the compensatory hypertrophy of the remaining tonsil so important that we were forced to reoperate. In the early stages of dysfunctional changes, especially if the patient is very young, the normalization of airways associated with functional training to obtain the neutralization of the functional matrix (behavior of neuromuscular system) was sufficient to resolve the structural problem and renormalize the growth pattern. If the problem was already consolidated, orthodontic treatment had to be combined with functional rehabilitation using the awareness training method. It is very important to underline that in a correction of a craniofacial problem, the three following steps must be performed in exact sequence in order to achieve success over the problem: (1) free airways in order to allow the patient to re-establish normal nasal breathing; (2) rehabilitation of normal function through awareness training in order to neutralize the functional matrix, and (3) orthopedic and/or orthodontic correction of the problem.

Free airway and nasal breathing are fundamental in order to be able to achieve functional matrix neutralization through functional and awareness training. Neutralization of the functional matrix represents the key to allow successful orthodontic and/or orthopedic treatment and its stability over time.

References

1   Brandtzaeg P: Immunopathological alterations in tonsilar disease. Acta Otolaryngol (Stockh) 1988(suppl)454:64–69.
2   Bluestone CD, Paradise JL, Kass EH, et al: Workshop on tonsillectomy and adenoidectomy: State of the art and current problems. Ann Otol Rhinol Laryngol 1975;84: 8–14.
3   Ricketts RM: Respiratory obstructions and their relation to tongue posture. Cleft Palate Bull 1958;8:3.
4   Ricketts RM: New prospectives on orientation and their benefits to clinical orthodontics. Angle Orthod 1975;45:4.
5   Gray LP: Unilateral tonsillectomy. Indications and results. J Laryngol Otol 1983;97: 1111.

R. Ghirardo, MD, Department of Otolaryngology, Via Forlanini 71,
I–31029 Vittorio Veneto (Italy)

Galioto GB (ed): Tonsils: A Clinically Oriented Update.
Adv Otorhinolaryngol. Basel, Karger, 1992, vol 47, pp 328–331

Pidotimod in the Prophylaxis of Recurrent Acute Tonsillitis in Childhood

P. Careddu, A. Biolchini, S. Alfano, G. Zavattini

First Department of Pediatrics, University of Milan, and
Medical Department, Poli Industria Chimica SpA, Milan, Italy

Recurrent acute tonsillitis is one of the most frequently met with respiratory infections in childhood. Immunologic immaturity is often the cause of this condition while recurrent infections change the cell-mediated immunity. Hence the need for a drug capable of inhibiting this interactive mechanism and stimulating immunity. Pidotimod is a synthetic oral biological response modifier (BRM) (3-*L*-pyroglutamoil-*L*-thiazolidin-4-carboxylic acid) proved capable of improving the lymphocytic blastogenesis index and the activation of neutrophil granulocytes as well as increasing the T helper/T suppressor ratio in longlasting treatment [1–3]. In the light of the above considerations, a clinical assessment of pidotimod effectiveness and tolerability in children affected with recurrent acute tonsillitis was deemed to be useful.

Patients and Methods

Thirty-eight outpatients (table 1) of both sexes, aged 2–14 years, were admitted to this randomized double-blind trial versus placebo according to the following inclusion criteria: (a) phlogistic episodes of recurrent acute tonsillitis occurred at least once a month during the past year, and (b) absence of severe hepatic, renal, cardiac or hematopoietic disorders.

Patients who received immunostimulants in the 2 months preceding the trial were excluded. Patients were treated at random with either two 400-mg pidotimod sachets or two indistinguishable placebo sachets every day for 20 consecutive days.

Clinical tests were made at baseline (T_0), at the end of the treatment (T_{20}), at the first (T_{50}) and the second (T_{80}) visit of the follow-up period to assess the following parameters:

Table 1. Characteristics of patients

	Pidotimod	Placebo
Patients	19	19
Male/female ratio	10/9	10/9
Age, years ($\bar{x} \pm SD$)	5.8 ± 3.22	7.3 ± 3.22
Age range, years	2–14	3–13
Body weight, kg ($\bar{x} \pm SD$)	21.8 ± 10.7	25.3 ± 10.7
Diagnosis		
Tonsillitis	10	8
Follicular tonsillitis	1	2
Pharyngeal tonsillitis	8	9
Tonsillitis during last winter ($\bar{x} \pm SD$)	4.5 ± 1.43	4.4 ± 1.3

the trend of basic disease (number, duration and severity of recurrences during the trial and their effect on antibiotic consumption and capability of attending school); the sign and symptom pattern (dysphagia, nasal stuffiness, cough, pharyngeal hyperemia, tonsillar hypertrophy); laboratory tests showing changes in blood composition, hemopoiesis, hepatic and renal function. At the end of the trial both the physician in charge and the patients were requested to rate the effectiveness and tolerability of the treatment.

Results

The patients showing no recurrences during the treatment and follow-up period were 12 (63.1%) in the pidotimod group and 5 (26.3%) in the placebo group. The difference between the two groups (36.8%) is statistically significant (p < 0.01) (fig. 1). There were 8 recurrences in the pidotimod group and 23 in the placebo group. The average length of the episodes (±SD) per group was 17 (±0.59) days between T_0 and T_{20}; 1.3 ± 0.48 days between T_{20} and T_{50}, and 2.2 (±0.67) days between T_{50} and T_{80}. The placebo figures referring to the same time intervals were 2.1 (±0.32), 3.3 (±0.54) and 3.3 (±0.49) days, respectively. In the pidotimod group, the proportion of subjects who required no antibiotic treatment was 73.7% between T_0 and T_{20}; 94.7% between T_{20} and T_{50}, and 73.7% between T_{50} and T_{80}. The placebo figures referring to the same time intervals were 57.9 and 36.8%, respectively (fig. 2). At T_{80}, 12 patients of the pidotimod group and 29 patients of the placebo group were prevented from attending school normally. As regards clinical parameters, it was found that the percentage

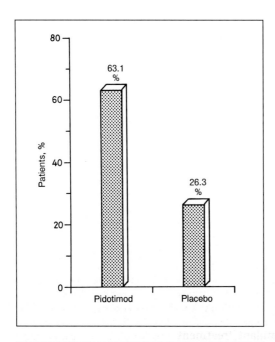

Fig. 1. Proportion of patients showing no recurrences between T_0 and T_{80}.

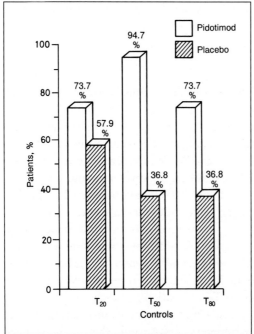

Fig. 2. Proportion of patients who received no antibiotics in the different controls.

increase of patients without cough was 84.2% in the pidotimod group and 31.6% in the placebo group and that of patients without dysphagia was 78.9% in the former and 31.5% in the latter group. Both differences are statistically significant (p < 0.05).

The physician in charge rated treatment effectiveness good or very good in 78.9% of the subjects belonging to the pidotimod group and in 15.7% of those of the placebo group. The difference is statistically significant (p < 0.01). Tolerability was good by both physician and parents.

Conclusion

The above results show that treatment with pidotimod of children affected with recurrent tonsillitis is effective both in checking the development of the disease and in reducing the number and severity of recurrences. The sustained effect of pidotimod, which goes well beyond the administration period, the good tolerability and compliance ensured by its oral formulation, fully qualifies this drug as a worthy therapeutic tool to be used whenever immunostimulant treatment in children becomes necessary.

References

1   Pugliese A, Girardello R, Martinelli L, Forno B, Pattarino PL, Biglino A: Valutazione degli effetti di pidotimod su alcuni parametri immunitari. Abstract Book of 6° Congresso della Associazione Italiana di Immunofarmacologia, Firenze 1990, pp 1–110.
2   Illeni MT, Bombelli G, Mailland F, Pattarino PL: Effetto del PGT/1A sulla blastogenesi con mitogeni: studio ex vivo. Atti XXIX Convegno Nazionale di Studi SIITS-AICT, Cernobbio 1990, No 36/2, pp 256–260.
3   Auteri A, Pasqui AL, Bruni F, Saletti M: Effect of PGT/1A, a new immunostimulating agent, on some aspects of immune response in vitro study. Abstract Book of Symposium of the International Association of Biological Standardization, Annecy 1991, pp 1–58.

Dr. G. Zavattini, Medical Department, Poli Industria Chimica SpA,
Via Volturno 48, I-20089 Quinto de' Stampi, Rozzano (Italy)

Galioto GB (ed): Tonsils: A Clinically Oriented Update.
Adv Otorhinolaryngol. Basel, Karger, 1992, vol 47, pp 332–337

Evaluation of Immune Response of Waldeyer's Tissues after Local Stimulation with Bacterial Ribosomal Extracts

B, T and NK Lymphocyte Phenotype and Function

Rita Maccario[b], Mara De Amici[b], Daniela Montagna[b],
Marco Benazzo[a], Attilio Ascione[b], Rosanna Pozzo[b],
Giorgio Romagnoli[c], Emilio Mevio[a]

Departments of [a]Otorhinolaryngology and [b]Pediatrics, University of Pavia,
IRCCS Policlinico San Matteo, Pavia, and [c]Simes Italia, Milan, Italy

Clinical and laboratory evidence has suggested that topical stimulation with bacterial ribosomal extracts (REs) induces an activation of local immune defences [1, 2] and therefore may be advisable as treatment of recurrent adenotonsillitis.

The aim of our study was to investigate B, T and NK lymphocyte phenotype and function in a group of children previously treated for 3 months with bacterial RE and successively undergoing tonsillectomy. Evaluation of the distribution of tonsillar lymphocyte subpopulations was performed by means of monoclonal antibodies (MoAbs) specific for differentiation antigens which are present on the surface of B, T and NK cells [3–6]. Tonsillar B lymphocyte capacity to secrete immunoglobulins (Ig) in vitro was assessed by culturing tonsillar mononuclear cells (TMC) with medium alone (spontaneous Ig production) or with pokeweed mitogen (PWM) which is a T-cell-dependent polyclonal activator of B cells, known to induce Ig production in vitro [7]. Tonsillar T-lymphocyte capacity to proliferate and secrete interleukin-2 (IL-2) and interferon (IFN)-γ – which are lymphokines known to be important in the induction and regulation of immune response [8, 9] – was assessed by culturing TMC with phytohemagglutinin (PHA), a mitogen capable of activating a large percentage of T cells [10]. NK cell activity was assessed in a cytotoxicity assay, using K562 erythroleukemia cell line as the target.

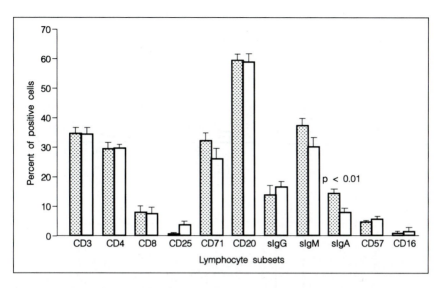

Fig. 1. Tonsillar lymphocyte phenotype evaluated by immunofluorescence and flow cytometric analysis. Mean values ± SE obtained from 10 patients treated with bacterial RE (▓) and 10 untreated patients (□) are reported.

Materials and Methods

Bacterial REs (Immucytal) were supplied by Simes SpA (Milan, Italy). TMC phenotype was evaluated by immunofluorescence and flow cytometric analysis. MoAbs specific for CD3 (anti-Leu4), CD4 (anti-Leu3a), CD8 (anti-Leu2a), CD25 (anti-IL-2R), CD71 (anti-transferrin receptor), CD57 (anti-Leu7), CD16 (anti-Leu11c), CD20 (anti-Leu16), surface (s) IgG, sIgM and sIgA were purchased by Becton-Dickinson (Mountain View, Calif., USA). For in vitro activation, TMC (1×10^6 cells/ml) were cultured in microwells in RPMI 1640 medium, supplemented with 2 mM L-glutamine, 50 µg/ml gentamicin, 10% fetal calf serum in the presence or absence of PHA or PWM. Proliferation was evaluated after 3 days' culture, cell-free supernatants were collected after 2 days' culture for IL-2, 6 days' culture for IFN-γ and 7 days' culture for IgG, IgM and IgA. IL-2 and IFN-γ secreted in the supernatants were measured by radioimmunoassay (Medgenix Diagnostics, Brussels, Belgium) and IgA, IgM and IgG by enzyme-linked immunosorbent assay.

Results

As shown in figure 1, about 60% of TMC were B lymphocytes, as defined by the expression of CD20 antigen. The majority of tonsillar B lymphocytes expressed sIgM, while B cells expressing sIgG and sIgA were

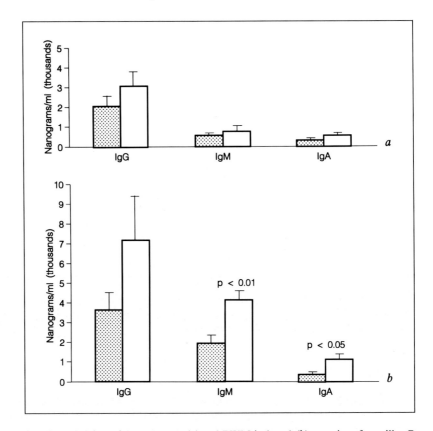

Fig. 2. Evaluation of spontaneous *(a)* and PWM-induced *(b)* capacity of tonsillar B lymphocytes to secrete Ig in vitro. Mean values ± SE obtained from 10 patients treated with bacterial RE (▓) and 10 untreated patients (☐) are reported.

less than 20%. The percentage of B lymphocytes expresssing sIgA was significantly higher in the group of patients treated with bacterial RE as compared with untreated children. TMC included about 30–40% of mature T lymphocytes, defined by the presence of CD3 antigen, most of which expressed CD4 antigen, while CD8-positive cells were less than 10%. Very few TMC expressed p55 chain of IL-2R (CD25) and about 30% of them expressed transferrin receptor (CD71). The percentage of NK cells was extremely low or undetectable in all patients tested.

Spontaneous (fig. 2a) as well as PWM-induced (fig. 2b) Ig production (especially IgG secretion) was elevated in the majority of patients; how-

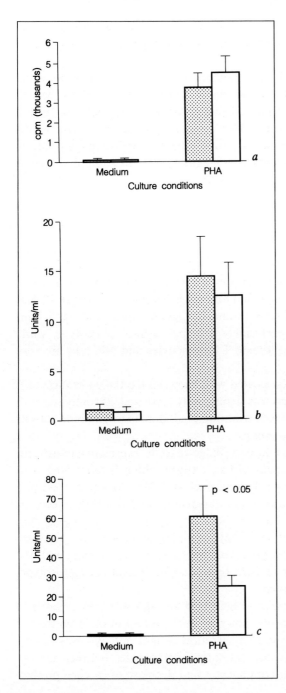

Fig. 3. Evaluation of the capacity of tonsillar T lymphocytes to produce IL-2 (a) and IFN-γ (b) and to proliferate (c) in vitro in response to PHA activation. Mean values ± SE obtained from 10 patients treated with bacterial RE (▨) and 10 untreated patients (☐) are reported.

ever, PWM-induced IgM and IgA production was significantly lower in the group of patients treated with bacterial RE, as compared to untreated controls.

TMC were unable to display spontaneous in vitro proliferation, while PHA-induced proliferation was detectable in all patients tested (fig. 3a). As shown in figure 3b and c, both IL-2 and IFN-γ were detectable in culture supernatants of PHA-activated TMC, and IFN production was significantly increased in the group of patients treated with bacterial RE, as compared with untreated children. NK activity was absent both in treated and untreated patients (data not shown).

Discussion

The evaluation of the distribution of tonsillar lymphocyte subpopulations showed that the majority of TMC are B lymphocytes, about 50% of them expressing sIgM and only a minority sIgG or sIgA. Tonsillar T lymphocytes express almost exclusively a helper surface phenotype, while CD8-positive suppressor/cytotoxic T lymphocytes and NK cells are very low or absent.

In the group of children treated with bacterial RE the percentage of B lymphocytes expressing sIgA was significantly increased, as compared with untreated patients, while the distribution of all the other lymphoid subsets was comparable in the two groups.

TMC included a sizeable percentage of cells expressing transferrin receptor, a nonlineage-specific surface antigen which is associated with activated/proliferating cells [5]. Nevertheless, TMC do not express p55 chain of IL-2 receptor which is usually associated with transferrin receptor on the surface of activated T lymphocytes [11]. These data suggest that transferrin receptor expression on TMC is mainly associated with the presence of activated B lymphocytes. This hypothesis is in keeping with the high levels of spontaneous in vitro Ig production, mainly of IgG isotype, observed in all patients tested.

PWM-induced production of IgG, IgM and IgA was also elevated in the majority of children tested, however in the group of children treated with bacterial RE, PWM-induced secretion of IgM and IgA was significantly lower than in untreated patients. Discrepancies between the enhancement of sIgA-bearing lymphocytes and decrease of in vitro production of IgA and IgM in treated children could be ascribed to recruitment of immature B-cell subsets.

In agreement with the presence of high percentages of helper T lymphocytes, TMC displayed a good level of PHA-induced lymphocyte proliferation and were able to secrete both IL-2 and IFN-γ. IFN-γ secretion in the supernatants of PHA-activated lymphocytes was significantly increased in children treated with bacterial RE as compared with untreated patients, thus suggesting that bacterial RE may improve the production in vitro of a lymphokine known to play an important regulatory role in both T- and B-cell-mediated immunity.

References

1   Vaquette C: Intérêt des fractions antigéniques purifiées dans le traitement des affections chroniques de la sphère ORL. NPN Méd 1982;1282:22–153.
2   Waldmen RH, Stone J, Lazzell V, Bergmann KCH, Khakov R, Jackowitz A, Howard S, Rose C: Oral route as method for immunizing against mucosal pathogens. Ann N Y Acad Sci 1983;409:510–516.
3   Ling NR: The relationship of B-lymphocyte surface marker phenotype to cell differentiation; in Bird G, Calvert JE (eds): B Lymphocytes in Human Disease. Oxford, Oxford University Press, 1988, pp 174–192.
4   Calvert JE, Cooper MD: Early stages of B cell differentiation; in Bird G, Calvert JE (eds): B Lymphocytes in Human Disease. Oxford, Oxford University Press, 1988, pp 77–101.
5   Reinherz EL, Kung PC, Goldstein G, Levey RH, Schlossman SF: Discrete stages of human intrathymic differentiation: analysis of normal thymocytes and leukemic lymphoblasts of T lineage. Proc Natl Acad Sci USA 1980;77:1588–1597.
6   Ritz J, Schmidt RE, Michon J, Hercend T, Schlossman SF: Characterization of functional surface structures on human natural killer cells. Adv Immunol 1988;42:1881–1890.
7   Greaves MF, Janossy G, Doenhoff M: Selective triggering of human T and B lymphocytes in vitro by polyclonal mitogens. J Exp Med 1974;140:1–12.
8   Dinarello CA, Mier JW: Lymphokines. N Engl J Med 1987;317:940–945.
9   Clemens MS, Morris AG, Garing ASH (eds): Lymphokines and Interferons: A Practical Approach. Oxford, IRL Press, 1987, pp 1–376.
10 Stites DP: Clinical laboratory methods of detection of cellular immune function; in Stites DP, Stobo JD, Wells JV (eds): Basic and Clinical Immunology. Los Altos, Lange Med Pub, 1987, pp 285–303.
11 Robb RJ: Interleukin-2: the molecule and its function. Immunol Today 1984;7:203–205.

Dr. Emilio Mevio, Department of Otorhinolaryngology, University of Pavia, IRCCS Policlinico San Matteo, P.le Golgi, 2, I–27100 Pavia (Italy)

Galioto GB (ed): Tonsils: A Clinically Oriented Update.
Adv Otorhinolaryngol. Basel, Karger, 1992, vol 47, pp 338–341

Antibiotic Diffusion in Tonsillar Tissue

R. Rondanelli[a], M.B. Regazzi[b], M. Sinistri[b]

[a] University of Pavia, and [b] Department of Pharmacology,
IRCCS-Policlinico S. Matteo, Pavia, Italy

The majority of throat infections (approx. 80–90%), whether accompanied by fever or not, is usually caused by viruses; however, the infection can also be caused by a variety of bacterial pathogens, the most important of which are the group A streptococci [1]. The primary objective of antimicrobial therapy is not only aimed at identifying the spectrum of antibacterial activity, but also at eradicating the microorganism involved in order to allow an adequate amount of drug to reach the focus of the infection. The dosages of antimicrobial drugs are usually determined by combining pharmacokinetic data with in vitro activity and, as a rule, the tendency is to keep the serum levels of the drug above the MIC and MBC for almost the entire dosage interval [2, 3].

This criterion is used to evaluate the adequateness of protocols employed in the treatment of tonsillitis, which is carried out with penicillin, cephalosporin and macrolide antibiotics. Indeed, among the various pharmacokinetic parameters considered, the one most closely correlated with efficacy – as far as penicillin, cephalosporin and erythromycin are concerned – seems to be the length of time that their levels remain above the MIC or the MBC. Frequent cases of relapsing streptococcal tonsillitis have been reported in the period immediately following antibiotic therapy, due to infections from β-hemolytic Streptococcus [1].

Wide variations in the serum levels of the drug employed have also been described during antibiotic treatment. Nevertheless, the significance of a possible relationship between such pharmacokinetic variability and therapy failure is still not clear. Penicillin is considered the drug of choice in bacterial tonsillitis. Serum levels of this drug vary greatly: the highest values found in one patient were 30 times larger than those registered in patients with the lowest concentrations of the drug. However, the pattern of the drug levels was not correlated with relapsing disease.

In general there is a good correlation, albeit variable, between serum levels and tissue concentration, and the relationship between tissue and serum does not appear to be influenced by time. The tissue levels of phenoxymethylpenicillin usually correspond to 19% of those in serum. High doses of phenoxymethylpenicillin result in sufficient tissue concentrations even in patients with low serum levels [4]. Nevertheless, various factors can influence the tissue distribution of the drug. For example, binding to plasma proteins may reduce antimicrobial activity, reduce tissue distribution and delay drug elimination. Craig and co-workers [2, 3] clearly demonstrate the effect of this protein binding in β_6-lactamide on the area under the serum concentration-time curve, both in serum and in the blister. The area under the curve of the free drug and of the total amount of drug in the blister decreased as the protein binding increased, and the reduction was most marked when the values of this binding exceeded 80%.

Plasma protein binding may also have a positive effect on the tissue distribution of the drug by showing down its rate of elimination and determining higher serum levels. This effect is not found in drugs that are eliminated by tubular secretion.

Figure 1 demonstrates how cefonicid, which is eliminated by tubular secretion, is excreted rapidly even though it is bound to the plasma proteins. On the other hand, ceftriaxone, which is equally bound to the plasma proteins but excreted by glomerular filtration, is eliminated more slowly and shows greater tissue distribution [5]. Such pharmacokinetic behavior influences the antibacterial efficacy of drugs. The mean MIC and MBC values for ceftriaxone with regard to *Haemophilus influenzae* are about 2–4 times lower than those reported for cefonicid. Examination of the curves of decline in bactericide quotients (BQ), which is the relationship between the concentration of antibiotic in the tissue (μg/g) and the MBC, reveals that at the second hour after administration ceftriaxone has BQ values of 39.1, while cefonicid presents values of 7.4. At 24 h cefonicid exhibits the tendency to lose its bactericidal properties; the BQ value drops below 1 beginning with the 18th hour. The BQ values for ceftriaxone, therefore, appear to be the better of the two drugs evaluated for the treatment of tonsil infections [5].

The lipophilic macrolides employed in the treatment of tonsillitis display excellent tissue penetration and a high tissue-plasma relationship.

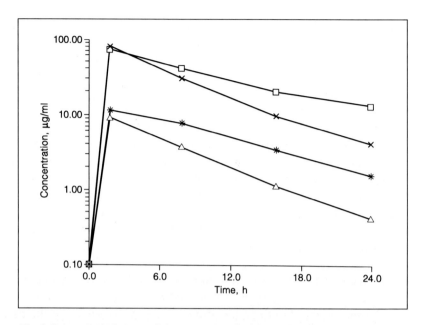

Fig. 1. Serum (µg/ml) (□ = ceftriaxone, × = cefonicid) and tonsillar (µg/g) (* = cef-triaxone, △ = cefonicid) levels of drugs after intramuscular (1 g) administration.

Roxithromycin is characterized by high serum and low tissue levels, while clarithromycin displays therapeutic serum levels and high tissue concentrations. The pharmacokinetics of roxithromycin is characterized by a strong degree of binding to the plasma proteins and a lesser amount of tissue diffusion. Furthermore, it should be noted that roxithromycin differs from the other macrolide antibiotics in its strong binding to acid α_1-glycoprotein. However, the tonsillar levels of roxithromycin are greater than the MIC for *Streptococcus pyogenes* and for many respiratory tract pathogens.

Most bacterial infections occur in the extracellular tissue fluid. Recently, microscopic examination of samples obtained from patients with tonsillitis revealed that the bacteria are localized almost exclusively on the surface of the tonsils and do not appear to penetrate the surface of the epithelium. Thus, the level of antibiotics in the tonsil surface fluid should be the clinically most important value. The level of antibiotics is higher in the tonsil surface fluid than in the tonsillar tissue. This concentration for many antibiotics is greater than the MIC for β-hemolytic Streptococcus for several hours. In this case too a more thorough investigation of the significance of the dosage interval in relation to the efficacy of treatment would be welcomed.

In general, from an analysis of the available data, the inability to reach the site of infection does not seem to be a probable cause of the relapsing cases that occur during the treatment of tonsillitis. Obviously the treatment of an infection with an antibiotic involves different pharmacokinetic variables; however, other factors should be considered when evaluating current and future therapy protocols. Quantitative experimental indicators of efficacy should not only include MIC or MBC, but also the postantibiotic effect in vitro and in vivo, the emergence of resistance in vitro and in vivo, and the relationship between plasma concentration profiles and efficacy [3].

References

1   Fisher SR, Gussack G: Medical management of common ear, nose and throat infections. Drug Ther 1984;14:99–102.
2   Craig WA, Vogelman B: Changing concepts and new applications of antibiotic pharmacokinetics. Am J Med 1984;31:24–28.
3   Mattie H, Craig WA: Determinants of efficacy and toxicity of aminoglycosides. J Antimicrob Chemother 1989;24:281–293.
4   Roos K, Brorson JE: Concentration of phenoxymethylpenicillin in tonsillar tissue. Eur J Clin Pharmacol 1990;39:417–418.
5   Fraschini F, Scaglione F: Distribuzione polmonare e tonsillare di ceftriaxone e cefonicid e risultante attività battericida d'organo. Recenti Prog Med 1990;81:41–46.

Dr. M.B. Regazzi, Department of Pharmacology, IRCCS-Policlinico S. Matteo, P.le Golgi, I–27100 Pavia (Italy)

Subject Index